D1062326

NSCA's Guide to Tests and Assessments

National Strength and Conditioning Association

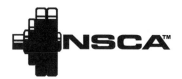

Todd Miller, PhD, CSCS*D

George Washington University

EDITOR

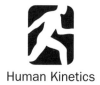

Human Kinetics

Library of Congress Cataloging-in-Publication Data

National Strength & Conditioning Association (U.S.)
  NSCA's guide to tests and assessments / National Strength and Conditioning
Association ; Todd Miller, editor.
    p. ; cm. -- (Science of strength and conditioning series)
  Includes bibliographical references and index.
  ISBN-13: 978-0-7360-8368-3 (hard cover)
  ISBN-10: 0-7360-8368-5 (hard cover)
  I. Miller, Todd, 1967- II. Title. III. Series: Science of strength and
conditioning series.
  [DNLM: 1. Athletic Performance--physiology--Guideline. 2. Physical
Fitness--physiology--Guideline. 3. Exercise--physiology--Guideline. 4.
Exercise Test--methods--Guideline. 5. Physical Examination--Guideline. 6.
Sports--physiology--Guideline. QT 260]

  613.7--dc23
                                      2011038488
  ISBN-10: 0-7360-8368-5
  ISBN-13: 978-0-7360-8368-3

The web addresses cited in this text were current as of August 2011, unless otherwise noted.

Developmental Editor: Kevin Matz; **Assistant Editors:** Steven Calderwood and Bethany J. Bentley; **Copyeditor:** Patsy Fortney; **Indexer:** Betty Frizzell; **Permissions Manager:** Dalene Reeder; **Graphic Designer:** Nancy Rasmus; **Graphic Artist:** Joe Buck; **Cover Designer:** Keith Blomberg; **Photographs (interior):** Neil Bernstein, all photos © Human Kinetics unless otherwise noted; **Photo Asset Manager:** Laura Fitch; **Visual Production Assistant:** Joyce Brumfield; **Photo Production Manager:** Jason Allen; **Art Manager:** Kelly Hendren; **Associate Art Manager:** Alan L. Wilborn; **Art Style Development:** Jennifer Gibas; **Illustrations:** © Human Kinetics; **Printer:** Sheridan Books

We thank the National Strength and Conditioning Association in Colorado Springs, Colorado, for assistance in providing the location for the photo shoot for this book.

Printed in the United States of America   10 9 8 7 6 5 4 3 2 1

The paper in this book is certified under a sustainable forestry program.

Human Kinetics
Website: www.HumanKinetics.com

United States: Human Kinetics
P.O. Box 5076
Champaign, IL 61825-5076
800-747-4457
e-mail: humank@hkusa.com

Canada: Human Kinetics
475 Devonshire Road Unit 100
Windsor, ON N8Y 2L5
800-465-7301 (in Canada only)
e-mail: info@hkcanada.com

Europe: Human Kinetics
107 Bradford Road
Stanningley
Leeds LS28 6AT, United Kingdom
+44 (0) 113 255 5665
e-mail: hk@hkeurope.com

Australia: Human Kinetics
57A Price Avenue
Lower Mitcham, South Australia 5062
08 8372 0999
e-mail: info@hkaustralia.com

New Zealand: Human Kinetics
P.O. Box 80
Torrens Park, South Australia 5062
0800 222 062
e-mail: info@hknewzealand.com

E4846

Science of Strength and Conditioning Series

NSCA's Guide to Sport and Exercise Nutrition

NSCA's Guide to Tests and Assessments

NSCA's Guide to Program Design

National Strength and Conditioning Association

Human Kinetics

Contents

Preface

If you can't measure it, you can't control it. One of my mentors repeated this "quality axiom" to me on a daily basis during my years as a graduate student, and this fundamental message has become ingrained in my approach to training. As strength and conditioning professionals, our primary goal is to design and implement programs that result in optimal athletic performance. At first glance, this appears to be a simple task. By following the principles of specificity, overload, and progression, we can design conditioning and resistance training programs that increase fitness and athletic performance.

Unfortunately, while our programs may bring about improved performance for athletes and clients, it is impossible to know whether these adaptations are optimal without incorporating some well-conceived testing and measurement schemes into a regimen. Indeed, it is common for a trainer to claim that his or her program works, but the design of strength and conditioning programs is not simply about improving performance. It is about safely improving performance *to the greatest degree possible* for a specific individual with a specific set of goals. Achieving this optimal level of improvement is simply not possible without a strategy for tracking changes in performance over time.

Historically, testing and measurement for the exercise sciences have been heavily slanted toward a clinical population and have been focused mainly through the lens of disease and disease prevention. Much less attention has been given to testing for athletic performance, and this is reflected in the paucity of literature on the topic. Tests for power, speed, agility, and mobility (all topics addressed in this text) lean heavily toward athletic performance and are rarely used in clinical settings. This book serves as a resource for coaches, trainers, students, and athletes of all skill levels and addresses the importance of testing and measurement for athletic performance.

The text begins by laying the foundation of testing and data analysis and the methods of interpreting results and drawing conclusions. The chapters that follow include tests from the rudimentary (such as body composition and blood pressure measurement) to the more complex, such as lactate threshold testing and aerobic power. While all of these tests vary in complexity, this variability is not indicative of their degree of importance. For example, measuring body composition is a relatively simple task, yet its implications in athletic performance are incredibly profound. It is clear that excess fat can be deleterious to performance in sports that rely on speed, acceleration, and rapid changes in direction. Despite this, coaches will often spend long hours on speed training but pay little attention to measuring or improving body composition. We hope that this text not only serves as an instructional tool for the mechanics of conducting specific tests but that it also helps coaches determine which tests are appropriate for specific populations. For example, a test of aerobic power may be inappropriate for a thrower, whose performance relies primarily on strength and power. Conversely, a coach of a distance runner would benefit little from conducting agility testing on athletes. Therefore, you should not assume that you need to read this text cover to cover, nor should you assume all tests are appropriate for all athletes.

As the field of strength and conditioning becomes increasingly sophisticated, so should the approach by which training programs are designed, implemented, and tested. A training program that lacks some type of progress tracking is grossly incomplete, yet it remains startlingly common among trainers of today. We are confident that this text will provide a solid foundation by which you can develop and implement your own testing and measurement programs, ultimately allowing you to grow as a coach and maximize the performance of your athletes.

1

Tests, Data Analysis, and Conclusions

Matthew R. Rhea, PhD, CSCS*D, and Mark D. Peterson, PhD, CSCS*D

Effective exercise prescription begins with an analysis to determine the needs of the client. Referred to as a needs analysis (National Strength and Conditioning Association 2000), this process involves determining the client's lifestyle and the demands of the sport, as well as identifying current and previous injuries and limitations, overall training experience, and the existing level of fitness and skill across a variety of fitness and athletic components. Without such data from which to provide baseline and follow-up evaluations, trainers and strength and conditioning professionals are inclined to design and implement cookie-cutter exercise programs created not for the individual, but for a large group of potential exercisers.

Conducting tests and assessing the collected data provides objective information regarding the strengths and weaknesses in a client's physiological and functional capacities. When done correctly, this process enables an exercise professional to develop the most effective and appropriate training program for the client. However, the process involves far more than simply collecting data. Gathering the appropriate data, analyzing it correctly, and presenting the information in a succinct and accurate manner are all important for the effective use of testing in a fitness or sport arena.

Sport Performance and Testing

Tests are conducted for a variety of reasons depending on the situation. Following are some examples in a professional setting:

- Identifying physiological strengths and weaknesses
- Ranking people for selection purposes
- Predicting future performances
- Evaluating the effectiveness of a training program or trial
- Tracking performance over time
- Assigning and manipulating training dosages (e.g., intensities, loads, volumes)

Exercise professionals can evaluate data to examine the overall effectiveness of an exercise routine. Specifically, strength testing data collected every month can be used to examine changes over time and to give an objective picture of the overall effectiveness of the strength training plan. If increases in strength are less than desirable, alterations may be made to enhance fitness adaptation during the subsequent training cycle.

Personal trainers may use test data to demonstrate and present improvements to clients and help them gain an understanding of the overall picture of the alterations in fitness brought about by their exercise programs. Alternatively, physical therapists might consult test data to determine appropriate rehabilitation progression timelines. When used properly, test data can help exercise professionals reach and maintain a higher level of practice.

Screening Tests

The first step in selecting components to include in the test battery is to determine the physiological components to be evaluated. Specific to the needs analysis, a preliminary assessment should include several additional tests to determine the client's exercise readiness. Depending on the client, this step requires a careful examination of potential sources of physical complications; this might involve a cardiovascular screening or an assessment of joint and posture mobility or integrity. Regardless of the client's age and training history, this pre-activity screening is a vital step in the needs analysis, and is necessary for identifying potential health risks of engaging in exercise, prior to the start of a program. Clearly, tests conducted to identify health risks are somewhat different from those used to simply gauge and monitor basic fitness. Nonetheless, these tests are all needed for creating effective programming and ensure client safety.

After the completion of a health risk appraisal, testing for current fitness is likely warranted. For personal trainers, this process is relatively straightforward, involving a thorough review of the client's health history and current health risk, as well as exercise and fitness goals. For strength and conditioning professionals, this step requires an intimate understanding of not only the tests needed for evaluating athlete preparedness, but also the fitness and performance benchmarks for that athlete to aspire to, to compete successfully in a given athletic endeavor.

To complete the testing process in a time- and energy-efficient manner, fitness professionals need to ensure that the tests are valid—that is, that they measure what they are intended to measure. A strength test should measure force production, whereas an endurance test should measure the ability to repeatedly exert force. From the many tests that have been developed and validated to measure specific health and fitness components, fitness professionals must select the most appropriate and valid one for a given client. They need to keep in mind that certain tests have been validated only for specific populations and may not be appropriate for people who are not in that classification. Therefore, caution must be used when selecting tests, because producing invalid results is very easy to do.

Tests must not only measure what they are supposed to measure, but also measure it consistently. Reliable tests result in consistent measures with a low opportunity for error. When using external raters or observers to measure performance measures, examiners should consider the reliability of each observer. To compare future test results to baseline results, fitness professionals must either ensure that the same observer conducts both tests or that multiple observers provide the same measure for a given performance. To verify consistency among raters, examiners can have all raters assess the same performance; this might reveal differences in ratings, or the extent of such differences.

Although many tests have been shown to be valid and reliable in a clinical or laboratory setting, some are not feasible in many work environments. Financial resources, time and space, as well as qualified staff to oversee testing are all factors that may determine the practicality of a specific test. However, examiners should consider alternatives for testing, because there are often multiple options for determining specific fitness and performance characteristics.

Validity, reliability, and feasibility should be the foremost considerations in test selection. Professionals who take all of these variables into account will get better, more useful information throughout their careers.

Data Evaluation and Statistical Analysis

Data collection represents only half of the overall process of testing and assessment. Once testing has been completed, data evaluation and interpretation must be conducted. Many fitness professionals are very good at conducting tests and storing information. However, where they frequently fall short is in the actual evaluation of the information they have collected, as well as in the subsequent use of those findings to inform their exercise prescriptions. Without an objective examination of the data, the full value of exercise testing cannot be realized.

Applied Statistics

Many fitness professionals view statistics as complex, useless mathematical equations. Although many complex equations and statistical procedures exist, and some of them do lack professional applications, applied statistics can offer an objective means for evaluating data. Developing a functional knowledge of statistics may require an investment of time and effort; however, the ability to perform even the most basic applied statistical analyses will greatly add to the fitness professional's toolbox of skills.

In statistics, very little emphasis is placed on one piece of data (e.g., one client's vertical jump score or one athlete's bench press 1RM). Instead, statistical evaluations focus on group dynamics. For instance, if one person in a group of 10 decreased performance after participating in an organized training program, but the other nine participants increased performance, we would not want to judge the program as ineffective simply because one person in the group did not experience a positive response. Yet, in the world of exercise prescription and programming, we must consider the individual responses. Although one treatment may work well for a large population, it may not be the most effective for a given person. However, if only one client improves, or if one client improves much more than the others do, promoting the training program as effective based on that one person is inappropriate (although many fitness professionals do this). Care is needed when applying statistical evaluations in the real world.

Probability Versus Magnitude

Two characteristics of collected data must be considered and understood when performing statistical evaluations. The first is the probability of the results. Probability represents the reproducibility of the findings and is presented as a probability value (α or the p value). This value can range from 0.0 to 1.0 in the research literature, and is often reported as $p \geq$ or ≤ 0.05. Further, this value represents the chance that the findings of the analysis were obtained erroneously. If the p value is equal to 0.05, then there is only a 5% risk of error and a 95% chance that the same findings would be achieved if the conditions were repeated.

The level of probability needed for reaching the predetermined significance level is set based on the amount of acceptable error. In medical research, in which decisions about drugs or treatment protocols carry life-altering consequences, less risk of error is allowed; α levels of .01 are generally used. In exercise science, in which differences in training programs or routines do not carry life-threatening consequences, it is common to accept levels of error at the 0.05 level. In either case, it is important to remember that the α level represents how many times we would expect different results if the study were repeated 100 times.

Probability is based on statistical power (most influenced by the number of people in the group being studied) and the variation in performance among the group. Although it is important to evaluate the reproducibility of a statistical analysis, it provides no measure of the actual magnitude of the change(s) in data. For instance, if 1,000 people were tested on the bench press 1RM, and then subsequently trained for three months to specifically improve bench press strength, examiners need to take into consideration the sample size and its influence on probability values to predict statistical difference, as well as the interpretation of the findings. If these people were retested and, as a group, demonstrated a 1-kilogram improvement in strength, the probability of generating the same results if the conditions were repeated would be high, because of the large number of participants in the group: perhaps even at $p < 0.01$. Assuming that this group was composed of members of the general population, even though a 1-kilogram improvement would be expected 99 times out of 100, and would therefore likely yield a statistically significant result, this improvement actually represents a very small increase in strength. Therefore, because it is not uncommon for average exercisers to see an increase of up to 15 kilograms in a three-month period, these findings would be clinically insignificant.

Ultimately, to describe and evaluate the magnitude of the improvement, we must rely on another calculation, usually the effect size (described later). The differences in these outputs must be understood because many errors have been made as a result of the incorrect assumption that probability is equal to magnitude.

Descriptive Analysis

The first step in evaluating a data set simply provides an overview of the data. This is done by calculating descriptive values such as the mean, median, mode, range, and variance. The average score (mean), which is calculated by summing all scores and dividing by the number of scores, represents the average score. The median represents the middle score and can be found by arranging scores in ascending order and finding the middle score. This represents the 50th percentile score, signifying that half of the scores fall above this score and half fall below it. The mode is the most frequently occurring score. These three measures of central tendency provide ample information for interpreting how a given subject's score compares to those of the group.

Measures of central tendency are often used to create normative data, calculated from tests conducted in a very large group. For instance, if we tested a group of 10,000 firefighters to see how many push-ups and sit-ups they can perform, and then calculated the average for the group (e.g., 50 in one minute), we could state that the norm for a firefighter is 50. We could then test other firefighters to see how they compared to the normative score measured in a larger group of firefighters. Although normative data provide a good comparison to peers, they provide no information regarding individuals' ability to perform a certain task. Do firefighters need to be able to perform 50 push-ups in one minute to do the job safely and effectively? Do they need to be able to do 100 push-ups in one minute? Measures of central tendency simply describe the typical performance of a group; they do not necessarily represent the optimal level of performance.

Another important consideration in comparing an individual's score to those of the group is the evaluation of the variability in the scores. As one example, a data range may be used (i.e., the high score minus the low score) to see how much of a spread exists among all scores. Another common measure of variability is the standard deviation, which is a calculation of how closely the data set clusters around the mean. In a normal distribution, in which scores are evenly distributed above and below the mean, 68.26% of all scores will fall within ±1 standard deviation from the mean, 95.44% will fall within ±2 standard deviations, and 99.74% will fall within ±3 standard deviations. Examining a single score, and subsequently determining how many standard deviations above or below the mean it falls, offers a greater perspective on the quality of that score.

Relationships Among Performance Variables

The ability to examine the relationship among variables is often of interest to exercise professionals. The way one variable changes in relation to another can provide valuable information. For instance, as cardiorespiratory fitness increases, the risk of heart disease decreases. This relationship has led to a greater focus on cardiorespiratory fitness promotion and the development of effective exercise programs.

Although a relationship among variables can be useful information, it is important to realize that such relationships do not represent a cause-and-effect situation. For instance, a strong correlation exists between shoe size and IQ: people with larger shoe sizes also tend to have higher IQ scores. However, having big feet does not impart intelligence. This relationship simply reflects the fact that as people grow and mature, they gain knowledge.

The correlation coefficient can be used to determine a linear relationship among variables. Consider the hypothetical relationship between body weight and vertical jump in the 10 subjects presented in table 1.1 and figure 1.1.

As body weight increases, gravitational force increases, making it more difficult to propel the body vertically. Therefore, people who are heavier are at a disadvantage. In the data provided, the correlation coefficient is $r = -0.85$. This calculation is made in the following way:

$$r = \frac{n(\Sigma XY) - (\Sigma X)(\Sigma Y)}{\sqrt{\left[n(\Sigma X^2) - (\Sigma X)^2 \right] \left[n(\Sigma Y^2) - (\Sigma Y)^2 \right]}}$$

in which
n = number of subjects,
X = variable 1, and
Y = variable 2.

The strength and direction of the relationship are important considerations when evaluating data. The strength of the correlation is determined

TABLE 1.1   Weight and Vertical Jump Data

Subject	Weight	Vertical jump
1	225	31
2	289	18
3	186	42
4	190	25
5	245	30
6	265	21
7	300	18
8	175	36
9	180	33
10	290	21

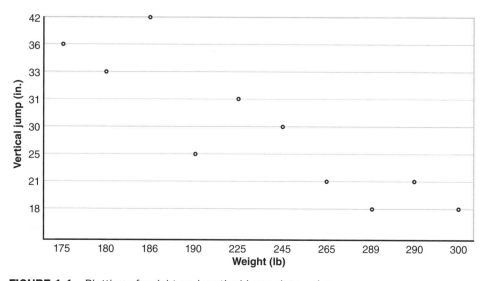

FIGURE 1.1   Plotting of weight and vertical jump data points.

TABLE 1.2 Scale for the Strength of a Correlation

Zero	0.0
Low	0.0–0.3
High	0.3–0.7
Perfect	1.0

by comparing the value to a scale ranging from 0 to 1.0 (see table 1.2; Morrow et al. 2000). The most frequently used statistic to evaluate the relationship between two variables on interval or ratio scales (e.g., the relationship between body weight in kilograms and vertical jump height in inches) is the Pearson product moment correlation coefficient. Calculation of the correlation coefficient relies on variance in both sets of data being analyzed for covariation (i.e., the degree to which the two variables change together). When two variables covary, they may be correlated to each other positively or negatively, which is indicated by a +/– designation. For the purposes of data interpretation, a larger correlation value (i.e., closer to 1.0 or –1.0) represents a stronger underlying association. Higher magnitudes of one variable occurring with higher magnitudes of another, and lower magnitudes on both variables, is a demonstration of a positive correlation. Conversely, two variables may covary inversely or oppositely, such as with a negative correlation (i.e., the higher magnitudes of one variable correspond with the lower magnitudes of the other, and vice versa). Thus, the relationship between weight and vertical jump from the sample data represents a strong negative correlation.

Differences Among Performance Variables

Determining differences among performance variables is often an important use of data collection and analysis. A variety of ways are available to objectively determine whether differences exist and to examine the magnitude of the actual difference. The technique used depends on the circumstances of testing. Examples of times when determining differences among measures might be desirable include a coach wanting to know whether athletes' strength levels are increasing, a physical therapist comparing two treatment strategies to see which is more effective, a trainer comparing changes in jump performance following a plyometric training program, and a researcher wanting to know the difference in performance level between major and minor league baseball players.

If the same group is compared, with measures taken before and after an intervention, a paired-samples t-test or a repeated measures analysis of variance would be used to examine changes. If different groups are placed on separate interventions, an independent-samples t-test or analysis of variance can be used. The statistical analysis evaluates the difference in scores and the variability between subjects or groups, as well as provides a probability value to help determine how consistently the measured difference could be expected. Examining the overall variability of the scores is important because, generally speaking, there will be individual differences within and between groups. However, it is important to determine whether those differences might be inferred to a larger population.

Determining the magnitude of the difference in performance measures is also important. If we simply calculate the change in the performance score (posttest minus pretest), and then calculate the average increase for the group, we get a crude measure of this magnitude. However, if one or several members of the group increase or decrease at a level much different from that of the rest of the group, the average increase may be misleading. For instance, if we measured bench press 1RM before and after a 12-week training program in a group of 10 clients, and then calculated the average increase in weight lifted, we would have a measure of the magnitude of the change. However, what if one client increased by 50 pounds (23 kg), while every other member of the group increased by only 5 pounds (2.3 kg)? The average increase for the whole group would be 10 pounds (4.5 kg). The large increase by one client doubled the consistent increase of 5 pounds (2.3 kg) by all other members of the group. Most likely, the correct magnitude of change would be approximately 5 pounds (2.3 kg), and the data from one client caused a skewed result.

This inconsistent increase in the one client may be the result of a difference in the starting point. If nine clients in the group started the program with a maximal bench press of approximately 300 pounds (136 kg) and a lengthy training background, and one client began at 100 pounds (45 kg) and a minimal training background, the potential for improvement in the one client is much greater. One way to deal with this confounding variable is to calculate percentage increases by dividing the difference in pre- and posttests by the pretest, and then multiplying the outcome by 100. A 50-pound (23 kg) increase in a client starting at 100 pounds (45 kg) would be equal to a 50% increase. A 5-pound (2.3 kg) increase by someone who started at 300 pounds (136 kg) represents a 2% increase. Although we have now considered the different starting points of the clients, the calculation of percentage increase actually makes the problem worse in this case. Without considering the variation in improvements, we risk skewing the results and making incorrect decisions regarding the test data.

One way to calculate group improvement in a way that considers the variation in improvement is to use effect size—a standardized value that depicts the improvements in performance in a group. Cohen (1988) suggested one method that may be of particular value for fitness professionals: calculating the mean absolute improvement in performance and dividing it by the standard deviation of the pretest. Referring back to the discussion of descriptive analysis, we can calculate the means for the pretest and

TABLE 1.3 Cohen's Scale

<.41	Small Effect
.41–.70	Moderate Effect
>.70	Large Effect

Based on Cohen 1988.

post-test, along with the standard deviation of the pretest, and use the following calculation to determine the magnitude of the change:

(Posttest mean – pretest mean) / pretest standard deviation

The outcome data, which are provided as standard deviation units, can be compared across groups. Several scales have been suggested to compare the calculated effect size. This determines the relative size of the effect. Cohen (1988) developed a scale (table 1.3) based on research in psychology with ranges depicting small, moderate, and large effects. Another scale (table 1.4), created specifically to evaluate strength development (Rhea 2004), can be useful for examining the magnitude of strength improvement among populations.

Normalizing Fitness Data

Field tests have become popular in applied exercise science and sport performance enhancement programs because of their simplicity and ability to generalize results. However, numerous confounding factors may influence the validity of test data from such evaluations. In addition to gender, age, level of physical fitness, and skill, body size is well recognized as a factor that influences both muscle fitness and the outcome of a number of functional performance tests (e.g., strength testing, vertical jump, sprint speed). Therefore, adjusting for body mass appears to be necessary when assessing these functional characteristics, especially when comparing to a norm-referenced standard (i.e., peer group).

For muscular strength capacity, the simplest way to normalize data is to divide strength by body mass. This ratio method provides a straightforward index of relative muscular strength abilities and is often considered superior to measuring absolute strength, especially when determining the contribution(s) to explosive movement performance (Peterson, Alvar, and Rhea 2006). It is important to note that this method is based on the assumption that the relationship between strength and body mass is linear.

However, some research has demonstrated that the relationship between strength and body mass tests may not be linear, but is, instead, curvilinear. Other ways to normalize strength are used in powerlifting (Wilks Formula) and Olympic-style weightlifting (Sinclair Formula), and allow the identification of a strength composite index relative to body mass. These formulas

TABLE 1.4 Rhea's Scale for Strength Effects

Magnitude	Untrained	Recreationally Trained	Highly Trained
Trivial	<.50	<.35	<.25
Small	.50–1.25	.35–.80	.25–.50
Moderate	1.25–1.90	.80–1.50	.50–1.0
Large	>2.0	>1.5	>1.0

Based on Rhea 2004.

minimize the risk of handicapping or recompensing the bigger athlete and smaller athlete, respectively, and provide for an equitable competitive environment. However, as in strength and conditioning for large team sports, it is often necessary to compare numerous people of differing body masses. Research pertaining to dimensional scaling suggests that such comparisons of muscular strength attributes among people of variable body sizes should be expressed relative to body mass, raised to the power of 0.67—for example, (kg lifted) / (kg body weight)$^{0.67}$ (Jaric, Mirkov, and Markovic 2005). Known as allometric scaling, this statistical transformation of the raw data is used to provide the appropriate relationship between body mass and the strength outcome of interest.

Allometric scaling is derived from the theory of geometric similarity and assumes that humans have the same basic shape, yet may still differ in size. Other investigations have demonstrated different requisite scaling exponents for performance in activities not related to maximal force production (e.g., aerobic power). Regardless of the performance outcome being assessed, allometric scaling is based on several assumptions, including the following:

- The relationship between body dimension (usually body mass, lean body mass, or muscle cross-sectional area) and performance is curvilinear.

- The relationship between performance (P) and body size (S) may be assessed by the equation: $P = aS^b$, where a and b are the constant multipliers and scaling exponent, respectively (Nevill, Ramsbottom, and Williams 1992).

- The curvilinear relationship must pass through the origin of both variables (e.g., an athlete with no lean body mass would have a strength score of 0).

Solving for the scaling exponent (b) allows for the removal of individual differences in the scaling factor (S) (i.e., body size) on the performance outcome (P) (e.g., strength).

Allometric scaling is necessary for any outcome in which body dimension and respective performance do not share a linear relationship. If strength and body mass shared a linear association, the scaling exponent would be equal to 1 (b = 1), and the aforementioned ratio method would sufficiently characterize relative strength—that is, (kg lifted) / (kg body weight)[1]. However, because this is not the case, a correction factor must be applied to accurately report or examine body mass–adjusted strength. Ultimately, using the correct scaling equation for a specific sample population for a particular performance-based test minimizes the confounding influence of body dimension.

Tracking Data Over Time

Tracking performance data over time can provide valuable feedback to fitness professionals and their clients. The ability to evaluate changes in performance in a group of peers, or with respect to an individual's previous performances, can enable the professional to alter training as needed or provide evidence that the given training program is working. In short, tracking performance over time can demonstrate that clients are reaching their goals or provide the necessary feedback for making alterations to ensure goal achievement.

Several factors must be considered when comparing changes in performance over time. The first is a learning effect, which occurs when people become accustomed to performing a particular test. Generally, tests should be performed on several occasions prior to gathering the initial data set, to familiarize clients with the test procedures. For instance, clients should be offered the chance to try the test after being taught the appropriate technique by a qualified instructor. If the bench press 1RM test were being used to track performance in upper body strength capacity, a qualified instructor should provide instruction on correct technique and progression in resistance. The instructor should also provide feedback during practice attempts to ensure that the client uses the appropriate technique. Several testing trials should be conducted to ensure that the client is familiar with the procedures and capable of completing them as required. Once this familiarization has occurred, a testing session should be completed to generate data to serve as the baseline performance for future comparisons.

Another factor that influences changes in performance over time is maturation. This is especially significant among children and young adults whose bodies are changing rapidly, because physiological growth factors can alter performance. These variables should be considered when evaluating performance, especially if comparisons are made over long periods of time (e.g., several years).

Tests, measurements, and data analysis may at times seem like unnecessary additions to the already heavy workload of fitness professionals. Moreover, understanding and interpreting statistics may seem outside of the scope of practice, or scope of understanding, for professionals in this line of work. However, the ability to gather appropriate information from clients, evaluate both group and individual data, and accurately interpret the findings is an important and valuable aspect of high-level practices. *Evidence-based practice* is a term often thrown around to gain the trust and confidence of potential clients. Professionals who use testing and data analysis to examine their own programs, evaluate new ideas and concepts, or compare training modalities can both profess to base their practices on scientific evidence and actually do so.

In addition to facilitating collecting data, crunching numbers, and evaluating statistics, a keen understanding of tests and measurements can enable fitness professionals to more accurately and confidently analyze and interpret published research. Many professionals glance over (or skip entirely) the methods and statistics sections of research papers because of their lack of familiarity with research terminology and methodology. As fitness professionals become more familiar with these procedures and this somewhat strange language, they will become more comfortable with and capable of taking valuable information from published research and implementing high-quality methods into their daily practices.

SUMMARY

- Performance tests and data evaluation can serve a variety of useful purposes for those working in exercise and health professions.
- Although the process must be conducted appropriately, and data evaluation requires a familiarization with various statistical procedures, using quality performance tests and objectively evaluating collected data will result in many benefits that are well worth the effort.
- Fitness professionals who become adept at the testing and evaluation process enhance their skills and become increasingly more effective.

2

Body Composition

Nicholas A. Ratamess, PhD, CSCS*D, FNSCA

Body composition is a term that describes the relative proportions of fat, bone, and muscle mass in the human body. *Anthropometry* is a term that describes the measurement of the human body in terms of dimensions such as height, weight, circumferences, girths, and skinfolds. Body composition and anthropometric tests have become standard practice for coaches, athletes, and fitness professionals. Valuable information regarding percent body fat (i.e., an estimate of the proportion of fat tissue within the human body), fat distribution, lean tissue mass (i.e., the mass of all nonfat tissue such as bones, muscles, and water), and limb lengths and circumferences may be gained through body composition testing.

Body composition tests may be useful for evaluating training, diet, or athletic performance, or for reducing the risk factors associated with musculoskeletal injury. For example, a body composition test may determine that an athlete is approximately 5 pounds (2.3 kg) over his desired weight and that his percent body fat is slightly higher (~1-2%) than normal. This information can help the coach and athlete determine training and dietary strategies. The coach may recommend a small reduction in daily kilocalorie intake (or just limitations in simple sugars or dietary fats), an increase in activity level to increase daily kilocalorie expenditure, or both, to reduce body fat. The athlete may add an additional 15 minutes of low- to moderate-intensity cardiorespiratory exercise at the end of a workout two or three days per week until he attains his ideal body mass and percent fat. Frequent testing will help him monitor his progress and assess the efficacy of the strategies used to attain his target body composition level.

Body composition is one of the five major health-related components of fitness (in addition to muscular strength and endurance, flexibility, and cardiorespiratory endurance), and its assessment has many benefits to children, adolescents and teenagers, adults, and elderly people, as well as performance benefits to athletes (American College of Sports Medicine 2008). In addition, body composition affects the other health-related components of fitness—that is, body mass, lean body mass, and fat content affect muscle strength and endurance, flexibility, and cardiorespiratory endurance. In general, knowledge of one's percent body fat serves as a starting point for comparison; people do not know how they rank compared to others of their gender and age (via classification standards) until their body composition is assessed. They can use this information as a tracking metric for subsequent weight loss, weight gain, or exercise-related training programs.

For example, body composition measurements are useful for athletes in some weight-controlled sports in which body fat levels and hydration (water content) can fall to low levels. Sports such as gymnastics, wrestling, and bodybuilding require athletes to compete at either low weight or low body fat levels. Athletes in these sports can benefit greatly from routine body composition evaluations.

Body composition analysis can also benefit the athlete who is training to increase muscle mass; lean tissue mass measurements can be used to evaluate training programs and measure progress. In addition, body composition tests are very useful for determining health and wellness. An excess amount of body fat, or obesity (especially in the abdominal area), is a risk factor linked to several diseases including type 2 diabetes mellitus, hypertension, hyperlipidemia, cardiovascular disease (CVD), certain types of cancer, low back pain, and osteoarthritis (Despres and Lemieux 2006; Liuke et al. 2005; Wearing et al. 2006).

Historically, some people have attempted to assess obesity via height–weight tables. One popular method involved the use of the Metropolitan Life Insurance table from 1983. This table established an optimal weight range for men and women with small, medium, and large frames. For example, a 6-foot (183 cm) male with a large frame would be considered overweight if he weighed more than 188 pounds (85 kg). Overweight is a weight in excess of the recommended range. However, overweight does not necessarily reflect obesity, because weight alone doesn't necessarily mean that one has a high percentage of body fat. Thus, *overweight* is a term more suited for sedentary populations and not athletes or those who exercise regularly. An athlete with greater lean tissue mass will also have a higher body weight; thus, height–weight tables have little value in the athletic world. Body weight itself is not a direct risk factor per se. However, an excessive amount of body fat poses major health risks. Determining percent body fat yields greater insight into health and fitness levels than body weight does.

Sport Performance and Body Composition

Sport performance is highly dependent on the health- and skill-related components of fitness (power, speed, agility, reaction time, balance, and coordination) in addition to the athlete's technique and level of competency in sport-specific motor skills. All fitness components depend on body composition to some extent. An increase in lean body mass contributes to strength and power development. Strength and power are related to muscle size. Thus, an increase in lean body mass enables the athlete to generate more force in a specific period of time. A sufficient level of lean body mass also contributes to speed, quickness, and agility performance (in the development of force applied to the ground for maximal acceleration and deceleration). Reduced nonessential body fat contributes to muscular and cardiorespiratory endurance, speed, and agility development. Additional weight (in the form of nonessential fat) provides greater resistance to athletic motion thereby forcing the athlete to increase the muscle force of contraction per given workload. The additional body fat can limit endurance, balance, coordination, and movement capacity. Joint range of motion can be negatively affected by excessive body mass and fat as well, and mass can form a physical barrier to joint movement in a complete range of motion. Thus, athletes competing in sports that require high levels of flexibility benefit from having low levels of body fat.

The demands of the sport require that athletes maintain standard levels of body composition. Some sports require athletes to be large in stature, mass, or both, whereas some athletes prosper when they are small in stature. For example, linemen in American football and heavyweight wrestlers need high levels of body mass. Although lean body mass is ideal, these athletes can benefit from mass increases in either form (fat included). Greater mass provides these athletes with more inertia, enabling them to play their positions with greater stability provided speed and agility are not compromised. Strength and power athletes such as American football players, wrestlers, and other combat athletes; powerlifters; bodybuilders; weightlifters; and track and field throwers benefit greatly from high levels of lean body mass. Endurance athletes such as distance runners, cyclists, and triathletes benefit greatly from having low percent body fat. Athletes such as gymnasts, wrestlers, high jumpers, pole vaulters, boxers, mixed martial artists, and weightlifters benefit greatly from having a high strength-to-mass (and power-to-mass) ratio. Training to maximize strength and power while minimizing changes in body mass (and keeping body fat low) is of great value to these sports. Gymnasts, pole vaulters, and high jumpers have to overcome their body weights to obtain athletic success. Thus, minimizing changes in mass enables greater flight height, time, and aerial athleticism.

Wrestlers, boxers, mixed martial artists, powerlifters, and weightlifters compete in weight classes. Because higher weight classes may denote more difficult competition, these athletes benefit from improving strength and power while maintaining their normal weight class. Athletes such as baseball and softball players benefit from increased lean body mass and reduced body fat. The additional lean mass can assist in power, speed, and agility, and keeping body fat low assists with endurance, quickness, speed, and agility as well (for performing skills such as throwing, hitting, fielding, and base running).

Basketball and soccer are two of several combination anaerobic and aerobic sports in which athletes need power, speed, quickness, agility, and strength yet also moderate to high levels of aerobic fitness. Athletes from both of these sports benefit from having low body fat while maintaining or increasing lean body mass. Although some athletes can tolerate higher levels of body mass and perhaps percent body fat, it is generally recommended that data obtained from frequent body composition measurements be used to develop training plans aimed at reducing body fat while maintaining or increasing lean body mass.

Practical Applications

The measurement and quantification of percent body fat is of great importance for fitness practitioners, coaches, trainers, and athletes for several reasons. The measurement of percent body fat allows athletes to identify where they rank (e.g., lean, average, high, obese) according to standards and can be used to identify athletes at the extremes (e.g., at risk for obesity or eating disorders, which are especially a concern for female athletes in weight-controlled sports).

Athletes can use body fat data to modify training, diet, or both, to achieve the desired body fat level for their sports. For example, an athlete with too high a level of body fat can increase aerobic exercise duration, increase volume and decrease rest interval length for resistance exercise (to increase the metabolic demand and energy expenditure), or reduce kilocalorie intake (primarily by decreasing saturated fat and simple carbohydrate intake) to favor a net energy deficit that can lower body fat. If an eating disorder (e.g., bulimia or anorexia nervosa) is identified in an athlete whose body mass and fat levels are lower than expected, attempts can be made to assist the athlete with nutritional and psychological counseling.

Body composition testing generates descriptive data of athletes for various sports and positions. This is particularly useful from a research perspective but can benefit a coach over time when norms are developed. Coaches can use these data to compare their athletes to other athletes in the league or conference and can compare their current athletes to former athletes in the program. This can be used to identify trends in player body composition over time.

Body composition testing also serves as a starting point for program evaluation. For example, if an athlete has 20.8% body fat at the beginning of a program, and after 12 weeks of training has 18.6%, the coach and athlete can conclude that the program resulted in a 2.2% reduction in body fat.

Athletes in weight-controlled sports or making weight for weight classes can use body composition testing to identify a safe percent fat low point, or minimal weight. Percent fat should not be lower than 4% in males and 10% in females for extended periods of time. If percent fat approaches these values, modifications can be made (i.e., no more weight loss or a change in weight class).

Some body composition tests (e.g., DEXA) can yield critical information such as bone mineral density, total body water, and lean tissue mass. Lean tissue mass can be calculated from skinfold analyses or any method used to determine percent body fat. These can be used to evaluate training adaptations particularly to a resistance training program targeting muscle hypertrophy.

Body fat measurement allows for the calculation of ideal body weight or fat mass. For example, an athlete who weighs 215 pounds (98 kg) with a percent fat of 15% targets a percent fat of 13% (or less) and a weight of 210 pounds (95 kg). Initially, this athlete has 32.3 pounds (14.7 kg) of body fat (215 lb × 0.15 = 32.3 lb; or 98 × 0.15 = 14.7). He knows he can safely reach this weight because he has 32.3 pounds (14.7 kg) of fat but only desires to lose 5 pounds (2.3 kg). On the other hand, his ideal body weight can be calculated when he sets a target body fat level (in this case, going from 15 to 13%). Ideal body weight (IBW) can be calculated as follows:

IBW = (body weight − fat weight) / (1.00 − desired % / 100)
IBW = (215 lb − 32.3 lb) / (1.00 − 13% / 100)
IBW = 182.7 lb / (1.00 − 0.13)
IBW = 182.7 lb / 0.87
IBW = 210 lb

Body Composition Measurement

There are no truly direct methods for measuring body composition. Rather, most body composition measurements involve indirect assessment, or estimation. Each method has advantages and disadvantages as noted in the many studies that have made direct comparisons. The decision of which method to use depends on several factors, including the needs of the client, the purpose of the evaluation, the cost of the measurements or equipment needed, the availability of each measurement tool, the training of the technician, and the weighted advantages and disadvantages of each. Several common and practical body composition measurement techniques are discussed in this chapter.

Measuring Height, Body Weight, and Body Mass Index

Height and body weight and mass measurements are easy to perform. They can provide useful body composition data. Height can change throughout the day (based on spinal loading and vertebral disc volume) and more significantly with aging. Because of its relatively low magnitude of daily fluctuation, height in adults does not need to be measured frequently. The measurement of body weight can be performed frequently especially during weight loss or weight gain training programs or when athletes are reducing weight to compete in a weight class.

HEIGHT

EQUIPMENT

Height should be measured with a stadiometer (a vertical ruler mounted on a wall with a wide horizontal headboard). Although many commercial scales have an attached vertical ruler, these devices are less reliable. Failure to follow accepted standards reduces reliability and accuracy.

PROCEDURE

1. The subject removes shoes.
2. The subject stands as straight as possible with heels together near the wall.
3. The subject takes a deep breath, holds it, and stands with head level, looking straight ahead.
4. The height of the subject is recorded in inches or centimeters (1 in. = 2.54 cm).

BODY WEIGHT AND MASS

Body weight and mass represent different kinetic variables. In biomechanics, body mass is the amount of matter an object or person consists of, whereas weight is a force measurement—that is, the product of mass and acceleration due to gravity ($9.81 \text{ m} \cdot \text{s}^{-2}$) depending on the effects of gravity. Both are measured the same way. However, body mass is expressed in kilograms, whereas body weight is expressed in pounds or sometimes Newtons (N). Clothing is also an issue, and the type and amount of clothing must be standardized. Body weight changes at various times of day as a result of meal and beverage consumption, urination, defecation, and dehydration, or water loss. Therefore, a standard time (e.g., early in the morning) is recommended.

EQUIPMENT

Body weight and body mass are best measured on a calibrated physician's scale with a beam and movable weights.

PROCEDURE

1. Clothing must be standardized and shoes must be removed. Accuracy is greatest with minimal clothing. A subject wearing clothing should empty pockets and remove jewelry.

2. The subject steps onto the scale and the weight is recorded upon stabilization of the beam. Body weight is recorded in pounds, or body mass is recorded in kilograms (1 kg = 2.2 lb; 1 N = 0.224 lb; 1 lb = 4.448 N).

BODY MASS INDEX

Body mass index (BMI) is used to assess body mass relative to height:

$$\text{BMI } (kg \cdot m^{-2}) = \text{body mass (kg) / height squared } (m^2)$$

BMI has been used to determine the risk of developing diseases such as type 2 diabetes, hypertension, and CVD and is very easy to calculate.

PROCEDURE

Body mass index may also be calculated using the following equation: BMI = body weight (lb) × 703 / height² (in.²). For example, a man who is 195 pounds (88.6 kg) and 6 feet 3 inches (190.5 cm, or 1.905 m) would have a BMI of 24.4 kg · m⁻² and would be considered normal when compared to BMI standards. The current BMI (kg · m⁻²) standards for men and women in the United States are as follows (American College of Sports Medicine 2007):

BMI < 18.5 indicates underweight

BMI of 18.5 to 24.9 is normal

BMI of 25 to 29.9 indicates overweight

BMI of 30 to 39.9 is obese

BMI > 40 indicates morbid obesity

Although simplistic in its calculation, BMI has greater practical relevance in sedentary and clinical populations. It strongly correlates with disease and is easy to use in large populations. Criticisms of the use of BMI are that it is a relatively poor predictor of body fat percent, is not indicative of weight distribution, and may result in inaccurate classifications (normal, overweight, obese) for muscular people, athletes, and those who play collegiate or professional sports. For example, one study that examined body composition in National Football League players in the United States showed that based on BMI, every player was classified as overweight, obese, or very obese despite having body fat percentages of 6.3 to 18.5% (with offensive linemen at 25.1%) (Kraemer et al. 2005). A recent study examining NCAA Division I American football players showed across all positions a mean BMI of 29.8 kg · m^{-2} despite an average percent body fat of ~15 ± 7% (Kaiser et al. 2008). Another study of American football players showed BMI to be an invalid measure because it overestimated being overweight and obese in more than 50% of the athletes (Mathews and Wagner 2008). This appears to be the case with strength and power athletes from other sports as well. Thus, BMI is not a particularly useful body composition measurement tool in resistance-trained populations.

WAIST-TO-HIP RATIO

The waist-to-hip ratio (WHR) compares the circumferences of the waist to that of the hip and is used as an indicator of body fat distribution (i.e., the apple or pear physique) or as a measure of general health. A high WHR has been recognized as a risk factor for disease. An advantage of this technique is that it is simple to administer and requires only a tape measure. In some cases, WHR may be a better predictor of mortality than BMI. However, because it is a circumference ratio, it does not provide an indication of percent body fat. Skinfold measurement (or other body fat technique) provides a more accurate estimation of percent body fat. Critical to the accuracy and reliability of WHR measurement is standardization of the circumference technique. Standards for WHR values are shown in table 2.1.

EQUIPMENT

A flexible tape measure (such as a Gulick II tape measure)

PROCEDURE

1. All that is needed for this procedure is a flexible tape measure. A Gulick II tape measure is beneficial because it applies a constant amount of tension to the tape, thereby eliminating variability among examiners.

2. The waist circumference should be taken around the smallest area of the waist, typically ~1 inch (2.54 cm) above the navel.

3. The hip circumference is taken around the largest area of the buttocks (with minimal clothing).

4. The WHR is calculated as the waist circumference (cm or in.) / hip circumference (cm or in.) and is expressed with no units because they cancel each other out during the process of division.

5. Multiple measurements should be taken until each is within ¼ inch (0.6 cm) of each other.

TABLE 2.1   Waist-to-Hip Measurement Standards for Men and Women

Population	Age	RISK			
		Low	**Moderate**	**High**	**Very high**
Men	20-29	<0.83	0.83-0.88	0.89-0.94	>0.94
	30-39	<0.84	0.84-0.91	0.92-0.96	>0.96
	40-49	<0.88	0.88-0.95	0.96-1.00	>1.00
	50-59	<0.90	0.90-0.96	0.97-1.02	>1.02
	60-69	<0.91	0.91-0.98	0.99-1.03	>1.03
Women	20-29	<0.71	0.71-0.77	0.78-0.82	>0.82
	30-39	<0.72	0.72-0.78	0.79-0.84	>0.84
	40-49	<0.73	0.73-0.79	0.80-0.87	>0.87
	50-59	<0.74	0.74-0.81	0.82-0.88	>0.88
	60-69	<0.76	0.76-0.83	0.84-0.90	>0.90

Reprinted, by permission, from V.H. Heyward, 2010, *Applied body composition assessment*, 6th ed. (Champaign, IL: Human Kinetics), 222.

SKINFOLD MEASUREMENT

Skinfold measurement is one of the most popular and practical methods for estimating percent body fat, and can be relatively accurate provided that a trained technician is performing the measurement with high-quality calipers (e.g., a Lange or Harpenden caliper that provides a constant pressure of ~10 g · mm^{-2}). Skinfold analysis is based on the principle that the amount of subcutaneous fat (fat immediately below the skin) is directly proportional to the total amount of body fat.

Following the collection of skinfold measurements, regression analysis (a statistical procedure used to predict a dependent variable based on one or more independent or predictor variables) is used to estimate total percent body fat. The sum of the skinfolds, along with gender and age (which are known significant predictors of body fat), are used in a regression analysis, which ultimately calculates a prediction equation to estimate body density and percent body fat. Variability in percent body fat prediction from skinfold analysis is approximately ±3 to 5% assuming that appropriate techniques and equations have been used (American College of Sports Medicine 2008). Body fat varies with gender, age, race or ethnicity, training status, and other factors. Therefore, numerous regression equations using a combination of skinfold sites have been developed to predict body density and fat from skinfold measurements.

Skinfold measurement is most accurate when prediction equations are used that closely match the population being tested. The number of sites needs to be predetermined based on the regression equation or methods used (i.e., three, four, or seven sites). Both seven- and three-site skinfold equations have shown similar standard errors of estimate in men (±3.4 to 3.6%) and women (±3.8 to 3.9%) (American College of Sports Medicine 2007).

EQUIPMENT

High-quality calipers (e.g., Lange or Harpenden)

PROCEDURE

1. The number of sites and equations should first be selected based on the population tested. Skinfold sites are shown in figure 2.1.

2. A fold of skin is firmly grasped between the thumb and index finger of the left hand (about 8 cm apart on a line perpendicular to the long axis of the site) and lifted away from the body while the subject is relaxed. Following are commonly used skinfold sites:

   - Abdomen: Horizontal fold; 2 centimeters to the right of the umbilicus
   - Biceps: Vertical fold on the anterior aspect of the arm over the belly of the biceps muscle
   - Chest or pectoral: Diagonal fold; half the distance between the anterior axillary line and the nipple (in men), or one third the distance between the anterior axillary line and the nipple (in women)
   - Midaxillary: Horizontal fold on the midaxillary line at the level of the xiphoid process of the sternum
   - Subscapular: Diagonal fold at a 45° angle, 1 to 2 centimeters below the inferior angle of the scapula
   - Suprailiac: Diagonal fold in line with the natural angle of the iliac crest taken in the anterior axillary line
   - Thigh: Vertical fold on the anterior midline of the thigh midway between the proximal border of the patella and the inguinal crease
   - Triceps: Vertical fold on the posterior midline of the upper arm midway between the acromion process of the scapula and the inferior part of the olecranon process of the elbow

3. A slight muscular contraction of the subject or a finger roll of the fold ensures that subcutaneous tissue is measured and not skeletal muscle. For obese people, a large grasping area (i.e., >8 cm) may be needed and could possibly exceed the measurement capacity of the caliper.

4. While the caliper is facing up, the jaws of the caliper are placed over the skinfold 1 centimeter below the fingers of the tester.

5. The caliper grip is released and the measurement is subsequently taken within three seconds.

6. All measurements are taken on the right side of the body in duplicate or triplicate for consistency among measurements to the nearest 0.5 millimeter. If there is more than a 3-millimeter difference between readings, a fourth measurement may be needed.

7. It is important to rotate through the sites as opposed to taking two or three measurements sequentially from the same site.

8. Each site is averaged and summed to estimate body density and percent body fat via a regression equation or prediction table. The total is viewed in a table relative to gender and age, and percent body fat is given.

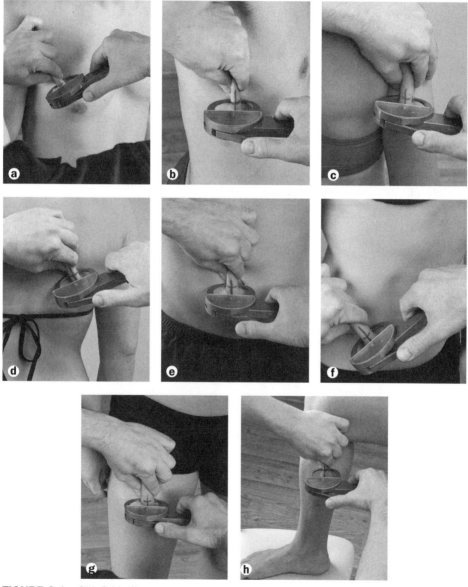

FIGURE 2.1   Skinfold sites.

Reprinted, by permission, from National Strength and Conditioning Association, 2008, Administration, scoring, and interpretation of selected tests, by E. Harman and J. Garhammer. In *Essentials of strength training and conditioning,* 3rd ed., edited by T.R. Baechle and R.W. Earle (Champaign, IL: Human Kinetics), 268-269.

Critical to skinfold analysis is the selection of an appropriate prediction equation. It is important to note that several equations are used to estimate body density, and a subsequent body density calculation is used to estimate percent body fat. Body density is described as the ratio of body mass to body volume. Table 2.2 depicts several equations used to estimate percent body fat from body density estimates. Since the early 1950s, more than 100 regression equations have been developed to predict body density and percent fat. Equations that have been cross-validated in other studies to support their efficacy should be chosen based on gender, age, ethnicity, and activity level. However, general equations have been shown to produce accurate estimates across all segments of the population (i.e., those with very high and low levels of body fat in addition to those whose body fat is near the population mean) and may be easier to use because only one or two equations are used as opposed to several (Graves et al. 2006). Because the relationship between body density and subcutaneous fat is curvilinear, quadratic and logarithmic terms have been added to most regression equations to increase their accuracy. Once body density has been determined, percent body fat can be calculated. Most often, the Siri (1956) or Brozek (Brozek et al. 1963) equations are used:

Siri equation: $(4.95 / B_d - 4.50) \times 100$

Brozek equation: $(4.57 / B_d - 4.142) \times 100$

*where B_d = body density

However, other population-specific equations (see table 2.3 on page 28) have been developed to estimate percent fat from body density based on ethnicity, gender, and age (Harman and Garhammer 2008). See table 2.4 on page 38 for information on when it is beneficial to perform BMI measurement. Table 2.5 on page 39 provides percent body fat classifications.

GIRTH MEASUREMENTS·

Girth measurements entail measuring the circumference of a body limb or region. In addition to providing useful information regarding changes in muscle size resulting from training, girth measurements, either alone or in combination with skinfold measurements, provide information regarding body composition. The advantages of taking circumference measurements is that doing so is easy, quick, and inexpensive and does not require specialized equipment. Accurate estimates of percent body fat (i.e., ±2.5 to 4%) can be made via girth measurements. Common sites measured include the right upper arm, abdomen, and right forearm for young men; buttocks (hip), abdomen, and right forearm for older men; abdomen, right thigh, and right forearm for young women; and abdomen, right thigh, and right calf for older women.

TABLE 2.2 Body Density Prediction Equations From Skinfold Measurements

Sites	Population	Gender	Equation	Reference
2: thigh, subscapular	Athletes	Male	$B_d = 1.1043 - (0.00133 \times \text{thigh}) - (0.00131 \times \text{subscapular})$	Sloan and Weir (1970)
2: suprailiac, triceps	Athletes	Female	$B_d = 1.0764 - (0.00081 \times \text{suprailiac}) - (0.00088 \times \text{triceps})$	Sloan and Weir (1970)
3: chest, ab, thigh	General	Male	$B_d = 1.10938 - 0.0008267$ (sum of 3 sites) $+ 0.0000016$ (sum of 3 sites)$^2 - 0.0002574$ (age)	Jackson and Pollock (1978)
3: triceps, suprailiac, thigh	General	Female	$B_d = 1.099421 - 0.0009929$ (sum of 3 sites) $+ 0.0000023$ (sum of 3 sites)$^2 - 0.0001392$ (age)	Jackson et al. (1980)
3: chest, triceps, subscapular	General	Male	$B_d = 1.1125025 - 0.0013125$ (sum of 3 sites) $+ 0.0000055$ (sum of 3 sites)$^2 - 0.000244$ (age)	Pollock et al. (1980)
3: triceps, suprailiac, ab	General	Female	$B_d = 1.089733 - 0.0009245$ (sum of 3 sites) $+ 0.0000025$ (sum of 3 sites)$^2 - 0.0000979$ (age)	Jackson and Pollock (1985)
4: biceps, triceps, subscapular, suprailiac	General	Male Female 20–29 years old	$B_d = 1.1631 - 0.0632$ (log sum of 4 sites)	Durnin and Womersley (1974)
4: biceps, triceps, subscapular, suprailiac	General	Male Female 30-39 years old	$B_d = 1.1422 - 0.0544$ (log sum of 4 sites)	Durnin and Womersley (1974)
7: thigh, subscapular, suprailiac, triceps, chest, ab, axillary	General	Female	$B_d = 1.0970 - 0.00046971$ (sum of 7 sites) $+ 0.00000056$ (sum of 7 sites)$^2 - 0.00012828$ (age)	Jackson et al. (1980)
7: thigh, subscapular, suprailiac, triceps, chest, ab, axillary	General	Male	$B_d = 1.112 - 0.00043499$ (sum of 7 sites) $+ 0.00000055$ (sum of 7 sites)$^2 - 0.00028826$ (age)	Jackson and Pollock (1978)

EQUIPMENT

Tape measure (preferably a Gulick II tape measure)

PROCEDURE

1. The tape measure (preferably a Gulick II tape measure) is applied in a horizontal plane to the site so it is taut and the circumference is read to the nearest half centimeter. Minimal clothing should be worn.

TABLE 2.3 Population-Specific Equations to Calculate Percent Body Fat From Body Density

Population	Age	Gender	Equation
Caucasian	7–12	Male	$(5.30 / B_d - 4.89) \times 100$
		Female	$(5.35 / B_d - 4.95) \times 100$
	13–16	Male	$(5.07 / B_d - 4.64) \times 100$
		Female	$(5.10 / B_d - 4.66) \times 100$
	17–19	Male	$(4.99 / B_d - 4.55) \times 100$
		Female	$(5.05 / B_d - 4.62) \times 100$
	20–80	Male	$(4.95 / B_d - 4.50) \times 100$
		Female	$(5.01 / B_d - 4.57) \times 100$
African American	18–32	Male	$(4.37 / B_d - 3.93) \times 100$
	24–79	Female	$(4.85 / B_d - 4.39) \times 100$
American Indian	18–60	Female	$(4.81 / B_d - 4.34) \times 100$
Hispanic	20–40	Female	$(4.87 / B_d - 4.41) \times 100$
Japanese	18–48	Male	$(4.97 / B_d - 4.52) \times 100$
		Female	$(4.76 / B_d - 4.28) \times 100$
	61–78	Male	$(4.87 / B_d - 4.41) \times 100$
		Female	$(4.95 / B_d - 4.50) \times 100$

Data from NSCA 2008; Heyward and Stolarczyk 1996.

2. Duplicate measures should be taken at each site, and the average is used. If readings differ by more than 5 millimeters, then an additional measurement is taken.

3. Subjects should remain relaxed while measurements are taken.

4. A large source of error is a lack of standardization of the measurement site. The correct placement of the tape measure per site is as follows:

   - Chest: The tape is placed around the chest at level of the fourth ribs after the subject abducts the arms. Measurement is taken when the subject adducts the arms back to the starting position and at the end of respiration.

   - Shoulder: The tape is placed horizontally at the maximal circumference of the shoulders while the subject is standing relaxed.

   - Abdomen: The tape is placed over the abdomen at the level of the greatest circumference (often near the navel) while the subject is standing relaxed.

   - Right thigh: The tape is placed horizontally over the thigh below the gluteal level at the largest circumference (i.e., upper thigh) while the subject is standing.

   - Right calf: The tape is placed horizontally over the largest circumference of the calf midway between the knee and ankle while the subject is standing relaxed.

- Waist and hip: The tape is placed around the smallest area of the waist, typically ~1 inch (2.54 cm) above the navel. The hip circumference is taken around the largest area of the buttocks (with minimal clothing).
- Right upper arm: The tape is placed horizontally over the midpoint of the upper arm between the shoulder and elbow while the subject is standing relaxed and the elbow is extended.
- Right forearm: The tape is placed horizontally over the proximal area of the forearm where the circumference is the largest while the subject is standing relaxed.

Estimations of percent body fat from circumferences can be made once values have been obtained. Age- and gender-specific equations have been developed to estimate percent fat. Equations for young and older men and women are based on a calculation of constants. Once constants are obtained, these values can be used in the following equations to estimate percent body fat. Circumference estimation of percent fat has an accuracy of ±2.5 to 4.0%. Table 2.4 on page 38 provides percent body fat classifications.

CIRCUMFERENCE PERCENT BODY FAT ESTIMATION EQUATIONS (AMERICAN COLLEGE OF SPORTS MEDICINE 2007; MCARDLE, KATCH, AND KATCH 2007)

Young men: Constant A + B − C − 10.2 = percent body fat

Young women: Constant A + B − C − 19.6 = percent body fat

Older men: Constant A + B − C − 15.0 = percent body fat

Older women: Constant A + B − C − 18.4 = percent body fat

HYDRODENSITOMETRY

Hydrodensitometry (underwater, or hydrostatic, weighing) has historically been considered the criterion method, or gold standard, for body composition analysis even though it is an indirect method. Hydrodensitometry is based on Archimedes' principle for determining body density where a body immersed in water encounters a buoyant force that results in weight loss equal to the weight of the water displaced during immersion. Subtracting the subject's body weight in water from the body weight on land provides the weight of the displaced water. Body fat contributes to buoyancy because the density of fat ($0.9007 \text{ g} \cdot \text{cm}^{-3}$) is less than water ($1 \text{ g} \cdot \text{cm}^{-3}$), whereas lean tissue mass ($\geq 1.100 \text{ g} \cdot \text{cm}^{-3}$) exceeds the density of water.

It is important to note that lean tissue density varies based on ethnicity and maturation. African Americans have been shown to have an average density of $1.113 \text{ g} \cdot \text{cm}^{-3}$, and Hispanics have shown an average value of $1.105 \text{ g} \cdot \text{cm}^{-3}$ compared to Caucasians ($1.100 \text{ g} \cdot \text{cm}^{-3}$) (McArdle, Katch, and Katch 2007). Children and older adults have lower lean tissue densities than young adults. In addition, disproportionately large increases in muscle mass (from resistance training) compared to bone mineral density changes can lower body density and result in an overestimate of percent body fat (McArdle, Katch, and Katch 2007). Body density (mass / volume) is calculated and then converted to percent body fat using an equation such as the Siri (1956) or Brozek (1963) equations. Population-specific equations (e.g., for African Americans, Indians, Hispanics, Japanese, and Caucasians) have been developed to more accurately convert body density data into percent body fat (American College of Sports Medicine 2007).

Because hydrodensitometry is considered a gold standard, other body composition measurement tools (e.g., skinfolds, bioelectrical impedance) are validated against it. Test–retest reliability is high when procedures are followed correctly. However, practical limitations can make hydrodensitometry difficult in certain situations. The cost and specialized use of the equipment needed is great, and may be impractical in certain facilities. The time involved in each measurement is lengthy, which could make other body composition measurements more attractive. Lastly, many subjects express fear and discomfort about needing to be fully submerged in water.

The following variables must be known when performing hydrodensitometry:

- *Residual volume*: The amount of air remaining in the lungs following full expiration. Residual volume can be measured or predicted using a combination of age, gender, and height. A substantial amount of air left in the lungs increases buoyancy, which may be mistaken as additional body fat.

- *Water density*: Water density varies with water temperature, because buoyancy decreases with warmer temperatures.

- *Amount of trapped gas in the gastrointestinal system*: Typically, a predicted constant of 100 milliliters is used.

- *Dry body weight.*

- *Body weight in water.*

EQUIPMENT

A tank made of stainless steel, fiberglass, ceramic tile, Plexiglas, or other material (or a swimming pool) that is at least $4 \times 4 \times 5$ feet ($1.2 \times 1.2 \times 1.5$ m). A seat suspended from a scale or force transducer is needed to allow subjects to be weighed while they are completely submerged in water.

PROCEDURE

1. Subjects should wear minimal clothing. A tight-fitting bathing suit that traps little air is recommended.

2. Subjects should remove all jewelry and have urinated and defecated prior to the procedure.

3. Subjects should be 2 to 12 hours postabsorptive and have avoided foods that increase gas in the gastrointestinal tract. Menstruation may pose a problem for females because of associated water gain; thus, women should try to avoid being tested within seven days of menstruation.

4. A seat suspended from a scale or force transducer is needed to allow subjects to be weighed while completely submerged in water. The temperature of the water should be between 33 and 36 °C (91.4 and 96.8 °F).

5. The subject is weighed on land to determine dry weight, and the mass is converted to grams.

6. The subject enters the tank, removes potential trapped air from the skin, hair, suit, and so on, and attains a seated position while supported by a belt to minimize fluctuations.

7. Once the subject is seated and the chair height has been adjusted, the subject fully expires as much air as possible prior to leaning forward to be weighed.

8. The subject is weighed 5 to 10 times while submerged underwater for 5 to 10 seconds. The highest of the weights or the average of the three highest weights are used for analysis. The weight of the chair and belt need to be considered in the calculation.

9. Residual lung volume (RV) can be measured directly (which increases accuracy) in some systems or estimated based on height and age:

Males: RV (L) = [0.019 × ht (cm)] + [0.0155 × age (yrs)] – 2.24

Females: RV (L) = [0.032 × ht (cm)] + [0.009 × age (yrs)] – 3.90

Body density is calculated using the following equation:

$$BD = \frac{\text{Mass in air (g)}}{[\text{Mass in air (g)} - \text{mass in water (g)}] - [\text{RV (mL)}]}$$
$$\text{Density of water}$$

10. Body fat can be calculated using the Siri, Brozek, or population-specific equations mentioned previously (p. 26). Table 2.4 on page 38 provides percent body fat classifications.

BIOELECTRICAL IMPEDANCE ANALYSIS

Bioelectrical impedance analysis (BIA) is a noninvasive and easy-to-administer tool for determining body composition. The underlying principle for BIA is that electrical conductivity in the body is proportional to the fat-free tissue of the body (American College of Sports Medicine 2007; McArdle, Katch, and Katch 2007). A small electrical current is sent through the body (from ankle to wrist), and the impedance to that current is measured. Lean tissue (mostly water and electrolytes) is a good electrical conductor (i.e., has low impedance), whereas fat is a poor conductor and impedes an electrical current. Thus, BIA can be used to measure percent body fat and total body water. Single- and multifrequency currents can be used to determine body composition; multifrequency currents are more sensitive to the body's fluid compartments (McArdle, Katch, and Katch 2007). Most studies examining BIA have used the equation $V = pL^2 \cdot R^{-1}$, where V is the volume of the conductor, p is the specific resistance of the tissue, L is the length of the conductor, and R is the observed resistance (Graves et al. 2006).

EQUIPMENT

A variety of BIA analyzers are commercially available and vary widely in price.

PROCEDURE

1. The BIA device should be calibrated according to the manufacturer's instructions.

2. The subject lies supine on a nonconductive surface with arm and legs at the side, not in contact with the rest of the body.

3. The right hand and wrist and right foot and ankle areas are prepared with an alcohol pad and then allowed to dry.

4. BIA electrodes are placed on the metacarpal of the right index finger and the metatarsal of the right big toe, and the reference (detecting) electrodes are placed on the right wrist (bisecting the ulnar and radial styloid processes) and the right ankle (midpoint on the line bisecting the medial and lateral malleoli).

5. The current is applied and the BIA analyzer computes the impedance and percent body fat.

6. New BIA devices are simpler to use than older ones and require only that the subject either stand on the machine (i.e., an electronic digital platform scale with built-in stainless steel foot pad electrodes) with both bare feet or hold the BIA analyzer in both hands. The device provides instructions to the subject (i.e., when to stand on the unit).

7. On occasion, a platform BIA device will produce an error if the subject's feet are dry. Adding some moisture to the feet can solve the problem.

Accuracy among BIA devices varies greatly. Most BIA machines use their own equations that account for differences in water content and body density based on people's gender, age, and race or ethnicity, as well as physical activity levels. The variation for BIA is ±2.7 to 6.3% (Graves et al. 2006), but this method can provide an accurate result when proper methods are used. The subject must not have eaten or consumed a beverage within four hours of the test, exercised within 12 hours of the test, or consumed alcohol or diuretics prior to testing; in addition, the subject must have completely voided the bladder within 30 minutes of the test and had minimal consumption of diuretic agents such as chocolate or caffeine (American College of Sports Medicine 2007). Dehydration can lead to overestimations in percent body fat. Glycogen stores can affect impedance and can be a factor during times of weight loss. If possible, BIA measurements should not be taken before menstruation to avoid the possible effects of water retention.

Although BIA is a valid measure of body composition, percent body fat is consistently overestimated for lean people and underestimated for obese people. In athletes, BIA has been shown to significantly underestimate percent body fat when compared to hydrodensitometry (Dixon et al. 2005). Subject factors, technical skill, the prediction equation used, and the instruments used all affect the accuracy of BIA. For best results, the same BIA unit should be used for multiple testing points. Table 2.4 on page 38 provides percent body fat classifications.

AIR DISPLACEMENT PLETHYSMOGRAPHY

Body volume can be measured by air displacement rather than water displacement. Air displacement plethysmography (ADP) offers several advantages over other methods including safety. It is quick and comfortable and noninvasive, and it accommodates all people. However, a major disadvantage is the cost of purchasing the ADP unit.

The BOD POD (a commercial ADP system) uses a dual-chamber (e.g., 450 L subject test chamber, 300 L reference chamber) plethysmograph that measures body volume via changes in air pressure within the closed two-compartment chamber. It includes an electronic weighing scale, computer, and software system. The volume of air displaced is equal to body volume and is calculated indirectly by subtracting the volume of air remaining in the chamber when the subject is inside from the volume of air in the chamber when it is empty.

Sources of error for ADP testing include variations in testing conditions, the subject not being in a fasted state, air that is not accounted for in the lungs or trapped within clothing and body hair, body moisture, and increased body temperature. Reliability of ADP in adults is good and has been shown to be valid in comparison to hydrodensitometry and dual-energy X-ray absorptiometry (DXA), which we discuss later.

ADP has been shown to produce similar (to DXA and hydrodensitometry) percent fat measurements in collegiate female athletes (Ballard, Fafara, and Vukovich 2004) and collegiate wrestlers (Dixon et al. 2005) and is an effective assessment technique for monitoring changes in percent fat during weight loss. However, some studies have shown that ADP overestimates percent body fat in collegiate female athletes (Vescovi et al. 2002) and underestimates percent body fat (by 2%) in collegiate American football players (Collins et al. 1999).

EQUIPMENT

An ADP unit such as the BOD POD

PROCEDURE

1. The subject's information is entered in the BOD POD computer.

2. The BOD POD is calibrated according to the manufacturer's instructions.

3. The subject is properly prepared. Similar to hydrodensitometry, minimal clothing is worn. Swimsuits, compression shorts, sport bras, and swim caps are recommended. Items such as jewelry and glasses are removed. Percent fat may be underestimated by nearly 3% if a swimming cap is not worn and hair covers a large portion of the face (Higgins et al. 2001).

4. The subject's mass is determined via the digital scale.

5. The subject enters the chamber and sits quietly during testing while a minimum of two measurements (within 150 ml of each other) are taken to determine body volume.

6. Thoracic gas volume is measured during normal breathing (i.e., via the panting method, in which the subject breathes normally into a tube connected within the chamber, followed by three small puffs after the airway tube becomes momentarily occluded at the midpoint of exhalation) or can be predicted via equations.

7. Corrected body volume (raw body volume – thoracic gas volume) is calculated, body density is determined, and percent body fat is calculated using similar prediction equations to hydrodensitometry via the system computer.

DUAL-ENERGY X-RAY ABSORPTIOMETRY

Dual-energy X-ray absorptiometry (DXA) is a body composition measurement tool that is increasing in popularity. In addition to percent body fat, regional and total-body measures of bone mineral density, fat content, and lean tissue mass are given. The principle of absorptiometry is based on the exponential attenuation of X-rays at two energies as they pass through the body. X-rays are generated at two energies via a low-current X-ray tube located underneath the DXA machine. The differential attenuation is used to estimate bone mineral content and soft tissue composition. A detector positioned overhead on the scanning arm and a computer interface are needed for scanning an image.

EQUIPMENT

DXA machine

PROCEDURE

1. The DXA machine must first be calibrated (quality assurance) with a calibration block; it is ready to use once all of the checks pass.

2. The subject's information is entered into the software program.

3. The subject is prepared. Regular clothing may be worn, but everything metallic must be removed. Shorts and a T-shirt will suffice.

4. The subject is placed supine on the scanning table and properly positioned. The body should be centered within the perimeter lines and aligned with the central demarcation line. The head should be at least 2 inches (5 cm) from the top perimeter line to allow the scanning arm a few blank cycles. Hands should be flat on the bed and may need to be placed underneath the hips to fit within the perimeter. Legs should be positioned in alignment with the central demarcation line (the line should be between the legs) and braced at two levels with Velcro straps, near the knees and at the feet, to minimize movement and allow the subject to relax comfortably without moving. Large (tall and heavy) people may have difficulty positioning their entire bodies within the perimeter lines because the scanning bed is designed for people under 6 feet 4 inches (193 cm) and 300 pounds (136 kg). Muscular subjects may also have difficulty fitting within the perimeter. In these cases, the technician must position the subject as best as possible. DXA can be uncomfortable for subjects who have to contract their muscles to constrict their bodies. A different body composition tool (e.g., hydrodensitometry, BIA) may be better for large people despite the loss of data.

5. The subject lies motionless on the bed as the test is initiated. Movement can cause irregularities on the scan.

6. The subject is scanned rectilinearly from head to toe for 5 to 25 minutes, depending on the type of scan and the person's size. Newer DXA units have greatly reduced total scan time making this procedure more practical and easier to administer.

7. Upon completion of the scan, the technician needs to denote the regions of interest (based on the manufacturer's or standardized guidelines) in the subject's software file to obtain accurate regional body composition information prior to analysis.

8. DXA reports give regional (head, trunk, limbs) and total-body bone mass, lean tissue mass, and fat mass (and percent) data.

DXA has many advantages. It is easy to administer, fast, accurate, and comfortable for most subjects; regional measurements are attractive for many populations. In addition, a whole-body measurement produces less than 5 µSv of radiation, which is much less than CT scans, chest X-rays, and lumbar spine X-rays.

However, DXA does have some limitations. The scanning bed is not designed for large people, and the machines (e.g., General Electric Lunar, Hologic, and Norland) are large and expensive. In some areas, a physician's prescription may be needed for a DXA scan. DXA assumes a constant hydration state and electrolyte content in lean tissue, and hydration status could affect the results. Body thickness problems may serve as a source of error, and user error can occur when delineating regional measurements, thereby demonstrating the importance of a single technician for sequential testing. Lastly, the lack of standardization among DXA equipment manufacturers poses a problem. Differences exist in hardware, calibration methodology, imaging geometry (pencil versus fan-beam), and software, which result in different body composition results among machines. Body fat measurements have been shown to vary by approximately 1.7% when repeated measurements are taken on different DXA machines from the same manufacturer (Tataranni, Pettitt, and Ravussin 1996), so it is important to use the same machine for repeated testing.

DXA has been shown to correlate highly with hydrodensitometry and other body composition measurements. However, DXA scans typically register higher body fat percentages (i.e., 2 to 5%) for total-body measurements than other procedures do (Clasey et al. 1999; Kohrt 1998; Norcross and Van Loan 2004). Although the results of most validation studies show DXA to be an accurate tool for body composition measurement, limitations preclude it from becoming a gold standard at the current time.

COMPUTED TOMOGRAPHY SCANS AND MAGNETIC RESONANCE IMAGING

Cross-sectional imaging of the whole body can be viewed with computed tomography (CT) and magnetic resonance imaging (MRI). These techniques produce scans that can noninvasively quantify tissue volume such as regional fat distribution. Total-body composition analysis is possible with sequential "slicing" through the body and assumptions for tissue densities. For CT scans, X-rays (ionizing radiation) pass through the subject and create cross-sectional slices approximately 10 millimeters thick. The image represents a 2-D map of pixels; each pixel has a numerical value (attenuation coefficient) that helps differentiate tissues based on the density and electrons per unit mass.

For MRI scans, electromagnetic radiation excites and aligns hydrogen atoms in water and fat molecules (via a magnet). Hydrogen protons then absorb energy and generate an image. Fat and lean tissue can be quantified by selecting regions of interest on the scan.

Both MRI and CT scans have been validated and are beneficial in that they provide the opportunity to perform relative analyses of muscle, bone density, and intra-abdominal fat. Because the use of radiation in CT scans is a concern, however, they may only be viable for medical or research purposes. In addition, scanning is costly (especially MRI) making it impractical for most people.

NEAR-INFRARED INTERACTANCE

Near-infrared interactance (NIR) is based on principles of light absorption and reflection using near-infrared spectroscopy. A light wand or fiber optic probe is positioned perpendicularly on a body part (typically on the anterior midline surface of the biceps brachii), and infrared light is emitted at specific wavelengths. The absorption of the infrared beam is measured via a silicon-based detector that is expressed as two optical densities. Prediction equations estimate percent body fat via optical density, gender, height, physical activity level, and body weight. Some commercial versions of NIR (e.g., Futrex-5000, -5500, -6000, -6100) are portable and require minimal technician training, making them attractive to the health and fitness industry. However, a major limitation is the small body sampling area.

NIR has been shown to be valid and reliable for determining the body composition of female athletes (Fornetti et al. 1999), but it does produce a higher error rate than other body composition procedures. NIR has been shown to overpredict percent fat by up to 14.7% in young wrestlers (Housh et al. 2004; Housh et al. 1996) and is least effective for monitoring body composition changes following resistance and aerobic training (Broeder et al. 1997). Thus, NIR is not recommended for routine use in healthy and athletic populations.

Body Fat Standards

Interpretation of body fat percent estimates is complicated because all methods are indirect (error needs to be considered) and there are no universally accepted standards for percent fat. Although national standards have been developed in the United States and have been accepted for BMI and WHR, none exist for percent fat estimates. Practitioners must choose from many classifications proposed by various authors. Table 2.5 presents some general percent fat classifications, although many other charts have been used.

A few points of emphasis need to be made. Human body fat may be categorized as essential or nonessential. Essential body fat fulfills several pertinent functions in the body and is needed for good health. It is found throughout the body but especially in the heart, lungs, liver, spleen, kidneys, intestines, muscles, bone, and central nervous system (McArdle, Katch, and Katch 2007). Essential body fat accounts for approximately 5% of body weight in males and 12% in females (this difference accounts for gender-essential fat primarily resulting from hormonal differences and childbearing factors). If percent fat falls below these levels, serious adverse health effects might ensue. This can become an issue for athletes such as wrestlers or bodybuilders who may keep their body fat levels low near competition time. Nonessential, or storage, body fat includes the subcutaneous adipose tissue as well as visceral fat tissue. This type should be kept low for health and athletic purposes because it contributes to the rest of the body fat percentage.

Comparison of Body Composition Techniques

Each body composition technique described has advantages and disadvantages, which are presented in table 2.4. The coach, practitioner, or athlete must weigh the positives with the negatives when determining which technique to use. Ultimately, practicality may be the determining factor. Cost, time, comfort, and accessibility are critical considerations when making this decision, especially when several athletes will be tested on multiple occasions.

TABLE 2.4 Percent Body Fat Classifications

	AGE (YEARS)						
Rating (male)	**<17**	**18–25**	**26–35**	**36–45**	**46–55**	**56–65**	**>66**
Very lean	5	4–7	8–12	10–14	12–16	15–18	15–18
Lean	5–10	8–10	13–15	16-18	18–20	19–21	19–21
Leaner than average	–	11–13	16–18	19–21	21–23	22–24	22–23
Average	11–25	14–16	19–21	22–24	24–25	24–26	24–25
Slightly high	–	18–20	22–24	25–26	26–28	26–28	25–27
High	26–31	22–26	25–28	27–29	29–31	29–31	28–30
Obese	>31	>28	>30	>30	>32	>32	>31
	AGE (YEARS)						
Rating (female)	**<17**	**18–25**	**26–35**	**36–45**	**46–55**	**56–65**	**>66**
Very lean	12	13–17	13–18	15–19	18–22	18–23	16–18
Lean	12–15	18–20	19–21	20–23	23–25	24–26	22–25
Leaner than average	–	21–23	22–23	24–26	26–28	28–30	27–29
Average	16–30	24–25	24–26	27–29	29–31	31–33	30–32
Slightly high	–	26–28	27–30	30–32	32–34	34–36	33–35
High	31–36	29–31	31–35	33–36	36–38	36–38	36–38
Obese	>36	>33	>36	>39	>39	>39	>39

Reprinted, by permission, from National Strength and Conditioning Association, 2008, Administration, scoring, and interpretation of selected tests, by E. Harman and J. Garhammer. In *Essentials of strength training and conditioning*, 3rd ed., edited by T.R. Baechle and R.W. Earle (Champaign, IL: Human Kinetics), 291.

TABLE 2.5 Advantages and Disadvantages of Body Composition Assessment Techniques

Assessment	Advantages	Disadvantages
BMI	Easy to assess Does not require special equipment Noninvasive clinical tool	Not valid tool for athletes Does not factor large muscle mass
Girth	Easy to administer Minimal training needed Minimal equipment (tape measure) Quick test time Many formulas to select from Good indicator of size changes	Girth size not always related to fat content Less accurate than other methods
Skinfold	Easy to use once trained Time efficient Noninvasive Inexpensive (cost of calipers) Many equations to choose from Can test many athletes in less time	Prone to technician error Less accurate for very lean or obese people Considers mostly subcutaneous fat Potential discomfort to subject (pinching or embarrassment)
Hydrodensitometry	Gold standard Very accurate, valid, and reliable	Time consuming Requires a lot of equipment and space High cost of equipment Requires in-depth examiner knowledge Water submersion can be uncomfortable Requires measure of lung volume
BIA	Requires little technical expertise Testing is very fast Very easy especially when using scale-type or handheld models Testing unit is easily transportable Does not require minimal clothing or much bodily exposure	Several confounding variables must be avoided High degree of error if procedures are not strictly followed
ADP	Relaxed atmosphere for subject Easy to operate Short measurement time Good for every population Accurate	Very expensive Equipment not very accessible Must wear minimal, tight clothing
DXA	Very accurate Radiation exposure is low Comprehensive measurements Can wear regular clothing Relatively quick measurement time Subject relaxed during test Gives regional measurements	Very expensive Less accurate when going from one DXA unit to another May require prescription from physician
NIR	Safe and noninvasive Fast and convenient Portable Little training needed	Least accurate assessment tool
CT/MRI	Very accurate Many applications	Very expensive Limited access Time consuming

Professional Applications

Strength and conditioning professionals should include frequent body composition measurements in athletes' general training macrocycles. Body composition measurements are easy to perform and are not fatiguing to the athlete the way performance tests can be. Two major issues may be encountered. The first is the cost of equipment. A few measurement tools are inexpensive, whereas some technology may be cost prohibitive. For example, DEXA, MRI, CT scans, and air displacement plethysmography units are expensive and may be beyond the budget of many athletic programs. In addition, a facility that has these technologies will typically have only one unit. Thus, testing a large group of athletes could be very time consuming. Bioelectrical impedance units are affordable and can be advantageous for testing athletes because they are quick and portable, and multiple units can be purchased to permit the testing of large groups of athletes in a short period of time. However, athletes' hydration status and activity level need to be carefully monitored prior to testing. Underwater weighing may be an option (although it could be cost prohibitive for some programs) but generally takes longer and requires longer testing sessions because only one athlete can be tested at a time. A period of familiarization is needed so athletes understand the importance of expelling as much air as possible, and some athletes may find holding their breath underwater uncomfortable.

The most practical solution for the strength and conditioning professional is to develop a body composition measurement program based on body weight, skinfold, and girth measurements. Body weight measurements require only a scale, which is not cost prohibitive. These can be performed frequently including multiple times a day. This is especially important when monitoring athletes who may be making weight (i.e., wrestlers and other athletes in combat sports) or monitoring hydration status, such as when weighing American football players before, during, and after practice in hot, humid conditions to quantify fluid weight loss. Skinfold calipers are relatively inexpensive, and multiple calipers can be purchased, which makes testing large groups of athletes in a short period of time easy. Population-specific equations (or tables) can be used for quick body fat percentage calculations. Using a spreadsheet to calculate the data increases the speed of testing; an assistant can immediately input data, obtain a fat percentage, and give the athlete rapid feedback. Tape measures can be purchased at low prices and are very useful for girth measurements. Girth measurements can also be useful for indirectly assessing muscle hypertrophy from a resistance training program. Thus, the strength and conditioning professional can be well equipped economically for large-scale body composition testing by having one or more accurate scales, skinfold calipers (preferably Lange), and tape measures (preferably Gulick tape measures because tension can be standardized) at their facilities.

The second issue facing the strength and conditioning professional is homogeneity of the testing staff and procedures. Because a large number of athletes may need to be tested, multiple staff members or personnel may be performing the tests. It is very important that technique be standardized among the staff.

In fact, one coach or assistant should be assigned to each athlete for consistent and accurate data acquisition. For example, with skinfold analysis two practitioners' techniques may be slightly different yielding two different values for the athlete. In this case, the body fat difference is due to tester error rather than physiological changes.

Calibration sessions for single athletes can be helpful. In such sessions, multiple testers perform the skinfold analysis on the same athlete, and the results are compared. Consistent results from staff members confirm data consistency. However, because athletes with more body fat have more variation, calibration sessions are most productive when small, medium, and large athletes are examined. This gives good practice to those learning proper technique. Thus, multiple athletes can be used as subjects, but the results must be compared among the same individual athletes. That is, athletes A, B, and C are tested, but testers compare results for A to calibrate technique, then compare results for B, and subsequently compare results for C. If the data vary glaringly, the staff must alter the technique to produce greater consistency.

With girth measurements, a slight variation in the location of the tape measure or a difference in tension applied to the tape measure can yield variable results. Body weight measurements, on the other hand, are standard provided the scale is functioning properly.

The head strength and conditioning coach must ensure that the staff uses consistent techniques. The most accurate system is to assign certain staff members to certain athletes. This standardizes the procedures per athlete and provides more accurate measurements of body composition over time.

SUMMARY

- Excess body fat is detrimental to health and performance, so measurement of body composition is of great importance for health professionals, fitness practitioners, athletes, and coaches.

- Several methods exist to indirectly measure body composition. Simple methods such as girth measurements, BMI, and skinfolds can be performed with little equipment and at low cost, and are fast and easy to perform, which is advantageous when testing large numbers of people over time.

- BIA is another simple body composition tool that can be attractive for use with athletic populations. However, equipment is more costly than that for skinfold and girth measurements, and BIA is prone to error.

- Advanced body composition estimates (hydrodensitometry, ADP, DXA, CT, and MRI) can be made when specific information is needed, equipment is available, and trained technicians perform the procedures. These methods are less practical for many athletes, but show greater accuracy, reliability, and validity than simpler methods.

Heart Rate and Blood Pressure

Daniel G. Drury, DPE, FACSM

Heart rate and blood pressure are two circulatory factors that ensure the proper distribution of blood throughout the body. As physiological demands change, each factor is adjusted to help perfuse the tissues with the right amount of blood. Changes in position, exercise intensity, mode of exercise, and state of arousal may result in an adjustment of heart rate and blood pressure. Although both factors can be altered independently, they are systemically interrelated so that an adjustment in one is often accompanied by an adjustment in the other.

Because active heart rate is an indirect indicator of exercise intensity, it is often used for monitoring, adjusting, and individualizing training programs. Heart rate monitors have become more accurate and readily available in recent years. Consequently, coaches and trainers have been able to help athletes fine-tune their training by making the intensity of workouts relative to their own physiological capabilities. Furthermore, chronic training adaptations can also be monitored by examining changes in the resting heart rate as well as during exercise at any given exercise intensity.

The pressure in the arteries is in a constant state of flux and is continually being adjusted and readjusted. The circulatory system provides just the right amount of blood pressure to meet the demands of a wide variety of activities. Although blood pressure is not commonly used as an indicator of fitness, it is important for trainers to understand blood pressure norms and the circumstances that may lead to rapid increases or decreases in blood pressure. Fluctuations in pressure enable athletes to circulate more blood to more tissues when needed. Because each activity requires a unique blood pressure response, trainers need to understand the mechanics of this dynamic system.

Heart Rate Control

Heart rate (HR) is a simple yet valuable indicator of cardiorespiratory function. At rest, the heart typically beats between 60 and 80 times per minute. However, in highly conditioned athletes, the physiological adaptations of endurance training can result in a resting HR as low as 28 beats per minute (Wilmore, Costill, and Kenney 2008). This decrease is thought to be a result of an increase in the stroke volume of the heart in combination with an increase in the parasympathetic influence of the nervous system. Conversely, a high resting heart rate could be a sign of poor cardiorespiratory function, overtraining, increases in stress, and a host of other factors that may be counterproductive to clients.

Heart rate measurements must be taken under certain physiological conditions. First, experts recommend that resting heart rate (RHR) be taken early in the morning on an empty stomach. During sleep and times of relaxation, the sympathetic nervous system has less drive, which allows the heart rate to better reflect the parasympathetic influence. The subject should be seated or recumbent and in an environment free of distraction. If RHR is being tracked over time, the measurement should be taken under similar circumstances each time.

During exercise, HR is a good indicator of relative exercise intensity and is used widely to monitor cardiorespiratory function in both health and disease (Ehrman et al. 2009). The heart muscle is one of the few tissues capable of generating its own impulse, and it does this at the sinoatrial (SA) node, which is located on the right ventricle (Marieb and Hoehn 2010). The SA node is considered the pacemaker of the heart. It is innervated by sympathetic and parasympathetic nerve fibers that emanate from the medulla oblongata and the cardiorespiratory control centers within the central nervous system (see figure 3.1). Both sets of nerve fibers innervate the SA node; the atrioventricular (AV) node provides a tonic influence that can be either enhanced or depressed. The sympathetic nerve fibers increase heart rate, whereas parasympathetic nerve fibers slow it down. At rest, parasympathetic influence usually dominates control of the HR by reducing the heart's natural, or inherent, rate of about 100 beats per minute (bpm) to somewhere between 60 and 80 bpm (Wilmore, Costill, and Kenney 2008). At the initiation of exercise, the removal of parasympathetic influence initially allows the heart rate to increase to about 100 bpm, followed by an increase in sympathetic activity that further accelerates HR based on circulatory demands (Wilmore, Costill, and Kenney 2008).

Exercise Intensity and Heart Rate

HR can be used as an indirect and noninvasive measure of exercise intensity because of its strong correlation with exercise intensity and oxygen

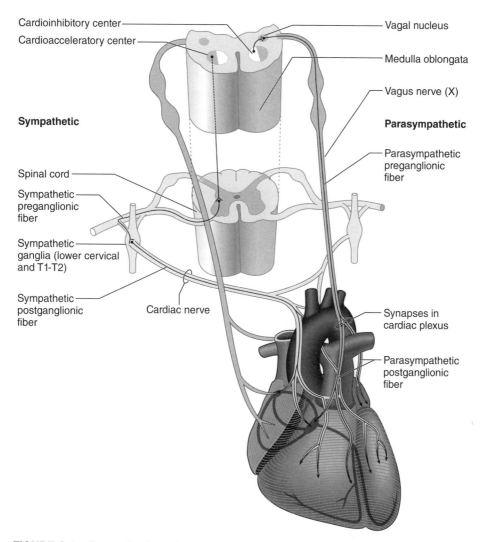

FIGURE 3.1   Sympathetic and parasympathetic nerve innervations of the heart.

consumption (Adams and Beam 2008). Numerous cardiorespiratory fitness tests use exercise HR to estimate or predict oxygen consumption by assessing a steady state HR (SSHR) at a given workload (Franklin 2000). SSHR is indicated when the circulatory demands of the current activity have been met by the circulatory system, and no further increases in HR are necessary (Wilmore, Costill, and Kenney 2008). At this point, because HR neither increases nor decreases substantially, it can be used to indicate the demands of that specific workload.

SSHR that occurs at any given absolute workload can vary significantly based on the person's fitness level. For example, if a sedentary person and a highly trained person of similar size and stature were walking together at 4 miles per hour (6.5 km/h), the sedentary person would likely have a much higher HR than the trained person, despite similar levels of oxygen consumption. This disparity in efficiency is also reflected in the way HR is adjusted between workloads. In short, an inefficient cardiorespiratory system relies on increases in HR more dramatically to meet the demands of an increased workload. Eventually, as exercise intensity increases, the sedentary person would approach maximal HR at a much lower workload compared to the trained person. Furthermore, after exercise has stopped, the trained person's HR would return to normal much more rapidly than that of the sedentary person, providing yet another way HR can be used to predict cardiorespiratory efficiency (Adams and Beam 2008). Given the relative ease of measuring HR, combined with the many ways HR can be used to predict cardiorespiratory efficiency, it is obvious why HR has been so widely used in the health and fitness industry.

Maximal Heart Rate

Maximal heart rate (MHR) is the greatest number of heart beats per unit of time that can be attained during an all-out effort to exhaustion. This number does not seem to be altered substantially by increases in cardio-respiratory efficiency or cardiorespiratory training. Rather, MHR seems to decline with age and is often predicted by subtracting one's age from 220 (Karvonen and Vuorimaa 1988). This value is appropriately called an age-predicted maximal heart rate (APMHR). For example, a 40-year-old male would estimate his APMHR as follows: 220 – 40 (age) = 180. Although this method of estimating maximal HR can vary considerably among people and is only an estimate, it is still used widely as a field method to establish the upper limits of HR, without exposing people to the maximal effort needed to measure a true maximal HR (Franklin 2000).

Heart Rate Reserve

Once APMHR has been calculated, this information can be used to establish exercise intensity guidelines based on heart rate reserve (HRR) (Franklin 2000). This prediction formula includes one variable that is affected by age (APMHR or maximal HR) and one factor that is affected by the state of fitness (RHR). Determining RHR and APMHR permits the calculation of the number of beats the person can potentially use to meet the demands of exercise (i.e., beats held in reserve). Heart rate reserve is found by subtracting RHR from APMHR.

Once the number of beats in reserve has been determined, a percentage of this reserve can be calculated by simply multiplying this number by the desired exercise intensity expressed as a percentage. By adding a percentage of the beats held in reserve onto RHR, a target HR can be determined to provide some objective criteria for monitoring training intensity. Both a minimum and a maximum training HR can be determined so that a desired training zone adaptation can be established. Athletes can train at a much higher percentage (70 to 85%) of their HRR as compared to sedentary or recreational athletes (55 to 70%). Often referred to as the Karvonen formula, this technique is based on research Dr. M. Karvonen conducted in the 1950s (Karvonen and Vuorimaa 1988). This formula is often used by having athletes maintain a certain HR intensity as they complete their cardiorespiratory training.

Here's an example of how to calculate training intensity using the heart rate reserve method. Begin by first determining the age-predicted maximal heart rate by subtracting the person's age from 220 (APMHR = 220 – 22 [age] = 198 bpm). Next, subtract the resting heart rate from this number to determine the number of beats that are held in reserve (198 [APMHR] – 72 [RHR] = 126 bpm [HRR]). In this case, the athlete literally needs a minimum of 72 beats per minute to meet the body's demands at rest and 198 beats to exercise at maximal intensity. Therefore, 126 beats are held in reserve. These beats can be added to the resting heart rate to increase the circulation of blood as needed. For a person wanting to train at approximately 70% of HRR, the calculation would look like this:

$$126 \text{ (HRR)} \times 0.70 \text{ (\%)} = 88.2 \text{ beats per minute}$$
$$\text{Target training HR} = 72 \text{ (RHR)} + 88.2 = 160 \text{ bpm (70\% of HRR)}$$

What truly makes this formula unique is the fact that a trained athlete with a low resting heart rate will increase this reserve by meeting the resting demands with fewer beats. This ultimately increases the heart rate reserve. At the same time, the natural decrease in maximal heart rate is also considered in the formula. Ultimately, the following formula can be used:

Target heart rate = [fractional intensity (maximal HR – resting HR)] + RHR

Sport Performance and Heart Rate

The intensity of training can be closely monitored to control and hopefully optimize the training regimen and adaptations (Franklin 2000). For example, if an athlete has a low degree of cardiorespiratory fitness, it might be appropriate to have her maintain a pace high enough to challenge her current cardiorespiratory efficiency, but not so high that she cannot sustain the exercise. As her fitness improves over time, the relative intensity of exercise that is reflected by HR can be increased so that she is constantly pushing herself to improve. The Karvonen method of maintaining exercise intensity provides a customized upper and lower HR limit that can be used to help the athlete remain motivated and focused on maintaining a specific relative intensity. If used religiously, monitoring HR can be a great way to quantify the difficulty of workouts over time, giving the coach or trainer some additional objective insight as to how the athlete is feeling.

Many practitioners establish target heart rate by simply calculating a percentage of the age-predicted maximal heart rate, although this method is not as robust as the Karvonen method. At first glance, this method appears rudimentary and generic because the formula does not consider anything but age. However, the exercise intensity established using this method is indeed specific to the person because each person requires a unique amount of work to reach any given target heart rate. Therefore, a sedentary 20-year-old and an athletic 20-year-old may have the same predicted values, but the exercise intensity needed to reach these values would be considerably different.

Figure 3.2 demonstrates the exercise heart rate range for a 35-year-old who wants to improve fitness (green zone). Because this person is not fit enough to handle the intensity required to increase performance (red zone), he should probably ease off on the intensity and choose a level more appropriate for his current state of fitness. Over time, the level can be adjusted, but it is probably best to be conservative when prescribing intensity so that the client remains motivated and develops a base of fitness to build on.

An athlete may use these target heart rates to cycle the intensity of training in a given workout or throughout the training season. Consider a soccer midfielder who has the physiological challenge of executing anaerobic bursts of speed throughout a game that lasts well over an hour. The training program for this athlete should most likely involve days focused on endurance as well as days that include high-intensity interval training.

Heart rate can be used in both of these situations. For long endurance training, the athlete may want to maintain a certain moderate intensity by monitoring his heart rate over the course of a long run. As cardiorespiratory improvements are gained over time, his heart rate will decrease at any given speed providing evidence that a faster pace may be needed to initiate additional improvements in fitness. Conversely, when the athlete engages in anaerobic interval training, heart rate can still be a valuable tool. Although heart rate is not an indicator of performance during sprinting activities, it can be an indicator of recovery between sprints. As the season approaches, the trainer can adjust the recovery interval to provide a customized challenge for the athlete or to slowly introduce a gamelike physiological challenge that will translate into improved performance.

Heart Rate Measurement

There are numerous ways to measure HR including palpation, auscultation, Doppler ultrasonic monitoring, and electrical monitoring. Although electrocardiography is considered the gold standard for HR measurement, other methods can be used with varying degrees of accuracy. The following sections provide brief descriptions of the techniques most often used in nonclinical settings.

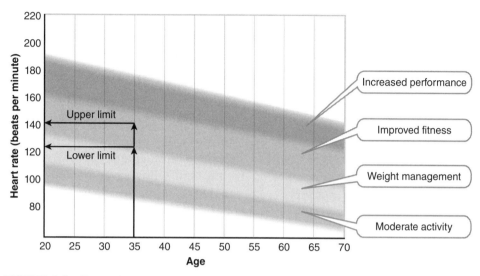

FIGURE 3.2 Target heart rate zones based on age-predicted maximal heart rate for males and females.

PALPATION

Palpation is the process of determining heart rate by feeling the distension of the arteries as a bolus of blood passes through the vessel. Numerous large arteries run close to the surface of the skin making them ideal for palpation. Two of the most commonly used locations for HR palpation are the radial artery on the palm side of the wrist (figure 3.3*a*) and the carotid arteries (figure 3.3*b*).

Deeper arteries and those surrounded by excessive adipose tissue can make palpating the pulse difficult. Also, exercises such as walking and running during measurement can confound the ability to count a pulse because the rhythmic body movements make distinguishing pulse waves difficult. Furthermore, it is important not to occlude (pinch) the artery with the pressure of the fingers. This is especially important when taking a pulse using the carotid artery; occluding the artery can hamper blood flow to the brain leading to syncope (dizziness) and possibly injury. The technique is to locate a relatively large artery, place the fingertips over it, and count the number of beats that occur in a given period of time.

PROCEDURE

1. The procedure begins by counting the first pulsation detected as zero and then counting the number of completed beats for the predetermined period of time.

2. Because HR is usually expressed in beats per minute (bpm), the amount of time a pulse is monitored is conveniently divisible into 60

seconds. For example, a pulse taken for 10 seconds can be multiplied by 6 to estimate bpm. Time increments of 15 seconds × 4) and 30 seconds (× 2) are also commonly used. It is important to note that smaller increments of monitoring time can amplify uncounted partial beats resulting in counting errors (Adams and Beam 2008).

3. Another palpation method for measuring HR involves determining the amount of time required for the heart to complete 30 beats and then dividing this time period into the constant of 1,800. This technique is based on the fact that 30 beats, or any given number of beats, will occur in a shorter period of time as the heart rate increases. The constant 1,800 is used so that smaller increments of one tenth of a second can be used for a 30-beat period to determine HR (Adams and Beam 2008). This test is simplified further by using a chart with the calculations already completed. This technique is often considered more accurate than time interval techniques because only completed cardiac intervals are counted. With the time interval techniques, a small error in counting or estimating partial beats can result in a large error when multiplied.

Example 1: 30 beats in 15.0 seconds   Example 2: 30 beats in 10.0 seconds
1,800 / 15 seconds = 120 bpm   1,800 / 10 = 180 bpm

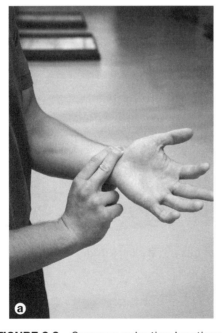
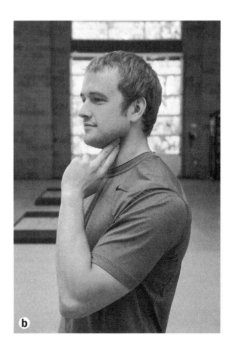

FIGURE 3.3 Common palpation locations.

AUSCULTATION

The counting techniques used for monitoring HR are very similar for auscultation and palpation. However, with auscultation the pulse waves that are felt are replaced by the sounds of the myocardium, large arteries, or both. A stethoscope facilitates hearing and counting the sounds associated with heart contractions.

PROCEDURE

1. The diaphragm of the stethoscope should be placed directly onto the subject with the entire diaphragm of the stethoscope flush with the surface of the skin. The diaphragm should be placed over the apical (apex) region of the heart or over the base of the heart between the second and third ribs just below the proximal end of the clavicle (Adams and Beam 2008). Slight pressure on the diaphragm may improve the quality of the heart sounds.

2. Once the stethoscope is in place, similar procedures to those of palpation can be used to count or time the beats of the heart. Both the palpation and the auscultatory methods are easier to conduct during exercise than at rest. Although the beats are occurring at a much faster pace during exercise, the strength of the pulse waves and of the contraction of the heart make the pulse easier to feel and hear.

ELECTROCARDIOGRAPHY

Although electrocardiography (ECG) is often reserved for clinical and research settings, calculating HR using this tool is not difficult and does not require extensive training. The ECG wave form is created by a unified moving wave of ions flowing through the heart as the signal to contract is passed from the SA node to the AV node and down the bundle branches (Guyton 1991). The normal electrocardiogram is composed of a P wave (atrial depolarization), a QRS complex (ventricular depolarization), and a T wave (ventricular repolarization). The specialized electrogenic system found in the heart conducts the rhythmic electrical impulse. Because cardiac tissue transmits electrical signals rapidly, the heart can contract in a coordinated and unified manner, which creates a detectable electrical impulse. A basic representation of the wave form associated with one cardiac cycle is depicted in figure 3.4. Note that the wave with the highest amplitude (R wave) is associated with the contraction of the ventricles. This wave is most often used to calculate HR in healthy people.

ECG strips are useful in a clinical setting because abnormalities in the timing (seconds) and amplitude (millivolts) of the basic wave form can be predictive of various forms of myocardial pathology. However, ECG analysis can also be used to establish an exact HR under resting and exercise conditions (Goldberg and Goldberg 1994).

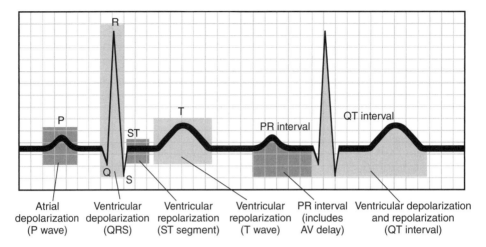

FIGURE 3.4   The phases of the resting electrocardiogram.

Reprinted, by permission, from W.L. Kenney, J. Wilmore, and D. Costill, 2011, *Physiology of sport and exercise,* 5th ed. (Champaign, IL: Human Kinetics), 147.

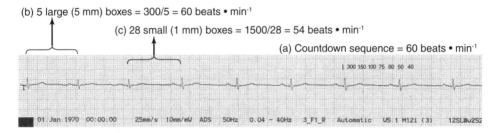

FIGURE 3.5   Procedure for heart rate determination using an ECG.

Reprinted, by permission, from G. Whyte and S. Sharma, 2010, *Practical ECG for exercise science and sports medicine* (Champaign, IL: Human Kinetics), 44.

Calculating HR using an ECG strip is possible because the standard ECG paper is printed with graph lines that represent specific time intervals. As the paper is produced from the electrocardiograph, the wave forms associated with each beat are printed on the paper. Because the paper is produced from the electrocardiograph at a consistent pace (25 mm/sec), the timing between heart beats can be used to determine HR by calculating the amount of time between two consecutive R waves using the standardized ECG graph paper (Goldberg and Goldberg 1994).

PROCEDURE FOR CALCULATING HEART RATE USING AN ECG STRIP

1. Indentify two consecutive R waves.

2. Count the number of small boxes (mm) on the graph paper between the R waves.

3. Divide the number of small boxes (mm) into 1,500 to obtain HR.

   ▪ Example: 1,500 / 20 (ECG squares) = 75 (see figure 3.5)

HEART RATE MONITORS

In recent years, the technology of personal HR monitoring devices has improved significantly (Boudet and Chaumoux 2001). These devices function using the same principles as ECG machines, but are made to detect only HR using small electrodes impregnated into a reusable chest strap. The electrical impulse generated by the heart is monitored by these electrodes, which are then sent, via telemetry, to a digital display worn on the wrist. A mean HR is reestablished and updated about every five seconds giving a valuable and objective way to determine relative exercise intensity. More advanced HR monitors interface with computer tracking programs that can display training HR over time. HR monitors are a useful addition to a comprehensive approach to monitoring an exercise regimen.

Monitoring HR can be valuable for gaining insight into this important cardiorespiratory variable both at rest and during exercise. Developing the skills for monitoring HR should be high on the list of any exercise professional, and these skills should be practiced frequently.

Blood Pressure

Blood pressure (BP) is the force that the blood exerts on the walls of all the vessels within the cardiovascular system (Venes 2009). Although the term *blood pressure* seems to refer to a singular factor, blood pressure is actually established and maintained by the working of numerous variables simultaneously to ensure the pressure necessary for blood circulation under a variety of conditions (Guyton 1991). Among other things, these factors include the elasticity of the vessels, the resistance to flow before and after the capillaries, and the forceful contraction of the left ventricle, as well as blood volume and viscosity (Smith and Kampine 1984). BP fluctuates throughout the day based on metabolic demands, body position, arousal, diet, and many other factors (Wilmore, Costill, and Kenney 2008). Furthermore, numerous hormonal, hemodynamic, and anatomical factors working together ultimately ensure the pressure needed for adequate circulation of the blood (Perloff et al. 1993).

Understanding the basic physiology of BP control and assessment is of critical importance to those involved in health promotion and health care. As one of the basic vital signs used to evaluate health, BP needs to be maintained within a certain range. At rest, normal systolic blood pressure is maintained between 100 and 120 mmHg, whereas diastolic blood pressure is maintained between 75 and 85 mmHg. BP that is chronically elevated (i.e., hypertension) can contribute to the development of cardiovascular disease. If BP drops too low (i.e., hypotension), blood delivery can be compromised, which may eventually lead to circulatory shock. During exercise and other strenuous activities, BP must be altered to deliver larger and larger amounts of blood and oxygen to the tissues. This section provides a basic summary of the factors associated with the physiological control and measurement of BP.

Hypertension

Hypertension is one of the most prevalent cardiovascular risk factors among Americans (Pickering et al. 2005b). This insidious disease is relatively easy to diagnose, but goes undetected primarily because symptoms are not readily apparent to the average person. The cause of primary hypertension remains elusive, yet the diagnosis and treatment of this condition are relatively inexpensive. Therefore, regular monitoring of BP can be an effective screening tool to help those at risk recognize this potentially life-threatening condition prior to a major coronary event. Although the etiology and physiology of hypertension are far beyond the scope of this chapter, table 3.1, from the American Medical Association, has been included indicating the various hypertension classifications for adults. Although the diagnosis of hypertension should be reserved for a medical professional, the day-to-day monitoring of BP can be self-performed at home or performed by another trusted health and wellness professional; proper procedures need to be followed (Pickering et al. 2005a).

Because BP tends to fluctuate throughout the day, hypertension may be incorrectly diagnosed or even undetected, based on the time and circumstances in which it has been measured. To ensure an accurate diagnosis, people need to monitor BP at different times during the day, preferably under the circumstances of natural daily living. This can now be performed with a 24-hour BP monitor (Clement et al. 2003), which can be worn under-

TABLE 3.1 Classification of Hypertension

	JNC 7		WHO/ISH		ESH/ESC	
Classification	SBP*	DBP*	SBP*	DBP*	SBP*	DBP*
Optimal	—	—	—	—	<120	<80
Normal	<120	<80	—	—	120-129	80–84
Prehypertension/ high normal	120–139	80–89	—	—	130-139	85–89
Stage 1/grade 1	140–159	90–99	140–159	90–99	140–159	90–99
Stage 2/grade 2	≤160	≤100	160–179	100–109	160–179	100–109
Grade 3	—	—	≤180	≤110	≤180	≤110
Isolated systolic hypertension	—	—	—	—	≤140	≤90

*Pressure measured in mmHg.

JNC 7 = *Seventh Report of the Joint National Committee on Prevention, Detection, Evaluation, and Treatment of High Blood Pressure;* WHO/ISH = World Health Organization/International Society of Hypertension; ESH/ESC = European Society of Hypertension/European Society of Cardiology.

Adapted from Chobanian et al. 2003; Mancia et al. 2007; and Whitworth et al. 2003.

neath clothing to work, around the house, and even during exercise. The primary advantage of these machines is that they permit people to monitor BP during real-life circumstances rather than only in a physician's office or other clinical setting. This may be helpful in preventing what is called white coat syndrome—that is, an artificially high BP due to the nervousness caused by visiting a physician's office.

Hypotension

Hypotension is experienced when the pressure in the system is compromised or insufficient to maintain the circulatory demand. A systolic pressure of less than 90 mmHg, a diastolic pressure of less than 60 mmHg, or both, generally indicate hypotension. This lack of pressure can leave the heart, brain, and muscles with an insufficient blood flow. Hypotension can occur from dehydration related to heat illness as well as other pathological conditions. Although much less common than hypertension, hypotension can be a very serious medical condition. The diagnosis of hypotension is highly individualized but is characterized by a significant drop in pressure from normal. What may be too low for one person, however, may be fine for another (www.ncbi.nlm.nih.gov/pubmedhealth/PMH0004536/).

Typically, signs of hypotension are dizziness, disorientation, or confusion. Other signs are blurry vision, fainting, and weakness. Hypotension may occur acutely with an orthostatic challenge (change in position) and may be caused by alcohol, certain medications, and a variety of medical conditions. People who experience hypotension on a regular basis should strive to identify the specific trigger and seek medical attention if necessary. Preventive measures include ensuring proper hydration, avoiding alcohol, and avoiding long periods of standing in one place. (www.ncbi.nlm.nih .gov/pubmedhealth/PMH0004536/).

Pressure Gradients and Blood Pressure

The movement of blood through the circulatory system depends on the development of pressure gradients (PG) (Venes 2009; Wilmore, Costill, and Kenney 2008). When blood is put under pressure, it automatically seeks an area of lower pressure in all directions. When an area of lower pressure is introduced, the blood flows in that direction based on how large the difference is between the pressure of the current compartment, the pressure of the new environment, and the resistance to flow within the vessel. Within the arteries, capillaries, and veins, PGs must be created to facilitate the movement of blood (Smith and Kampine 1984) . Blood moves from the heart into the circulation based on the PG created by the forceful contraction of the heart in relation to the pressure in the aorta. Initially, the blood that leaves the left ventricle of the heart and enters circulation is under relatively high pressure as the heart rhythmically contracts and relaxes

(Marieb and Hoehn 2010). As the heart beats, every cardiac cycle is composed of a low-pressure filling phase (diastole), followed by a higher-pressure ejection phase (systole) (Smith and Kampine 1984). Therefore, the volume of blood as well as the pressure of the blood that enters the aorta are constantly changing according to the cardiac cycle and the rhythmic creation of PGs (Powers and Howley 2007).

As the aorta and other large arteries receive this blood, they expand and store some potential energy in the elastic fibers in the walls of the arteries and arterioles (Tanaka, DeSouza, and Seals 1998). After systole has concluded and the aortic valve closes, these

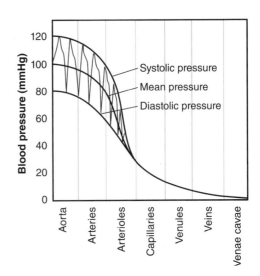

FIGURE 3.6 Blood pressure throughout the vascular system.

Adapted, by permission, from D.L. Smith and B. Fernhall, 2010, *Advanced cardiovascular exercise physiology* (Champaign, IL: Human Kinetics), 8.

vessels recoil and squeeze the blood, creating yet another PG that moves the blood to vessels downstream. In each case, the blood moves down its PG seeking an area of lesser pressure while moving closer to the capillaries where the exchange of gasses and nutrients can take place (figure 3.6).

Once the blood has entered the capillaries, the majority of the pressure created from the heart itself has been dissipated, and the blood entering the venous side of the circulatory loop is under very low pressure as it travels back to the heart (Smith and Kampine 1984; Wilmore, Costill, and Kenney 2008). To facilitate this flow in an environment of very low pressure, the venous circulation is supported by three mechanisms that also create PGs. The first mechanism lies in the anatomical configuration of one-way valves located within the veins. These valves are arranged to promote unidirectional flow to combat the pull of gravity on the blood as it travels back to the heart. These structures allow blood to travel in only one direction, preventing backflow and venous pooling.

The skeletal muscles work in conjunction with the one-way valves by increasing intramuscular pressure within the active muscles. These contractions help create a PG by squeezing the blood in the veins of the muscles. Finally, the respiratory system facilitates venous blood movement by creating a cyclic pressure difference within the thorax that corresponds to the rising and falling of the diaphragm. Both the skeletal muscle and respiratory pumps help "milk" the blood through the veins so that it returns to the heart under the influence of almost no pressure. PGs are essential for the movement of blood through the circulatory system. Anatomically, the human body is designed to circulate blood by creating PGs to facilitate blood movement (Marieb and Hoehn 2010).

Arterial Blood Pressure

BP varies considerably in different parts of the cardiovascular loop. The term *blood pressure* is often used generically to refer to arterial blood pressure (ABP), which is expressed in millimeters of mercury (mmHg) (Adams and Beam 2008). The arterial portion of the cardiovascular loop begins at the aorta and ends at the arterioles, just prior to the capillaries. Because of their elastic nature, these vessels can accommodate the dynamic pressure changes during systole and diastole. ABP is not a static pressure within the system, but a dynamic relationship between the upper and lower values achieved between beats and over time. It is also important to note that ABP is not representative of the pressure throughout all of the arteries, but is more of a reflection of the pressure in the large arteries that are subject to the greatest degree of pressure fluctuation. Therefore, ABP is expressed as two pressures. The highest pressure created in the vessels during left ventricular contraction is referred to as the systolic blood pressure (SBP) (Pickering et al. 2005b). Conversely, the lowest pressure occurs during the relaxation phase of the cardiac cycle and is called the diastolic blood pressure (DBP) (Pickering et al. 2005c). It is important to note that these pressures represent only the extremes of pressure at any given time and that ABP is truly in constant flux between these two pressure measurements.

The mathematical difference between SBP and DBP is termed pulse pressure (PP). At rest, an elevated PP may be used as an indicator of arterial compliance (Adams and Beam 2008). During exercise and other vigorous activities, one would expect the PP to increase as the need for additional flow is increased. Theoretically, SBP is an indicator of the pressure of blood entering the arterial circulation, whereas DBP represents the resistance of blood to leaving. Therefore, if the difference between these pressures increases during exercise, more blood must be both entering and leaving the arterial circulation indicating a greater flow through the tissues.

Mean arterial pressure (MAP) can be calculated using SBP and DBP. Although ABP is always in transition within the arterial system, MAP represents the average pressure in the arteries at any given time. At rest, the pressure generated during systole represents approximately one third of the entire cardiac cycle, whereas the diastolic phase is approximately twice as long (Adams and Beam 2008). Therefore, the formula for calculating resting MAP must account for the fact that the heart is in the diastolic relaxation phase for a longer period of time as compared to the contraction phase. The formula for calculating MAP at rest is as follows:

$$\text{Resting MAP} = 2/3 \text{ DBP} + 1/3 \text{ SBP}$$
Example: 120/80 (120 systolic and 80 diastolic)
$$80 \text{ DBP} \times 0.666 = 53 \text{ mmHg}$$
$$120 \text{ SBP} \times 0.333 = 40 \text{ mmHg}$$
$$\text{MAP} = 53.28 + 39.96 = 93 \text{ mmHg}$$

During exercise, the diastolic phase of the cardiac cycle is reduced as the heart rate increases making the systolic and diastolic phases approximately equal. Consequently, the formula for MAP changes slightly to account for this change:

$$\text{Exercise MAP} = 1/2 \text{ DBP} + 1/2 \text{ SBP}$$
Example: 140/80 (140 systolic and 80 diastolic)
$$80 \text{ DBP} \times 0.50 = 40 \text{ mmHg}$$
$$140 \text{ SBP} \times 0.50 = 70 \text{ mmHg}$$
$$\text{MAP} = 40 + 70 = 110 \text{ mmHg}$$

Arterial Blood Pressure Regulation

Under resting conditions, the volume of blood on the arterial side of the circulatory loop is relatively small (13%) compared with the volume contained in the capacitance vessels of the venous circulation (64%) (Wilmore, Costill, and Kenney 2008). At rest, this distribution of blood is sufficient to meet the pressure and circulatory demands of the body. However, when an increase in ABP is needed, it can be achieved by mobilizing the blood from the venous side of the loop and redistributing it over to the arterial side (Powers and Howley 2007). Arterial blood pressure is dynamically altered by manipulating the factors that control the volume of blood within the system. Arterial blood volume can be changed by increasing or decreasing cardiac output ($\dot{Q}$), increasing or decreasing total peripheral resistance (TPR), or changing both factors simultaneously.

Cardiac output is the total amount of blood that leaves the left ventricle each minute. It is calculated by considering the stroke volume multiplied by the number of cardiac cycles (HR) completed in one minute. Total peripheral resistance represents the resistance the blood encounters while flowing from the arterial side of the cardiovascular loop over to the venous side. The interplay between the amount of blood entering the arterial circulation and the amount of blood allowed to leave ultimately determines whether ABP increases, decreases, or stays the same (Smith and Kampine 1984).

Acute Arterial Blood Pressure Regulation

The cardiovascular system is equipped with a negative feedback system that detects ABP changes and reports them to the central nervous system, which responds with adjustments to blood pressure. These reports are sent to the central nervous system by specific pressure or stretch receptors called baroreceptors (Smith and Kampine 1984; Marieb and Hoehn 2010). Strategically located in the aortic arch and carotid arteries, baroreceptors provide a tonic flow of information to cardiovascular centers within the medulla (Marieb and Hoehn 2010). Under low-pressure circumstances, afferent input to the brain is decreased, and the brain responds by increasing and decreasing sympathetic and parasympathetic drive, respectively (Marieb and Hoehn 2010; Wilmore, Costill, and Kenney 2008). Consequently, heart rate (HR) and stroke volume (SV) increase leading to increases in blood volume in arterial circulation. A concurrent increase in TPR prevents too much blood from exiting the arterial circuit, which ultimately expands arterial blood volume and pressure. Under higher nonexertion-based pressure situations, adjustments are made in exactly the opposite manner (Marieb and Hoehn 2010).

Exercise and Arterial Blood Pressure Regulation

As the result of an acute bout of aerobic exercise, SBP will typically increase to meet the metabolic demands of the tissues. DBP will most likely stay the same, leading to an expansion of both MAP and PP (Wilmore, Costill, and Kenney 2008). A release of the sympathetic neurotransmitters epinephrine (EPI) and norepinephrine (N-EPI) causes an increase in both HR and SV contributing to an expansion in arterial blood volume and ultimately ABP. At the same time, this sympathetic response causes a temporary vasoconstriction of the peripheral vessels allowing relatively less blood to exit the arterial circulation in comparison to the amount flowing in from the increase in $\dot{Q}$. Together, these variables temporarily expand arterial blood volume, increase ABP, and promote a greater distribution of the blood to active tissues.

Consider the blood pressure requirements of cycling on a flat surface and of cycling up a 5-mile (8 km) hill. While a person is cycling on flat ground, a slight increase in blood pressure will easily provide the leg muscles with the additional pressure needed to supply the active tissues with more blood. However, when the intensity of exercise increases while cycling up a hill, more blood flow will be needed to supply the oxygen requirements of the leg muscles. More of the leg muscles will be active, and more blood will be delivered. But this cannot be achieved without an increase in ABP.

Prolonged, vigorous activity resulting in excessive sweating leads to a decrease in plasma volume resulting in dehydration, an increase in hemoconcentration, and a decrease in blood pressure. Under these conditions, antidiuretic hormone (ADH) is produced and then secreted by the hypothalamus. Also known as vasopressin, ADH acts on the kidneys to help retain water in an effort to dilute the hemoconcentration (Wilmore, Costill, and Kenney 2008).

During acute bouts of intense anaerobic activity (e.g., weight training), SBP is likely to increase substantially along with a concomitant increase in DBP. Pressures as high as 480/350 mmHg have been recorded during maximal lifts (MacDougall et al. 1985). For this reason, weight training has historically been contraindicated for many people with cardiovascular disease. However, the American Heart Association has recently acknowledged the safety and potential value of strength training as a mode of therapeutic exercise if contemporary recommendations are followed (Thompson et al. 2007).

The degree to which both SBP and DBP will be elevated seems to be linked to the relative intensity of the exercise. In this context, *relative intensity* refers to the amount of weight being lifted in comparison to the person's maximal capabilities (MacDougall et al. 1992). During maximal or near-maximal lifting efforts, people often hold their breath, initiating the Valsalva maneuver (VM) (Venes 2009). Although this tends to stabilize the core, it can also cause spikes in SBP and DBP (Sale et al. 1994; Sjøgaard and Saltin 1982). For this reason, people at risk for cardiovascular disease should avoid it.

Long-Term Regulation of Arterial Blood Pressure

Arterial blood pressure is largely regulated by the kidneys and several key hormones. Recall that the kidneys filter the blood continuously and help balance the extracellular fluids within the body (Robergs and Roberts 1987). When the body becomes dehydrated, the kidneys conserve water to maintain fluid balance. Conversely, when the body has an excess amount of water, the kidneys determine how much to excrete (Kapit, Macey, and Meisami 1987). The process of fluid balance becomes very important to the understanding of blood pressure because excess fluid held in the blood can contribute to hypertension (Robergs and Roberts 1987). Furthermore, excessive fluid loss from the blood can also be extremely dangerous. Because arterial blood volume ultimately dictates arterial blood pressure, fluid balance within the extracellular fluid and blood can be of critical importance for regulating blood pressure.

When the body loses excessive amounts of fluid, the kidneys secrete the enzyme renin, which activates the plasma protein angiotensinogen. After several enzymatic conversions, angiotensinogen is converted into angiotensin I, which is converted to angiotensin II in the lungs; angiotensin II has two primary effects that can elevate blood pressure. First, it is an extremely powerful vasoconstrictor that increases TPR. Second, it decreases the excretion of Na+, which ultimately increases extracellular fluid. Furthermore, this process triggers the minerlocorticoid aldosterone, which promotes sodium reabsorption enabling the body to retain fluids as they pass through the kidney. Therefore, the renin-angiotensin-aldosterone mechanism helps to maintain blood pressure by increasing TPR while simultaneously attempting to balance the extracellular fluid that in turn affects blood volume.

ARTERIAL BLOOD PRESSURE MEASUREMENT

Early methods for measuring ABP used water columns to measure pressure, but these systems were very large and were subject to significant fluctuations on a beat-by-beat basis (Adams and Beam 2008). Eventually, mercury columns were created resulting in a much more compact and manageable fluid column. Today, ABP is universally reported in millimeters of mercury (mmHg) regardless of the apparatus used for measuring (Pickering et al. 2005a). Despite their accuracy, sphygmomanometers that use mercury are susceptible to breaking and exposing the mercury, which is a toxic substance that is very dangerous to humans. For this reason, many health professionals have switched to automated BP cuffs or to aneroid devices. These devices can be highly accurate if calibrated regularly (Canzanello, Jensen, and Schwartz 2001; Clement et al. 2003; Pickering et al. 2005a).

Although ABP can be measured using indwelling catheters inserted into arterial vessels, this is a very invasive form of measuring ABP and is reserved for the clinical setting (Pickering 2002). A much more common technique using a sphygmomanometer can measure ABP at rest and during vigorous exercise (O'Brien, Beevers, and Lip 2001). Often referred to as the cuff method, this technique uses an inflatable tourniquet to temporarily occlude blood flow through the brachial artery. As the pressure is bled from the cuff, the technician listens to the artery below the cuff through a stethoscope and auscultates the various Korotkoff sounds.

Arterial blood pressure can be measured using Korotkoff sounds based on how the blood flows through the brachial artery. Initially, the cuff is inflated to a pressure that literally prevents any blood flow through the artery. Because no blood is passing through the artery, no sounds or vibrations are detected beyond the cuff by the stethoscope. As the air pressure in the cuff is slowly released, the technician listens for the initial bolus of blood to pass through the previously occluded artery. This first Korotkoff sound is indicative of systolic blood pressure (SBP) because the pressure in the artery must be higher than the pressure in the cuff if the blood in the artery has the PG needed to flow forward past the cuff through the semiconstricted artery (Franklin 2000).

As the cuff continues to be deflated, greater amounts of blood pass through the artery and the cuff during the systolic phase of each heartbeat. The classic lub-dub sound is heard while auscultating the heart directly. However, the sounds heard during blood pressure measurement are created by the blood that passes through the cuff when the pressure in the system exceeds the pressure in the bladder of the cuff. Because the cuff is still impeding *some* of the flow that would naturally pass through the brachial artery, vibrations can still be auscultated during this phase. Eventually, as the pressure in the cuff continues to fall, normal blood flow is restored. The pressure at which the restoration of normal blood flow and the concurrent disappearance of sound heard through the stethoscope occur is the diastolic blood pressure (DBP).

PROCEDURE

1. Have paper and pencil available to record SBP and DBP.

2. The subject should be seated in a quiet environment with the arm resting on a table approximately at heart level.

3. Apply the appropriate-sized cuff around the midpoint of the upper arm centering the bladder over the brachial artery approximately 2 centimeters above the antecubital fossa. The aneroid gauge should be at eye level for visual inspection.

4. Place the stethoscope ear pieces in the ear canals so that they are angled forward. Be sure that the bell of the stethoscope is rotated to the low-frequency position by lightly tapping on the diaphragm.

5. Place the head of the stethoscope over the brachial artery below the cuff and medial to the antecubital fossa. Press the head of the stethoscope so that the entire circumference of the diaphragm is in contact with the skin.

6. Inflate the bladder rapidly by squeezing the bulb to a pressure that is approximately 30 mmHg above the suspected or previously recorded systolic pressure.

7. Open the release valve on the bulb and slowly (3 to 5 mm/sec) deflate the air from the bladder listening for the initial appearance of the Korotkoff sounds (see table 3.2 for Korotkoff sounds).

8. Continue to reduce the pressure listening for the sound to become muffled (fourth phase of DBP) and finally disappear (fifth phase of DBP). Normally, the fifth phase is recorded as DBP.

9. Once the sounds disappear, continue to slowly deflate the cuff for another 10 mmHg to ensure that no further sounds are audible; then release all of the air from the bladder and wait a minimum of 30 seconds before repeating these procedures.

10. Average the two trials together and record these values for future reference.

Modified from Perloff et al. 1993.

TABLE 3.2   Korotkoff Sounds

Phase I	First appearance of clear, repetitive, tapping sounds. This coincides approximately with the reappearance of a palpable pulse.
Phase II	Sounds are softer and longer, with the quality of an intermittent murmur.
Phase III	Sounds again become crisper and louder.
Phase IV	Sounds are muffled, less distinct, and softer.
Phase V	Sounds disappear completely.

Reprinted, by permission, from D. Perloff et al., 1993, "Human blood pressure determination by sphygmomanometry," *Circulation* 88(5): 2460-2470.

The measurement of ABP is a relatively easy procedure that can be performed accurately without extensive medical training if standardized procedures are followed closely. Although the procedural steps are relatively easy to understand, it often takes years of experience to learn how to take blood pressure accurately and reliably (Canzanello, Jensen, and Schwartz 2001). Methods and procedures for taking blood pressure have been published by the American Heart Association (Pickering et al. 2005a).

Professional Applications

As described earlier in the chapter, resting heart rate can be used as a measure of fitness. Typically, a lower resting heart rate is indicative of better cardiovascular health. Although this adaptation is common among those who have achieved a high level of cardiorespiratory efficiency, it is possible that a highly trained athlete will maintain a normal resting heart rate (60 to 80 bpm). Furthermore, untrained people can also have relatively low heart rates that are not the result of cardiorespiratory training. The important factor here is that the fitness professional have a baseline measurement that can be used for future comparison. Both increases and decreases in resting heart rate can be important.

It is also important to note that a variety of external factors can affect resting heart rate. Stress, caffeinated drinks, various medications, and overtraining are all factors that can elevate resting heart rate. Fitness professionals must recognize why someone might have an elevated resting heart rate and consider ways to help the person reduce this number. A chronically elevated resting heart rate (100+ beats per minute) may require medical attention. Teaching athletes to monitor their own resting heart rates during periods of intense training may be helpful in determining a potential problem.

The use of heart rate as a training tool is a skill that all fitness professionals should master. This relatively simple skill is easy to execute and can be of great value to both the client and the trainer. The primary reason this technique is so widely used is that heart rate is a reflection of how the body is responding to the current physiological challenge. People can report verbally how they are feeling, but this is of limited value when they are influenced by other nonphysiological factors. For example, an ex-athlete may wish to appear strong and tough during a vigorous workout that actually exceeds his current physical condition. His verbal response may be that he is feeling fine when in reality he is on the edge of exhaustion. This may also happen in a group exercise class in which a client does not want to be identified or perceived as the weakest link. The social pressure to keep up with the group may cause people to overextend themselves. A simple measurement of heart rate can provide some objective feedback that may tell the trainer and the client what's really going on. Consequently, the intensity of the workout can be altered so that the client can continue to exercise rather than having to quit once undeniable fatigue has set in. This is a safer approach for everyone involved.

(continued)

(continued)

Finally, it is important to acknowledge the relatively new technology related to heart rate monitors. Not only has the price of these devices come down, but also the usability and technical programming have also improved. One particular feature that can be very useful is the pacing feature in which an audible beeping sound is triggered when the person reaches a predetermined target heart rate zone. Heart rate monitors can give audible feedback when the exercise intensity is too high or too low. This is a great feature for distance athletes as well as for people who want to monitor their pace closely. Once the workout is complete, many new systems allow users to download results for tracking purposes. This is an affordable and accurate way to provide some objective data and analysis to what has traditionally been a subjective process.

SUMMARY

- Resting heart rate can be used as a measure of cardiovascular health.
- Maximal heart rate can be estimated by subtracting the person's age from 220.
- Training intensity can be monitored using heart rate because of the correlations among oxygen consumption, workload, and heart rate.
- Training intensity can be established using exercise heart rate. The Karvonen method is a valuable formula for determining the minimal and maximal heart rate that should be achieved during a workout.
- Measuring heart rate is an easy, inexpensive, and valuable skill to learn for fitness professionals.
- Arterial blood pressure is the pressure that the blood exerts against the arterial walls.
- Although the arterial blood pressure is in constant flux, it is typically reported by writing the systolic pressure over the diastolic pressure.
- Systolic pressure is the pressure in the system while the heart is pumping, whereas diastolic pressure is the pressure in the arterial system between heartbeats.
- Arterial blood pressure can be either too high (hypertension) or too low (hypotension). Fitness professionals should be familiar with both extremes.

Metabolic Rate

Wayne C. Miller, PhD, EMT

The capacity of the body to exercise or do physical work depends on its ability to produce, use, and regulate energy. *Metabolism* is the term used to describe this all-encompassing use of energy in the body. Although metabolism includes both the building up and the breaking down of biological compounds, or the sum of the balance between food intake and energy expenditure, we generally refer to the metabolic rate as the rate of energy expenditure. The rate of energy expenditure (metabolism) required by the body or any one of its cells can vary from high-power output to low-power output. Exercise scientists classify the biochemical processes used to expend energy during exercise into categories, depending on the power output demand. Terms such as *fast glycolysis, slow glycolysis, aerobic metabolism, anaerobics,* and others, are used to describe rates of metabolism.

Other chapters in this book describe how the capacity for energy expenditure in the various biochemical pathways affects exercise performance. The focus of the current chapter, however, is on the body's total metabolic rate at rest, during exercise, and throughout the day. This chapter addresses what constitutes the 24-hour energy expenditure, how energy expenditure is measured, how physical activity is monitored, and how energy expenditure can be predicted.

Knowledge about energy expenditure and how it is measured can be helpful to both the practitioner and the client. For example, knowing the 24-hour energy expenditure of a client can help the practitioner structure a diet plan that can help the client lose weight, gain weight, or maintain weight. This knowledge of metabolic rate would be particularly important for the overweight client attempting weight loss or the ultra-endurance athlete trying to maintain weight during a competitive season. Knowledge about metabolic rate may also be helpful as a diagnostic tool to identify possible reasons for decrements or improvements in exercise performance.

Staleness or decrements in athletic performance can often be traced to a chronic energy imbalance, particularly in sports such as gymnastics, wrestling, and cycling.

Components of Energy Expenditure

The body's 24-hour energy expenditure can be broken down into three components: the thermal effect of food, the resting metabolic rate, and the energy cost of physical activity.

Thermal Effect of Food

The thermal effect of food (TEF) is defined as the amount of energy required to digest, absorb, and further process the energy-yielding nutrients in food (i.e., fat, protein, carbohydrate). These energy-expending processes for preparing food prior to its use in the body are collectively called the thermal effect of food, or alternatively, dietary-induced thermogenesis. The contribution of the TEF to the total 24-hour energy expenditure is 5 to 10% (Miller 2006). From a practical or intervention standpoint, the TEF is rather insignificant—individual variance in the TEF does not seem to make a difference in body composition among people; and changes in diet composition do not alter the TEF appreciably (Miller 2006).

Resting Metabolic Rate

The amount of energy expended to sustain the basic body functions is called the resting metabolic rate (RMR) and is generally expressed as kilocalories (kcal). The RMR amounts to about 1 kcal · kg^{-1} of body weight per hour, or roughly 1,800 kcal per day for the average 75-kilogram (165 lb) man. The RMR accounts for approximately 60 to 75% of the total daily energy expenditure, and therefore, anything that alters the RMR has the potential to significantly affect the body's energy balance. Factors that have been implicated in the variance found for RMR within and among people are body composition, gender, race, restrictive dieting, and exercise. Some of these factors are interrelated, some are subject to behavior modification, and some are nonmodifiable (e.g., race).

Individual differences in body composition, particularly in lean body mass, account for most of the 25 to 30% variation in RMR among people. Muscles, organs, bone, and fluids make up most of the lean body mass. The tissues and organs that contribute most to the RMR are the liver, skeletal muscles, brain, heart, and kidneys. The size of each of these is directly related to body size. The size of the skeletal muscle mass is also related to body type, muscle development, and age. People with greater amounts of lean body mass generally have higher RMRs than those with less lean body mass (Cunningham 1982). Although the metabolic rate of fat mass contributes only 2% to the total RMR, obese people generally have a higher absolute RMR than lean people. The proportionately larger tissue and organ size of obese people gives them a greater total lean body mass than lean people. Similarly, the generally larger body size and greater muscularity in men gives them a greater total lean body mass than women. The salient point to remember, then, is that the RMR for people of all sizes and shapes is strongly related to their lean body mass, because lean body mass is positively related to body size or body surface area.

Variation in RMR within a person is predominantly attributed to fluctuations in lean body mass. When an overweight or obese person loses weight, the RMR decreases in proportion to the amount of lean body mass that is lost, not the amount of fat lost. People who gain muscle mass (and other lean tissue) through athletic training experience an increase in RMR in proportion to the lean mass gained.

The fact that RMR is largely determined by lean body mass has led many professionals (and unfortunately, some quacks) to heavily promote unproven products, programs, supplements, and aids that are purported to boost metabolism by increasing lean body mass. Even well-intentioned professionals often get caught up in the notion that exercise is going to make a huge difference in RMR by dramatically increasing lean body mass. It is true that exercise will increase lean body mass, which will ultimately elevate RMR, but the resultant changes in RMR are modest and will not overshadow the effects of poor health behaviors.

For instance, the metabolic rate of 1 kilogram (2.2 lb) of lean body mass is approximately 20 kcal/d (McArdle, Katch, and Katch 2001). Therefore, exercise would have to induce an increase in lean body mass of 5 kilograms (11 lb) to elevate RMR by 100 kcal/d. Although an elevation in RMR of 100 kcal/d may have a significant effect on body composition over a long period of time, a person can easily overcompensate for that 100 kcal by consuming half of a chocolate chip cookie or 8 ounces (240 ml) of soda.

Exercise physiologists have contended for years that aerobic, or endurance, exercise training increases RMR. The research, however, suggests that aerobic exercise training does not necessarily increase RMR significantly. For example, Wilmore and associates (1998) showed that RMR remained unchanged following 20 weeks of aerobic exercise training in men and women of all ages, in spite of an 18% increase in maximal aerobic capacity. Because it is well accepted that strength training can increase muscle mass, and that muscle mass is very active metabolically, Byrne and Wilmore (2001) investigated how strength training may differentially affect RMR in comparison to aerobic, or endurance, exercise training. This cross-sectional study revealed no significant difference in RMR among strength-trained, endurance-trained, and untrained women. Thus, it appears that neither aerobic nor strength training increases RMR significantly.

In spite of the research, many professionals insist and continue to promote the notion that exercise training, particularly resistance training, will greatly increase lean body mass and consequently RMR substantially. This viewpoint is frequently endorsed by professionals working with overweight clients desiring to lose weight. The weakness in this line of thinking lies in the fact that a decrease in lean body mass almost always accompanies a significant drop in body weight (Stiegler and Cunliff 2006). Nonetheless, the loss in lean body mass can be minimized by including exercise in a weight loss program (Hunter et al. 2008).

Even if a person were able to gain lean body mass through an exercise program, how much would this affect RMR? The average amount of lean body mass gained during several weeks of resistance training is variable. However, the obesity research suggests that the increase in lean body mass during exercise training with obese people amounts to only about 2 to 3 kilograms (4.4 to 6.6 lb). Similarly, the resting metabolic rate of muscle tissue is variable, but several reports suggest that the value ranges from 20 to 30 kcal $\cdot$ kg^{-1} $\cdot$ day^{-1}. Taking the average of these estimates, the energy expenditure of an additional 2.5 kilograms of muscle, at 25 kcal $\cdot$ kg^{-1} $\cdot$ day^{-1}, would be 63 kcal $\cdot$ day^{-1}. This would be the equivalent in energy value to about 3 kilograms (6.6 lb) of body fat in one year. The obese person who may need to lose 10 times this amount of fat to become normal weight will need more motivation to resistance exercise train than the promise that resistance exercise training will increase the lean body mass and RMR enough to appreciably alter body fat content. On the other hand, resistance training for the obese person will help maintain the observed decrease in lean body mass and RMR seen with restrictive dieting.

Bray (1983) was the first to demonstrate that a reduction in energy intake results in a decline in RMR. He found that this decrease in RMR was about 15% when subjects were removed from a maintenance diet of 3,500 kcal $\cdot$ day^{-1} and placed on a very-low-calorie diet of 450 kcal $\cdot$ day^{-1}. Although RMR drops while a person is on a very-low-calorie diet, most scientists agree that when energy intake is restored to predieting levels, the RMR also returns to predieting levels, unless there is a decrease in lean body mass. In this case, the postdiet RMR-per-lean-body-mass ratio (RMR:LBM) would be equivalent to predieting levels. However, an early research paper revealed that severe energy restriction lowers RMR:LBM significantly (Fricker et al. 1991). During this study, obese women were placed on a very-low-calorie diet for three weeks. RMR:LBM declined to 94%, 91%, and 82% of the original value on days 3, 5, and 21 of the diet, respectively.

In a randomized controlled clinical trial, moderately obese men and women were assigned to one of three groups: diet plus strength training, diet plus endurance training, or diet only (Geliebter et al. 1997). The exercise protocols were designed to be isoenergetic, meaning that the energy expenditures for the two types of exercise training were equivalent. The average weight loss among the three groups did not differ significantly after eight weeks, but those in the strength-trained group lost less lean body mass than those in the other two groups did. The RMR declined significantly in each group, with no difference among groups. These data indicate that neither strength training nor endurance exercise training prevent the decline in RMR caused by restrictive dieting.

These studies on the effects of restrictive dieting and RMR suggest that the metabolic activity of the lean tissues themselves may be reduced with restrictive dieting. The consequence of such an adaptation would be a greater weight gain when energy consumption returns to predieting levels, greater difficulty maintaining a reduced weight postdiet, or both. More research needs to be done to determine whether this reduction in metabolic rate due to severe dieting is permanent. For now, maintaining exercise training while attempting weight loss, and avoiding periods of extensive and extreme dieting, are recommended.

African Americans have a lower RMR than Caucasians, and the magnitude of difference between the races is similar for both men and women. Investigators have measured the RMR for African Americans to be anywhere from 5 to 20% below that of Caucasians (Forman et al. 1998; Sharp et al. 2002). The range of difference in the RMR over a 24-hour period amounts to 80 to 200 kcal. This metabolic discrepancy cannot be attributed to differences in age, body mass index (BMI), body composition, daily activity levels, menstrual cycle phase, or fitness level. The mechanism underlying this metabolic discrepancy has not yet been identified, and it is still controversial as to whether this difference in RMR between races is the cause of the higher prevalence of obesity in African Americans. Nonetheless, research has also shown that African Americans respond the same physiologically to weight loss intervention as do Caucasians (Glass et al. 2002).

One promising finding is that aerobic exercise may prevent the common age-related decline in RMR. Endurance-trained middle-aged and older women presented a 10% higher RMR than sedentary women, when RMR was adjusted for body composition (Van Pelt et al. 1997). Although descriptive in nature, these data suggest that exercise may help prevent the age-related weight gain seen in sedentary women, and that the protective mechanism may be an altered RMR.

TEF and RMR are not subject to voluntary perturbations that would cause changes in the 24-hour energy expenditure considerably enough to affect body energy balance in the short term (weeks to months). Therefore, it must be concluded that these two components of metabolism are relatively fixed, and that we cannot voluntarily do much to change them. At best, a healthy diet and exercise regimen can help maintain a normal RMR and possibly prevent the slow decrease in RMR seen with aging. On the other hand, the energy expenditure associated with physical activity, whether in the form of structured exercise or not, is quite variable and under voluntary control.

Energy of Physical Activity

Even though skeletal muscle contributes less than 20% to the RMR, skeletal muscle can cause the most dramatic increase in metabolic rate. During strenuous exercise, the total energy expenditure of the body may increase to over 20 times the resting levels. This enormous elevation in the body's metabolic rate is the result of a 200-fold increase in the energy requirement of exercising muscles. In terms of comparison, the RMR of a 70-kilogram (154 lb) person is approximately 1.2 kcal per minute, whereas the energy cost during strenuous exercise can be up to 25 kcal per minute.

A 30-minute exercise bout at moderate intensity may account for 10% or more of daily energy expenditure. This amount of energy expended during exercise can easily offset the energy balance of the body. A 10% or more increase in daily energy expenditure may be desirable for an overweight person, but may be detrimental to performance for an athlete who is not taking in adequate energy. Furthermore, exercise may have a metabolic effect beyond what is accounted for during the exercise session itself.

It is well established that metabolic rate remains elevated for some time following exercise. This phenomenon has been termed excess postexercise oxygen consumption (EPOC). Studies have shown that the magnitude of EPOC is linearly related to the duration and intensity of exercise, and that EPOC following a moderate-intensity exercise bout accounts for about 15% of the total energy cost of the exercise (Gaesser and Brooks 1984). The time for metabolism to return to baseline following an acute exercise session can vary from as little as 20 minutes to more than 10 hours, depending on the duration and intensity of the exercise. Increments of EPOC may play a significant role in the energy balance of the body. Unfortunately, EPOC is insufficiently predictable as a measurable variable in exercise prescription.

The 24-hour energy expenditure, therefore, consists of TEF, RMR, and the energy of physical activity. TEF cannot be easily manipulated and therefore is not considered a viable mechanism to voluntarily affect change in body composition. RMR is strongly related to lean body mass and is depressed during restrictive dieting, while being elevated in response to exercise training that increases lean body mass. The changes in RMR that are seen with either dieting or exercise training are relatively small, but they can affect body composition over an extended period of time. The changes in RMR due to diet and exercise can either augment or hinder weight loss attempts by obese people. An acute exercise bout can increase metabolism by as much as 20-fold, and can contribute as much as 20% or more to the 24-hour energy expenditure. Exercise is the only voluntary behavior that positively affects metabolic rate.

Sport Performance and Metabolic Rate

Knowledge of metabolic rate can help athletes as well as health-conscious people improve their exercise performance or obtain the fat-to-lean-mass ratio optimal for their personal situations. Metabolic knowledge can be used to create a personal training plan, to design an eating schedule for an ultra-endurance event, to monitor body composition during the off-season, and to lose weight to improve health status; it can also be applied to other needs. Two examples of how this works follow.

A personal trainer, who is also a dietitian, is working with an athlete who wants to increase lean body mass during the off-season. The professional obviously knows how to structure the off-season training regimen and how to design a diet to meet specific nutritional needs. What the professional will need to know to make this program most effective is the client's metabolic rate—specifically, the client's 24-hour energy expenditure. Because this client is an athlete who expends a great deal of energy when training, the professional will need to determine the athlete's exercise energy expenditure as well as the resting energy expenditure to calculate the athlete's 24-hour energy expenditure. If the athlete's RMR is 2,300 kcal per day, and the athlete will expend an additional 700 kcal a day in exercise, the athlete's 24-hour energy expenditure would be 3,000 kcal per day. The personal trainer would then have to design a nutritional plan for the athlete that surpasses 3,000 kcal per day for the athlete to increase lean body mass.

A second example is of a competitive cyclist planning to compete in an ultra-endurance event lasting several days (e.g., the Tour de France). The goal for the dietary prescription during the event is to ensure adequate energy intake to meet the metabolic demands of the competition. Otherwise, the athlete will become fatigued prematurely. Again, knowing the athlete's 24-hour energy expenditure is critical to the design of the diet plan. If the athlete's RMR is 2,000 kcal per day, and the athlete expends an additional 6,000 kcal per day in activity, the goal would be to consume 8,000 kcal per day during the event. Knowing this, the professional can now structure the composition of the diet and the timing of dietary intake to match the exercise needs and meet the 8,000-kcal-per-day requirement.

In the two preceding examples, accurate measures of RMR and exercise energy expenditure were necessary prior to the design and implementation of a diet and exercise regimen. There are several ways to measure energy expenditure. The method of choice will depend on equipment availability, cost, and desired accuracy.

Measurement of Energy Expenditure

Heat is released as a by-product in cellular metabolism. Because the rate of heat release is directly proportional to the rate of metabolism, metabolic rate can be determined by measuring heat release. The process of measuring this metabolic heat release is termed direct calorimetry.

Direct Calorimetry

Direct calorimetry can be used to measure the heat emission from a person enclosed in an insulated chamber. The change in chamber temperature as a result of the heat released from the body is measured in units with which we are all familiar, kilocalories (or kcal). The machines for measuring body heat loss are called calorimeters.

Several types of direct calorimeters have been used in studying human metabolism: room-sized, booth- or closet-sized, and body suit calorimeters. Room-sized direct calorimeters allow for the study of energy expenditure in "freely living" subjects. However, the room measurements are that of a small bedroom (3 by 3 meters, or yards), and it is debatable whether a person is truly "freely living" in a room this confined. Closet-sized and body suit calorimeters further confine the movement of a person and therefore can be used only to estimate the person's 24-hour resting energy expenditure.

Direct calorimeters are usually not available in health clubs or sport settings because of their high cost. A body suit may cost several thousand dollars, and a room calorimeter may cost several hundred thousand dollars. However, professionals who work in conjunction with hospitals, clinics, or university research labs may have access to direct calorimeters.

Indirect Calorimetry

The heat liberated from the body is the result of the metabolism of food. The metabolism of food can be simplified into the biochemical equation:

$$food + O_2 \rightarrow usable\ energy + heat + CO_2 + H_2O$$

This equation indicates that oxygen use and heat release are directly related. That is, as more food is metabolized and heat release increases, oxygen use increases as well. Most clinics and laboratories do not measure energy expenditure (heat production) directly, because direct calorimetry equipment is not universally available and is very expensive. Therefore, a technique called indirect respiratory calorimetry is more commonly employed in clinics and laboratories to measure metabolic rate. This form of calorimetry directly measures the oxygen consumption ($\dot{V}O_2$) in metabolism through the measurement of respiratory gases. The $\dot{V}O_2$ data are then converted to an equivalent energy cost in kcal.

Metabolic rate is derived indirectly in respiratory calorimetry by first measuring the $\dot{V}O_2$ and converting this value to a calorie value. This is possible because $\dot{V}O_2$ can be converted to heat equivalents when the type of nutrients undergoing metabolism is known. The energy liberated when only fat is metabolized is 4.7 kcal $\cdot$ L^{-1} oxygen consumed, and 5.05 kcal $\cdot$ L^{-1} oxygen when only carbohydrate is metabolized. Because the energy source for metabolism in the body is generally a combination of fat and carbohydrate, an average caloric expenditure is usually estimated as 5 kcal $\cdot$ L^{-1} of oxygen consumed. For example, if a person exercises at a $\dot{V}O_2$ cost of 1.0 L $\cdot$ min^{-1} of oxygen, the approximate energy expenditure equals 5 kcal $\cdot$ min^{-1}.

Indirect respiratory calorimetry may be performed by either closed-circuit spirometry or open-circuit spirometry. With closed-circuit spirometry systems, the person breathes 100% oxygen from a prefilled cylinder connected to a recording apparatus to account for the oxygen removed from the cylinder and the carbon dioxide produced and collected by an absorbing material. By calculating the ratio of the volume of oxygen consumed to the carbon dioxide produced, a more exact calorie value for $\dot{V}O_2$ can be determined, rather than using the average value of 5 kcal $\cdot$ L^{-1} of oxygen.

The ratio of oxygen consumed to carbon dioxide produced is called the respiratory exchange ratio (RER). The RER will be 0.70 when the food metabolized is 100% fat and 1.00 when the food metabolized is 100% carbohydrate. A mixture of half fat and half carbohydrate yields an RER of 0.85. The biochemical formula for protein metabolism is not as simple as that for carbohydrate and fat, so indirect respiratory calorimetry methods ignore protein's contribution to the metabolic rate. Ignoring protein's metabolic contribution presents some inaccuracy of measurement, but it is well known that protein contributes almost nothing to resting metabolism and very little to exercise metabolism (Brown, Miller, and Eason 2006).

The closed-circuit method of indirect respiratory calorimetry is most commonly used to measure energy expenditure in clinical laboratories. Its usefulness during exercise conditions is limited because of the resistance to breathing offered by the closed circuit and the large volumes of oxygen consumed during exercise.

To accommodate the exercising subject, the open-circuit technique is most commonly used. In this method, the patient inspires air directly from the atmosphere, and measurements of the fractional amounts of oxygen inspired and oxygen expired are made. The respiratory volume is also measured. By calculating the difference between the percentage of oxygen that comprises both inspired and expired air, as well as the respiratory volume, the $\dot{V}O_2$ can be determined. For example, at a respiratory volume of 80 L $\cdot$ min^{-1}, an inspiratory oxygen concentration of 20.93% (0.2093), and an expiratory oxygen concentration of 18.73% (0.1873), the difference in oxygen concentration for the respiratory gas is 2.2%, or 0.022. The corresponding $\dot{V}O_2$ is 1.76 L $\cdot$ min^{-1} ($\dot{V}O_2$ = 80 L $\cdot$ min^{-1} × 0.022, or 1.76 L $\cdot$ min^{-1}). At an average calorie value of 5 kcal · L^{-1} of oxygen, the exercise energy expenditure would be 8.8 kcal · min^{-1} ($1.76 \times 5 = 8.8$).

The costs of open-circuit spirometry and closed-circuit spirometry are about the same; they range from around $15,000 to $40,000, depending on the peripherals and added features that come with the system. The fact that RER can be determined with indirect calorimetry makes this type of metabolic measurement particularly useful for exercise tests and prescriptions. For example, it is well known that muscle glycogen (carbohydrate) depletion is a major cause of fatigue during endurance events. Indirect calorimetry can be used to determine how much fat versus how much carbohydrate is being burned during exercise (the event). Then, after a dietary intervention or change in training routine is implemented, indirect calorimetry can be used to determine whether the manipulation slowed the rate of carbohydrate use for energy, which would theoretically prolong the onset of fatigue.

Doubly Labeled Water

Another method for measuring metabolic rate through gas exchange is through the use of doubly labeled water. The doubly labeled water method of indirect calorimetry works on a similar principle as indirect respiratory calorimetry—gas exchange. However, with doubly labeled water, carbon dioxide (CO_2) production is calculated rather than oxygen consumption. An oral dose of the stable isotopes of ^2H and ^{18}O is taken. The ^2H labels the body water pool, and the ^{18}O labels both the body water pool and the bicarbonate pool. The disappearance rates of the two isotopes measure the turnover of water and the turnover of water plus CO_2. The CO_2 production is calculated by the difference. Because CO_2 production and oxygen consumption are directly related (food + O_2 → usable energy + heat + CO_2 + H_2O), oxygen consumption becomes known once CO_2 is determined. Once CO_2 and the corresponding oxygen consumption are known, energy expenditure can be calculated by the same calorimetric equations that are used for indirect respiratory calorimetry.

The doubly labeled water technique is a clinical method for determining energy expenditure over prolonged periods of time. The advantage of this method is that the client can live freely for days and weeks without any perception that a metabolic measurement is being taken. However, the calculated result is the average energy expenditure over the entire measurement period (days to weeks). Thus, this method is not suitable for measuring energy expenditure during a single exercise bout. Doubly labeled water is almost exclusively used to assess metabolism in hospital and clinical settings in which the focus is on obesity research and treatment.

TABLE 4.1 Common Prediction Equations for RMR

Name	Equation
Harris and Benedict equations	RMR (men) = 13.75 × BM + 500.3 × H – 6.78 × Age + 66.5 RMR (women) = 9.56 × BM + 185.0 × H – 4.68 × Age + 655.1
Kleiber equation	RMR = 73.3 × BM$^{0.74}$
Livingston and Kohlstadt equations	RMR (men) = 293 × BM$^{0.4330}$ – 5.92 × Age RMR (women) = 248 × BM$^{0.4356}$ – 5.09 × Age
Mifflin equations	RMR (men) = (10 × BM) + (625 × H) – (5 × Age) + 5 RMR (women) = (10 × BM) + (625 × H) – (5 × Age) – 161

RMR = kcal · day^{-1}; BM = body mass in kg; H = height in meters; Age = age in years.

Harris and Benedict 1919; Kleiber 1932; Livingston and Kohlstadt 2005; Mifflin et al. 1990.

Prediction of Energy Expenditure

Direct and indirect calorimetry methods for measuring energy expenditure are too complex, time consuming, and costly for most settings. Therefore, major efforts have been made to derive equations for predicting energy expenditure. The most common prediction equations for RMR are those of Kleiber (1932) and Harris and Benedict (1919). Both of these prediction models are based on the relationship between body mass and metabolic rate. Kleiber (1932) demonstrated that RMR, relative to body mass raised to the exponent of 0.74, was consistent for mature mammals, ranging in size from rats to steers (see table 4.1). Harris and Benedict (1919) included variables other than body mass in their equation; namely, height and age (table 4.1). These two equations are less predictive for the obese, because obese people were not included in the original data sets.

Mifflin and coworkers (1990) included men and women of varying body sizes and body compositions in their data set, and derived valid RMR prediction equations based on weight, height, and age. More recently, Livingston and Kohlstadt (2005) derived RMR prediction equations from a large data set containing both normal weight and obese people (table 4.1). These two newer prediction equations are best suited for clients who are overweight, whereas any of the equations presented are viable for normal weight people.

During the middle of the 20th century, much research was performed to determine the energy cost of various physical activities. Tables and charts were published that gave energy expenditure values (kcal) for activities of daily living, work activities, recreational activities, and sport activities. The accuracy of these predictors of physical activity energy expenditure is similar to that of predicting RMR. The American College of Sports Medicine (2010) published metabolic equations for predicting energy expenditure in

TABLE 4.2   Common Prediction Equations for Exercise Energy Expenditure

Activity	Equation
Walking	kcal · min⁻¹ = [(0.1 × S) + (1.8 × S × G) + 3.5] × BM × 0.005
Running	kcal · day⁻¹ = [(0.2 × S) + (0.9 × S × G) + 3.5] × BM × 0.005
Leg cycle ergometer	kcal · day⁻¹ = [(10.8 × W × BM⁻¹) + 3.5] × BM × 0.005
Arm cycle ergometer	kcal · day⁻¹ = [(18 × W × BM⁻¹) + 3.5] × BM × 0.005
Stepping	kcal · day⁻¹ = [(0.2 × F) + (1.33 × 1.8 × H × F) + 3.5] × BM × 0.005

Speed = meters · minute⁻¹; G = percent grade expressed as a decimal; BM = body mass in kg; W = watts; F = stepping frequency per minute; H = step height in meters.

Data from ACSM 2010.

clinical settings (table 4.2). These equations were derived from metabolic measurements taken during ergometer work while subjects were walking, running, leg cycling, arm cycling, and stepping; and therefore would be the preferred calculations for people exercising on any one of these ergometers.

Estimation of 24-Hour and Physical Activity Energy Expenditure

It is very costly, and in most cases impractical, to measure 24-hour energy expenditure or to monitor physical activity energy expenditure through either direct or indirect calorimetry. These two methods of measurement are used only for research and clinical applications. Therefore, most professionals use energy expenditure prediction equations, movement analysis devices, or both, to estimate the energy cost of physical activity and the 24-hour energy expenditure for their clients. Tools used to monitor physical activity and estimate energy expenditure range from expensive and sophisticated machines, which are found only in health centers, to inexpensive gadgets and activity diaries, which can be found in almost any setting.

Activity Monitors

The most plausible tools for measuring either 24-hour energy expenditure or physical activity energy expenditure in the field are pedometers, accelerometers, and heart rate monitors. Pedometers are more suited for monitoring physical activity than 24-hour energy expenditure, whereas accelerometers and heart rate monitors are well suited for both.

Pedometers

Pedometers have been around for several decades. The pedometer itself measures the number of steps taken during the day. The summation of these steps is converted to a distance, and energy expenditure is estimated based on the distance traveled. Pedometer estimates for physical activity energy expenditure correlate moderately well with indirect calorimetry measures (Brown, Miller, and Eason 2006). However, only the total distance traveled is recorded on the pedometer, and there is no indication of the intensity of the physical activity. Therefore, pedometers are useful for gaining insight into 24-hour energy expenditure, but do not offer any reference to exercise intensity or activity patterns throughout the day. An advantage of pedometers is that they are relatively inexpensive; even children can learn how to use them.

Accelerometers

Accelerometers work on a principle that is different from that of pedometers. Accelerometers contain tiny force transducers that continuously measure the intensity, frequency, and duration of movement for extended periods of time. The forces measured by the accelerometer are summed and recorded as counts per time frame. There is no consensus about the accelerometer count thresholds for defining mild, moderate, and high exercise intensities. Nonetheless, accelerometers are valid and reliable for monitoring physical activity counts in both children and adults. Correlation coefficients between accelerometer counts and indirect calorimetry measures range from about 0.60 to 0.85, which represent fairly high correlations (Brown, Miller, and Eason 2006).

The advantage of accelerometers over pedometers is that accelerometers can measure the intensity of energy expenditure throughout the day, and this information can be downloaded to a computer. The computer then generates the data and pinpoints the fluctuations in energy expenditure at any time of day. The computer also uses regression equations to calculate the actual energy expenditure from recorded activity counts.

Heart Rate Monitors

Heart rate is strongly related to respiratory rate and energy expenditure across a wide range of values. Heart rate monitors are similar to accelerometers in that they can accumulate data from short or long bouts of activity throughout the day. Heart rate data can also be downloaded to a computer, and the magnitude of fluctuations in heart rate during the day can be pinpointed. Regression equations are used to convert heart rate measures to energy expenditure.

Activity Surveys and Diaries

Activity diaries necessitate that the participant (or an adult observer in the case of young children) make a record of every activity undertaken throughout the day. The person describes the nature of the activity and the time spent participating. This record includes activities that are sedentary as well as those that require physical exertion. Predetermined values for the energy expenditure of each activity noted in the diary are applied, and the energy expenditure is summed across time and throughout the day.

Activity surveys are similar to activity diaries, but rather than record the actual events at the time they occur (or shortly thereafter), recorders estimate the activity of an average day or an average week or month. In other words, people describe their usual routines over a period of many days, rather than recording actual events over a period of a few days. Calculations for energy expenditure are performed as with activity diaries to get the estimated energy expenditure.

The accuracy of physical activity surveys and diaries is variable; they range from being rather poor indicators of actual physical activity to being relatively good measures of physical activity. Activity surveys and diaries for children tend to be less accurate than those intended for adults. Nonetheless, physical activity surveys and diaries are commonly used to determine physical activity levels in both children and adults, because they are inexpensive, unobtrusive, and easily administered.

Many physical activity surveys have been designed for adults. Some of these have been intended for specific populations, or constructed specifically for independent research studies. The reliability and validity of these surveys is variable. The most popular of these surveys were collected and published by the American College of Sports Medicine (1997) several years ago.

One of the most popular physical activity surveys is the International Physical Activity Questionnaire (Craig et al. 2002; IPAQ 2011). The IPAQ comes in a long and short version, and in several languages, and can be downloaded (IPAQ 2011). Both versions ask respondents to record their health-related physical activity for the past seven days. Both versions can be either administered by a professional (in person), or self-administered. The long version consists of 27 questions that focus on job-related physical activity, transportation-related physical activity, housework, recreation and sport activity, and sedentary or sitting time. The short version of the form asks only seven questions about time spent in vigorous physical activity, moderate intensity activity, walking, and sitting.

A popular physical activity diary for older children and adolescents is the Previous Day Physical Activity Recall (PDPAR; Children's Physical Activity Research Group 2011). The PDPAR was designed to provide accurate data on the type, frequency, intensity, and duration of physical activities; these are then used to estimate physical activity energy expenditure (Weston, Petosa, and Pate 1997). The PDPAR is an activity diary that is segmented into seventeen 30-minute intervals. Participants are given a list of 35 numbered activities in which youth normally engage. They record the number of the activity in which they participated for any given 30-minute interval of the previous day. For the selected activity, they also record the intensity as being very light (slow breathing and little or no movement), light (normal breathing and movement), medium (increased breathing and moderate movement), and hard (hard breathing and quick movement). An estimated energy expenditure value is then calculated for each activity within the given time frame.

Relevance of and Applications for Metabolic Testing

Once a client's metabolic data are available, the fitness professional can use them to prescribe a diet intervention, an exercise intervention, or both, or to monitor energy balance. The metabolic data from indirect calorimetry measurements taken during a graded exercise test can also be used to set a safe and appropriate exercise intensity.

Resting Metabolic Rate (RMR) Testing

The measurement of RMR is most valuable in clinical practice, but it also has applications to athletic performance. The clinical application for RMR testing usually lies on two extremes of the spectrum—obesity and malnutrition or anorexia. The obvious use for RMR in obesity treatment is to determine the client's metabolic rate so that dietary interventions, exercise interventions, or both, can be implemented to create an energy deficit that will favor weight loss. The opposite is true for malnutrition or anorexia. In this case, the RMR helps in the design of dietary practices that will create a positive energy balance favoring weight gain.

The RMR test can also be used as a diagnostic tool. Because the average RMR for adults is 3.5 milliliters of oxygen consumed per kilogram of body weight per minute (American College of Sports Medicine 2010; $3.5 \text{ ml} \cdot \text{kg}^{-1} \cdot \text{min}^{-1}$), an RMR measure that varies significantly from this average can be seen as abnormal. If an abnormal RMR is discovered, further medical testing, psychological testing, or both, can be done to determine whether the aberrant RMR is to the result of a physical condition, such as hypothyroidism, or an eating disorder. A client with an abnormal RMR should be referred to the appropriate health care professional for follow-up testing and diagnosis. The predominant use for nonclinical RMR testing in athletics is to ensure that adequate nutrition is maintained for the energy demands of athletic competition.

The procedures for measuring RMR are fairly standardized and consistent from one facility to the next, although testing centers do not use the same time frames for taking metabolic measurements. Whether the time frame of metabolic measurement is several minutes or several hours, the estimated RMR is calculated by averaging the minute-by-minute metabolic rate measurements across the time of measurement.

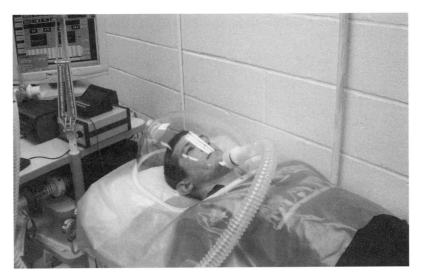

FIGURE 4.1 RMR testing using indirect respiratory calorimetry.

RMR testing is almost exclusively performed by indirect calorimetry. The general procedure is that the client reports to the laboratory in the morning as soon as possible after waking and after fasting for 8 to 12 hours. The subject is not to have taken any stimulants, such as coffee, or been agitated emotionally. The test begins with a run-in period of 30 to 60 minutes of supine rest in a dimly lit room; no metabolic measurements are recorded. This run-in period allows the person to adjust to the testing environment and for metabolism to return to the resting level following any possible stimulating effects incurred by coming to the testing facility. Following the run-in period, metabolic rate is measured using indirect calorimetry. Respiratory gasses are collected using a respiratory gas mask or respiratory hood that is draped over the client (see figure 4.1). Minute-by-minute measures are summed and averaged to derive the RMR.

Theoretically, if the RMR of an obese person were measured at 1,700 kcal · day^{-1}, and the person wanted to lose weight at a rate of 0.5 kilogram (1 lb) per week; an energy intake of 1,200 kcal · day^{-1} would be prescribed (1 lb fat = 3,500 kcal). If the client were to exercise, the rate of weight loss would be increased by the energy cost of the exercise. Alternatively, the dietary intake could be increased above 1,200 kcal · day^{-1} by the energy cost of the exercise to keep the predicted weight loss consistent with 0.5 kilogram (1 lb) per week.

Metabolic Prediction Equations

Quite often, fitness professionals do not have access to the equipment needed for measuring metabolic rate through indirect respiratory calorimetry. In these cases, prediction equations are used to estimate the RMR or the energy cost of exercise. Once an estimate of metabolic rate is derived, the application is the same as described. An example of how this is done is given next.

The client is a 50-year-old obese woman who weighs 100 kilograms (220 lb) and is 169 centimeters (5 feet 6.5 inches) tall. The woman desires to lose weight at a rate of 0.5 kilogram (1 lb) a week. Using the Harris and Benedict equation (see table 4.1), her RMR is estimated at 1,700 kcal · day^{-1} [RMR (kcal · day^{-1}) = $9.56 \times 100 + 185 \times 1.68 - 4.68 \times 50 + 665.1$]. Comparatively, her predicted RMR using the equation of Livingston and Kohlstadt (table 4.1) is estimated at 1,588 kcal · day^{-1} [RMR (kcal · day^{-1}) = $248 \times 100^{0.4356} - (5.09 \times 50)$]. The slight discrepancy between the values derived from the two equations demonstrates that prediction equations are less accurate than real metabolic measurements. Nonetheless, for this woman to lose weight at a rate of 0.5 kilogram (1 lb) a week, she should consume only 1,088 to 1,200 kcal · day^{-1}. Such a low energy intake may seem too restrictive for this woman. Alternatively, she could consume between 1,338 and 1,450 kcal · day^{-1} and expend 250 kcal · day^{-1} in exercise to meet her goal.

If the woman decides to exercise, the question becomes how much exercise must she perform daily to meet her exercise energy expenditure goal? The answer is found by using the exercise metabolic calculations provided in table 4.2. If the woman selects walking for her physical activity, at a rate of 3 miles per hour (80.5 m · min^{-1}), then she should walk for 43 min · day^{-1} to meet her goal of 250 kcal · day^{-1} spent in exercise [(kcal · min^{-1}) = $(0.1 \times 80.5) + (1.8 \times 80.5 \times 0) + 3.5) \times 100$ kg body weight $\times 0.005$ kcal · ml^{-1} oxygen, yields 5.77 kcal · min^{-1}]. If the woman chooses to ride a cycle ergometer for exercise, at a rate of 50 watts, she would need to ride for 56 min · day^{-1} to meet her goal of 250 kcal · day^{-1} spent in exercise [(kcal · min^{-1}) = $10.8 \times 50 \times 100^{-1} + 3.5 \times 100$ kg body weight $\times 0.005$ kcal · ml^{-1} oxygen, yields 4.45 kcal · min^{-1}].

Pedometers

Pedometers estimate energy expenditure similar to the way metabolic prediction equations do. However, the metabolic prediction equations in pedometers are based on distance traveled rather than the speed and grade of travel. Therefore, the pedometer output is usually expressed as kcal per mile (or kilometer), rather than kcal per minute. The metabolic calculations used in pedometers are based on the energy cost of walking 1 mile (or kilometer). Sophisticated pedometers allow the user to enter body weight and stride length into the device, whereas inexpensive pedometers use a predetermined average value for these variables. Pedometers are more accurate estimating energy expenditure when the person is walking on level ground with a consistent stride length, than when the person is walking on a grade, has an intermittent stride length, or both. Therefore, pedometers are more accurate at estimating energy expenditure during a formal exercise bout than over a 24-hour period. Although pedometers may not be that accurate at determining actual energy expenditure, they are very useful for making relative comparisons for the same person (e.g., day-to-day step counts; Harris et al. 2009).

Accelerometers

Accelerometers are electronic motion sensors that quantify the volume and intensity of movement over time. The raw acceleration signal of an accelerometer is specific to the brand name or model of the device, meaning that counts from one brand or model accelerometer cannot be directly compared to counts from another brand or model. Consequently, the raw acceleration signal of an accelerometer is usually translated into a variable that has some common meaning (e.g., kcal). Because accelerometer technology is based on biomechanical principles and metabolic rate is based on biological measures, it is difficult to accurately translate accelerometer signals to metabolic rates. The process is further complicated when individual differences in body mass and biomechanical efficiency are taken into consideration.

Indirect calorimetry is used to calibrate each brand or model of accelerometer for determining the metabolic rates of children, adolescents, and adults. The manufacturers provide software programs that default to metabolic calculations for adults; however, because the metabolic cost of movement in children changes as they grow, a common metabolic parameter for children has not been agreed on. Therefore, accelerometer users either use the software default calculations for children and adolescents or construct their own conversion programs using the data they find for children in the scientific literature.

The accelerometer can be worn at the hip, wrist, or ankle. However, most users find that measurements are the least variable when the unit is worn on the hip (Heil 2006; Respironics 2008). Before using the accelerometer, the user or clinician programs the device to take measurements in epoch lengths ranging from a few seconds to several minutes. The gender, age, height, and weight of the wearer are also programmed into the accelerometer at this time. Most accelerometers are waterproof and can record data 24 hours a day for a few weeks at a time. At the end of the trial period, the data are downloaded to a computer and analyzed with the manufacturer-provided software. As mentioned earlier, the benefit of accelerometers is that they can register the intensity of exercise within a given time frame. Furthermore, accelerometers can be used to estimate 24-hour expenditure as well as the energy expenditure of physical activity.

Heart Rate Monitors

Sophisticated heart rate monitors (figure 4.2) collect data in time epochs similar to the way accelerometers do. Rather than accumulate accelerations, though, heart rate monitors record heartbeats. Generally, the more heartbeats in a time epoch, the higher the metabolic rate. Heart rates are converted into metabolic measures in the same way that they would be correlated to energy expenditure during a graded exercise test using indirect respiratory calorimetry (see chapter 5). In other words, metabolic rate is determined by knowing the relationship between heart rate and aerobic metabolism. Data from sophisticated heart rate monitors can be downloaded to computers, as with accelerometers.

Less expensive heart rate monitors do not interface with computers and cannot be programmed. The usefulness of these monitors, therefore, is limited to immediate observation or manual recording of heart rate at various time points. Many people use low-cost heart rate monitors to help them main-

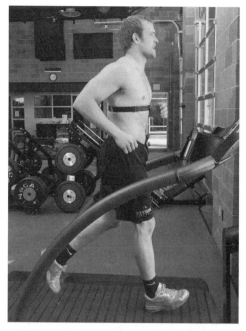

FIGURE 4.2   Training with a heart rate monitor can be useful for making relative energy expenditure comparisons from day to day.

tain their heart rate in a predetermined range during an exercise bout. Observations and recordings of personal heart rates during exercise can be used later to calculate whether the desired exercise intensity was met to achieve the prescribed metabolic rate. On the other hand, the person can determine ahead of time the target heart rate necessary for meeting any desired metabolic rate during exercise, and then during the exercise bout bring the heart rate to the predetermined level for the desired time frame. Regardless of how heart rate monitors are used to estimate metabolic rate, it must be remembered that they are not accurate in estimating the energy cost of anaerobic exercise.

International Physical Activity Questionnaire (IPAQ)

As mentioned earlier, the IPAQ comes in a long and short version (IPAQ 2011). Both versions ask respondents to record their health-related physical activity for the past seven days. Both versions ask about physical activity undertaken across four domains:

- Leisure time physical activity
- Domestic and yard physical activity
- Work-related physical activity
- Transport-related physical activity

The IPAQ short version asks for three specific types of activity within these four domains: walking, moderate-intensity activity, and vigorous activity. The IPAQ long version asks for details on activities within the four domains. Both versions of the IPAQ can be scored as continuous measures of physical activity. The calculations are made by multiplying the energy cost of each activity in METs (metabolic equivalents or multiples of the RMR) by the minutes the activity is performed. For example, an activity with an energy cost of 3.0 METs performed for 25 minutes has a MET-minute value of 75. Alternatively, the energy cost of the activity (MET) can be multiplied by the quotient of the body weight (kg) divided by 60 to yield an energy cost in kcal per minute.

The usefulness of the IPAQ is to determine the energy cost of physical activity in various settings, and not to determine RMR or 24-hour energy expenditure. However, by combining the values for the energy cost of physical activity obtained from the IPAQ with a value for the RMR obtained from one of the prediction equations detailed earlier, a person can derive an estimate of the 24-hour energy expenditure. Guidelines for scoring and comparing IPAQ scores among individuals and populations are provided with the questionnaires (IPAQ 2011).

Previous Day Physical Activity Recall (PDPAR)

The PDPAR captures the habitual physical activity of older children and adolescents. The PDPAR uses a time-based recall approach to record and measure physical activity levels. Each day is divided into 34 time blocks of 30 minutes going from 7:00 a.m. to midnight. Adolescents are asked to record their specific activity (35 common activities are listed for them to select from, each with a numeric code) and the intensity of the activity for each block of time. The energy cost of physical activity is then determined using the metabolic equivalent (MET) value for each activity. MET values can be converted to kcal using standard conversion factors.

Comparing Metabolic Rate Measurement Methods

Although accelerometers, pedometers, heart rate monitors, and question-naires are not as accurate as direct and indirect calorimetry in determining metabolic rate, these less expensive tools can be used to create exercise plans, particularly those focused on health promotion and fitness. For example, if a person wants to increase her fitness level by doing aerobic exercise four times a week at a predetermined intensity, a heart rate monitor would be an excellent tool to use for monitoring intensity. The fitness professional could help the client determine the appropriate target heart rate, and then show the client how to use the heart rate monitor safely to achieve the

TABLE 4.3 Comparison of Tests and Measures for Metabolic Rate

Test or measure	Metabolic application	Difficulty of access and adminis-tration	Validity	Reliability	Cost	Client burden
Direct calorimetry	RMR, PAEE, 24-hEE	High	High	High	High	High
Closed-circuit indirect calorimetry	RMR, 24-hEE	Moderate	High	High	Moderate	Moderate
Open-circuit indirect calorimetry	RMR, PAEE, 24-hEE	Moderate	High	High	Moderate	Moderate
Doubly labeled water	RMR, 24-hEE	High	High	High	High	Low
Prediction equations	RMR, PAEE, 24-hEE	Low	Low to moderate	High	Low	Low
Pedometers	24-hEE	Low	Low to moderate	Low to moderate	Low	Low
Accelerometers	RMR, PAEE, 24-hEE	Moderate to high	High	High	High	Low
Heart rate monitors	RMR, PAEE, 24-hEE	Low	Moderate	Moderate	Low	Low
Surveys and diaries	PAEE, 24-hEE	Low	Low to moderate	Low to moderate	Low	Low

RMR = resting metabolic rate; PAEE = physical activity energy expenditure; 24-hEE = 24-hour energy expenditure.

intensity goal. Table 4.3 provides a summary of measurement methods for metabolic rate.

A pedometer might be the tool of choice for a previously sedentary person who wants to increase physical activity levels to lose weight or decrease disease risk. In this instance, the fitness professional could use the pedometer to get a baseline measure of steps per day for the client, and then help the client set a goal to increase the number of steps per day in a safe progression.

Accelerometers and questionnaires might be used to give clients feedback on how their activity levels fluctuate during the day or from day to day. These tools provide a diary or history of the client's activity that can be reviewed with the client. Goals can be set to increase overall physical activity, physical activity during specific time periods, or the intensity of activity at certain points. All of this information could be mapped out, depending on the client's needs and objectives.

As shown throughout this chapter, fitness professionals can use information about clients' metabolic rates to help them achieve their performance or health-related goals. Problems can arise, however, when the metabolic data generated do not seem to coincide with what would be expected from the client's demographics, behavior or training patterns, or predicted physiological outcome(s). Under these situations, the professional needs to know how to interpret metabolic data and how to determine whether metabolic data and predictions are valid for that particular client. The two case studies that follow demonstrate how the professional can overcome what initially seem to be unsolvable inconsistencies.

Case Study 1: John's Inability to Lose Weight

John is a client requesting an exercise program to help him lose weight. He is an accountant, is 40 years old, and has not exercised since college. He is 6 feet 0 inches tall (183 cm) and weighs 220 pounds (100 kg). You calculate John's BMI to be 29.9, which is borderline obesity. You also perform a body composition assessment on John and find him to be 31.0% body fat. John does not have any health risk factors, except his weight. John selects walking as his mode of exercise, and agrees to exercise for 30 minutes a day. You complete your exercise prescription for John by teaching him how to safely monitor himself while walking.

Your facility does not have equipment for measuring metabolic rate, so you decide to use prediction equations to estimate John's 24-hour energy expenditure. You will subsequently use that predictive data to design a modest restriction in John's energy intake that will allow him to feel satisfied when eating, but still lose weight (because he is not really interested in dieting). You decide to use the Mifflin equation (see table 4.1) to predict John's 24-hour resting metabolism, because John is overweight. The results calculate to be 1,948 kcal per day. You next use the prediction equation in table 4.2 to calculate John's walking energy expenditure. At John's selected speed of 3.0 miles per hour (4.8 km/h), he should expend 5.98 kcal per minute or 179 kcal per exercise bout. John's total energy expenditure each day is predicted to be 2,127 kcal.

You and John next sit down with your coworker, who is a dietitian, to design John's eating plan. Because John does not want a restrictive diet, the dietitian prescribes a healthy diet containing 1,800 kcal per day. This means that John's energy deficit should be 327 kcal per day, causing a predicted weight loss of 1 pound (0.45 kg) every 11 days.

You track John's progress, and at the end of two months, John is feeling discouraged because he has lost only 3 pounds (1.4 kg). His predicted weight loss should be 5.5 pounds (2.5 kg). Your initial instinct is that John has lost 5.5 pounds (2.5 kg) of fat, but gained 2.5 pounds (1.1 kg) of lean mass from the exercise. You repeat the body composition assessment and find that John is still 31.0 % body fat. Your next speculation is that John has not kept his diet.

However, John is an accountant and very particular about numbers. He has not only adhered to his diet, but also actually weighed his food and calculated the energy content of everything he ate. He provides dietary diaries that show he averaged 1,800 kcal a day for the past 60 days. The dietitian concurs that John's records are correct. The only conclusion you can make is that the prediction equations for metabolic rate were not accurate for John.

Fortunately, you have access to an accelerometer. John agrees to wear an accelerometer 24 hours a day for the next week. The results from the accelerometer reveal that John's average 24-hour energy expenditure is 1,981 kcal. This means that the prediction equations underestimated John's daily energy expenditure by 146 kcal per day (7% discrepancy). Multiplied by 60 days, this error is equivalent to the caloric value of 2 pounds (0.9 kg) of fat. The discrepancy, or apparent inconsistency, has been resolved. You can now adjust John's regimen to meet his weight loss goal.

Case Study 2: Jill's Deteriorating Gymnastics Performance

Jill is a competitive gymnast. Her coach is very adamant about the team's maintaining a rigid training schedule. The end of the season is approaching, and Jill's performance has deteriorated over the season. Moreover, Jill has been plagued with minor injuries and constant aches and pains all season. Jill's coach has sent her to you, the strength and conditioning coach for the team. Your job is to find out why Jill's performance has deteriorated, and to fix the problem.

Your initial interview with Jill reveals that she has interpreted her coach's strict training schedule to mean that she is too fat and needs to lose weight. Jill's reaction to this perceived message was to diet throughout the season. She has been seeing a clinical psychologist this year because of some emotional problems she is having. She gives you permission to speak with her psychologist. The psychologist assures you that Jill does not have an eating disorder, but that Jill does have a long history of dieting. The psychologist has been working on Jill's body perception, and asks if you have any objective information that may help change Jill's perception.

Your plan is to perform a diet analysis, measure resting metabolic rate, and determine Jill's percent body fat. The clinical psychologist refers Jill to a dietitian, and you perform the tests for body fat content and metabolism. Jill's body fat content is 15.2%, which is lean for a female athlete. Jill's measured RMR comes out to be 1,600 kcal per day. Using the Harris and Benedict equation (table 4.1), you get a similar prediction. So, you assume that the RMR measure is a valid metabolic measure for Jill's small body size.

Jill's diet analysis reveals that she is consuming only 1,250 kcal a day. Thus, there is an energy deficit of 350 kcal a day between Jill's intake and her 24-hour RMR, and you have not yet accounted for her daily exercise energy expenditure.

(continued)

(continued)

It is also enlightening to see that when you calculate Jill's metabolic rate in relation to her lean body mass, you find that the value is 18 kcal · kg LBM^{-1} · day^{-1}. Given that the normal value is about 25 kcal · kg LBM^{-1} · day^{-1}, with a range of 20 to 30 kcal · kg LBM^{-1} · day^{-1}, you conclude that Jill's history of dieting may have reduced her metabolic rate.

You bring all of this information to Jill's psychologist and explain the following:

- Jill is consuming several hundred kcal below what she needs to maintain her health.
- Jill's history of restrictive dieting may have reduced the metabolic rate of her lean tissues.
- Jill's body fat content is low, but not dangerously low for a female athlete. Nonetheless, Jill does not need to lose weight.

Rather than prescribe a rigid diet plan for Jill, the psychologist decides to work with the dietitian to help Jill learn to eat intuitively. This means helping Jill learn to eat with intention while paying attention to body cues of hunger and satiety. The metabolic information you provided to Jill's psychologist will help both the psychologist and Jill to view Jill's problematic behaviors more objectively. You now need to report back to Jill's coach that the problem has been identified and that Jill is on the road to recovery; however, the recovery will not be completed before the end of the season.

SUMMARY

- *Metabolism* is the term used to describe the body's ability to produce, use, and regulate energy.
- The overall energy expenditure of the body is a summation of TEF, RMR, and the energy cost of physical activity. RMR contributes from 60 to 75% of the 24-hour energy expenditure. RMR is almost exclusively a reflection of the lean body mass (Cunningham 1982). Severe restrictions in energy intake reduce RMR significantly, and can even reduce the RMR:LBM ratio. Increases in lean body mass raise the RMR slightly, but most people do not gain enough lean body mass through exercise training to appreciably affect the RMR or overall energy balance in the body.
- The energy cost of physical activity or exercise energy expenditure is the only component of the 24-hour energy expenditure that can be voluntarily controlled.
- Energy expenditure, or metabolic rate, can be measured through direct calorimetry and indirect respiratory calorimetry; or estimated by using activity monitors, prediction equations, and surveys. Once a

client's metabolic rate is known, the fitness professional can use the information to prescribe diet interventions, exercise interventions, or both, or monitor the energy balance of the client.

■ Knowledge about exercise energy expenditure can be used to prescribe the proper intensity and duration of exercise to meet the preventive, therapeutic, or performance goals of the client.

5

Aerobic Power

Jonathan H. Anning, PhD, CSCS*D

Aerobic power refers to the ability of the muscles to use oxygen received from the heart and lungs to produce energy. As this process becomes more efficient, aerobic power improves. Therefore, improvements in aerobic power are usually monitored by determining $\dot{V}O_2$max, or the maximal volume of oxygen a person consumes and uses with the active muscles during exercise.

Developing aerobic power is a lower training priority for athletes participating primarily in anaerobic activities (i.e., for which oxygen is not necessary for energy production) than it is for athletes participating in aerobic activities such as long-distance events. Obviously, long-distance walking, running, cycling, swimming, and even cross-country skiing are highly aerobic activities and thus require oxygen to produce energy. Yet, long-distance athletic potential is not entirely related to maximal aerobic power because improvements in anaerobic threshold result in competitive differences among athletes (see chapter 6) (Bosquet, Léger, and Legros 2002).

Consider the fact that sedentary people can improve aerobic power by training near the anaerobic threshold, whereas trained athletes must train above the anaerobic threshold (Londeree 1997). Nonetheless, tests specifically designed to measure maximal aerobic power during walking, running, cycling, or swimming competitions appear to be best suited for comparing endurance capabilities with performance outcomes. Conversely, aerobic power tests are not appropriate for sports performed at high intensities because these activities are predominantly anaerobic.

Because anaerobic activities are associated with greater fatigue, the value of aerobic power is limited to facilitating energy recovery during repeated efforts of such activities. Although there is no set formula for determining aerobic power needs within a sport, the repetitive high-intensity demands combined with game duration highlights a need for anaerobic system recovery. Sports that may require aerobic power to facilitate continuous recovery include field hockey, ice hockey, lacrosse, mixed martial arts, downhill skiing, soccer, wrestling, and to a lesser extent, basketball and American football (Baechle and Earle 2008). Athletes in these sports must switch instantaneously from high- to low-intensity activities, and vice versa, over the course of a game.

The additional challenge placed on athletes in anaerobic sports is recovery from dependence on the anaerobic glycolytic system, which breaks down carbohydrate to produce energy while decreasing pH levels in the body. The decrease in pH is referred to as metabolic acidosis, and this interferes with the athlete's ability to continue performing at a high level. For the athlete to overcome the fatigue associated with metabolic acidosis, the recovery process must include removing the prohibitive by-products while replacing the energy stores. Therefore, athletes involved in interval training, or the manipulation of exercise and rest ratios to maximize these metabolic pathways, are improving the aerobic and anaerobic systems simultaneously.

Another aspect of anaerobic activities experienced in sport is the foundational fitness, or progression, aspect. Even though the aerobic demand of sports such as baseball, field events, golf, and weightlifting are minimal (Baechle and Earle 2008), the proper progression of muscle adaptations begins with establishing a strong fitness foundation that includes cardiorespiratory and musculoskeletal health components during the off-season. Consequently, aerobic power need only be measured at the beginning and end of the off-season to confirm an athlete's training commitment and fitness foundation prior to preseason conditioning.

The advantage of selecting aerobic power tests for predominantly anaerobic sports is that they offer more choices, whereas individuals competing in long-distance events are limited by the specificity principle. Choosing aerobic power tests and protocols for endurance athletes should begin with knowing the person's training preferences. The next step is to ensure that the administration of the test will meet general maximal or submaximal assessment criteria. The primary criterion for ensuring the accuracy of the results of a maximal aerobic power test is that the person reaches volitional fatigue within 8 to 12 minutes. Submaximal aerobic power tests, on the other hand, should be based on research literature recommendations for protocol intensities that achieve a heart rate steady state (American College of Sports Medicine 2010). The heart rate steady state is the plateau at which the heart rate and rate of oxygen consumption tend to remain relatively stable at a given workload. An examiner can verify steady state by measuring the heart rate during the final two minutes of a protocol stage to determine whether those two measurements are within six beats per minute (bpm) of each other. Nonetheless, unless the examiner is trying to determine an athlete's ability to perform longer than 12 minutes, the recommendation is to select the maximal or submaximal aerobic power test that best matches the demands of the sport.

Tables 5.1 and 5.2 summarize the maximal and submaximal exercise tests, respectively, described in this chapter. To facilitate the selection of an appropriate cardiorespiratory test, population-specific correlations and standard errors reported in the referenced literature are included in the tables. Correlation coefficients between predicted and observed $\dot{V}O_2$max values have been proposed at a minimum of .60 by Mayhew and Gifford (1975), but it should be noted that correlations above .80 are much more preferable (Baumgartner and Jackson 1991). In addition, a value of ±4.5 mL · kg⁻¹ · km⁻¹ as a standard error of estimate is considered an acceptable range for predicting aerobic power (Dolgener et al. 1994; Greenhalgh, George, and Hager 2001). After identifying the cardiorespiratory test that appears to address the athlete's goals accurately, the fitness professional should refer to the textbook page identified in the table for more details about the specific protocols.

Regression Equation Variables

Tables 5.1 and 5.2 consist of regression equations that require the data variables in table 5.3 to perform the calculations. Some data require little skill to collect, such as age, height and weight, elapsed time (measured with a stopwatch), the distance traveled on a track, the speed and grade of the belt on the treadmill, and the cycle ergometer workload (e.g., revolutions each minute along with resistance). Conversely, collecting other forms of data requires technical proficiency. For instance, using the regression equation to determine the maximal mile run for healthy youth (Buono et al. 1991) requires a sum of skinfolds in addition to the elapsed time. Another technical proficiency is determining heart rate because it is essential for almost all of the testing protocols, especially the submaximal testing protocols used to measure improvements in aerobic power. Chapter 2 describes the techniques used to measure tricep and subscapular skinfold sites. Chapter 3 describes the palpation, heart rate monitor, and electrocardiograph methods for determining heart rate.

Maximal Exercise Testing Methods

The maximal laboratory exercise tests in table 5.1 are optimal for assessing aerobic power because they offer the best opportunity for gas measurements. Oxygen and carbon dioxide analyzers permit the collection of gases while facilitating the performance goal prescription and monitoring process. Although these gas analyzers have a high degree of sophistication in measuring cardiorespiratory fitness, the technical expertise necessary for administering and interpreting the data exceeds the scope of this chapter. Hence, only the heart rate methods for performing a maximal exercise test

TABLE 5.1 Maximal Exercise Tests Used to Predict Aerobic Power ($\dot{V}O_2$max)

		MODE: TREADMILL		
Test protocol	**Population (age)**	**Regression equations** ($\dot{V}O_2$max = mL · kg^{-1} · min^{-1}; *r* value; SEE)	**Textbook page**	**Resource**
Bruce	Healthy adults (18-29)	Males: 3.88 + 3.36 (time in minutes) Females: 1.06 + 3.36 (time in minutes) *r* = .91; SEE = 3.72	104	Spackman et al. 2001
	Healthy females (20-42)	4.38 (time in minutes) – 3.9; *r* = .91; SEE = 2.7	104	Pollock et al. 1982
	Healthy adults (29-73)	Males: 3.88 + 3.36 (time in minutes) Females: 1.06 + 3.36 (time in minutes) *r* = .92; SEE = 3.22	104	Bruce, Kusumi, and Hosmer 1973
	Healthy males (35-55)	4.326 (time in minutes) – 4.66	104	Pollock et al. 1976
	Healthy males (48.1 ± 16.3)	14.76 – 1.38 (time) + 0.451 (time²) – 0.012 (time³); *r* = .977; SEE = 3.35 *Note:* Time is expressed in minutes.	104	Foster et al. 1984
	Healthy sedentary and active males (48.6 ± 11.1)	Sedentary: 3.288 (time in minutes) + 4.07 Active: 3.778 (time in minutes) + 0.19 *r* = .906; SEE = 1.9	104	Bruce, Kusumi, and Hosmer 1973
Balke	Healthy females (20-42)	1.38 (time in minutes) + 5.2; *r* = .94; SEE = 2.2	105	Pollock et al. 1982
	Healthy males (35-55)	1.444 (time in minutes) + 14.99	104	Pollock et al. 1976

		MODE: CYCLE ERGOMETER		
Test protocol	**Population (age)**	**Regression equations** ($\dot{V}O_2$max = L · min^{-1} except 5K cycle ride; *r* value; SEE)	**Textbook page**	**Resource**
Storer-Davis	Sedentary adults (20-70)	9.39 (workload in watts) + 7.7 (weight in kg) – 5.88 (age in years) + 136.7 *r* = .932; SEE = 1.47 L · min^{-1} *Note:* Watts = resistance in kp × 300 / 6.12	106	Storer, Davis, and Caiozzo 1990
Andersen	Healthy adults (15-28)	0.0117 (workload in watts) + 0.16 *r* = .88; SEE = 10% *Note:* Watts = resistance in kp × 300 / 6.12	106–107	Andersen 1995
5K cycle ride	Healthy adults (27 ± 5)	316 – 97.8 (log of cycle time in seconds) *r* = -.83; SEE = 14%	107	Buono et al. 1996

MODE: TIMED FIELD TESTS				
Test protocol	Population (age)	Regression equations ($\dot{V}O_2max = mL \cdot kg^{-1} \cdot min^{-1}$; r value; SEE)	Textbook page	Resource
5-minute run	Healthy youth (12-15)	12 years: 0.024 (distance in meters) + 22.473; $r = .672$ 13 years: 0.034 (distance in meters) + 15.257; $r = .751$ 14 years: 0.022 (distance in meters) + 26.165; $r = .534$ 15 years: 0.035 (distance in meters) + 16.197; $r = .685$	107–109	MacNaughton et al. 1990
	Sedentary and active males (18-46)	3.23 (run velocity in km · hr⁻¹) + 0.123 $r = .90$; SEE = 5% Note: Run velocity = 12 (distance in km).	107–109	Berthon et al. 1997b
	Trained athletes (19-38) and runners (20-46)	Athletes: 1.43 (run velocity in km · hr⁻¹) + 29.2; $r = .56$; SEE = 4.6% Runners: 1.95 (run velocity in km · hr⁻¹) + 26.6; $r = .69$; SEE = 6.6% Note: Run velocity = 12 (distance in km).	107–109	Berthon et al. 1997a
Cooper's 12-minute run	Military males (17-52)	35.97 (distance in miles) – 11.28; Outdoor ¼-lap = 0.0625 miles 35.97 (distance in meters / 1,609) – 11.28; Outdoor ¼-lap = 100 meters $r = .897$ Note: Best accuracy ≥ 1.4 miles.	107–109	Cooper 1968
Cooper's 12-minute swim	High school swimmers (13-17)	Run $\dot{V}O_2max = 10.69 + 0.059$ (distance in yards) $r = .47$; SEE = 6.82	107–109	Huse, Patterson, and Nichols 2000
	Healthy males (18-32)	Swim $\dot{V}O_2max = 0.028$ (distance in meters) + 34.1 $r = .40$; SEE = 5.7 Run $\dot{V}O_2max = 0.023$ (distance in meters) + 43.7 $r = .38$; SEE = 5.14	107–109	Conley et al. 1991
	Healthy females (18-34)	Swim $\dot{V}O_2max = 0.026$ (distance in meters) + 24 $r = .42$; SEE = 4.5 Run $\dot{V}O_2max = 0.026$ (distance in meters) + 29.8 $r = .34$; SEE = 6.0	107–109	Conley et al. 1992

(continued)

TABLE 5.1 *(Continued)*

		MODE: TIMED FIELD TESTS (CONTINUED)		
15-minute run	Healthy youth (12-15)	12 years: 0.01 (distance in meters) + 19.331; $r = .881$ 13 years: 0.012 (distance in meters) + 18.809; $r = .851$ 14 years: 0.013 (distance in meters) + 18.756; $r = .671$ 15 years: 0.015 (distance in meters) + 16.429; $r = .881$	107–109	MacNaughton et al. 1990
20-minute run	High school students (14-17)	Males: 22.85 + 8.44 (distance in miles) + 3.98 Females: 22.85 + 8.44 (distance in miles) $r = .80$; SEE = 4.36	107–109	Murray et al. 1993

		MODE: DISTANCE FIELD TESTS		
Test protocol	**Population (age)**	**Regression equations** ($\dot{V}O_2$max = mL · kg^{-1} · min^{-1} unless noted; *r* value; SEE)	**Textbook page**	**Resource**
Mile (1,600 m) run	Endurance-trained children (8-17)	Combined: 96.81 – 8.62 (time) + 0.34 (time^2) Male: 98.49 – 9.06 (time) + 0.38 (time^2) Female: 82.2 – 6.04 (time) + 0.22 (time^2) $r = .70$; SEE = 3 *Note:* Time in minutes.	109	Castro-Pinero et al. 2009
	Healthy males and females (8-25)	Combined: 96.81 – 8.62 (time) + 0.34 (time^2) Male: 98.49 – 9.06 (time) + 0.38 (time^2) Female: 82.2 – 6.04 (time) + 0.22 (time^2) $r = .72$; SEE = 4.8 *Note:* Time in minutes.	109	Cureton et al. 1995
	Healthy youth (10-12)	22.5903 + 12.2944 (speed in m · sec^{-1}) – 0.1755 (weight in kg) $r = .804$; SEE = 5.54	109	Massicotte, Gauthier, and Markon 1985
	Healthy youth (10-18)	Males: 86.1 – 0.04 (time) – 0.08 (sum of skinfolds) – 4.7 – 0.15 (kg wgt) Females: 86.1 – 0.04 (time) – 0.08 (sum of skinfolds) – 9.4 – 0.15 (kg wgt) $r = .84$; SEE = 9% *Note:* Time in seconds; refer to chapter 2 for skinfold procedures.	109	Buono et al. 1991
	College students (18-30)	Males: 108.94 – 8.41 (time) + 0.34 (time)^2 + 0.21 (age) – 0.84 (BMI) Females: 108.94 – 8.41 (time) + 0.34 (time)^2 – 0.84 (BMI) $r = .7$-0.84; SEE = 4.8-5.28 *Note:* Time in minutes; refer to chapter 2 for BMI calculation procedures.	109	Plowman and Liu 1999
	Trained male runners (27.5 ± 10.3)	2.5043 × (0.84 (run velocity in km · hr^{-1}) $r = .95$; SEE = 2.3% *Note:* Run velocity = 96.558 / time in minutes.	109	Tokmakidis et al. 1987

MODE: DISTANCE FIELD TESTS (CONTINUED)				
1.5-mile (2,400 m) run	Healthy youth (13-17)	$22.5903 + 12.2944$ (speed in m · sec^{-1}) $- 0.1755$ (weight in kg) $r = .804$; SEE $= 5.54$	109	Massicotte, Gauthier, and Markon 1985
	College students (18-26)	Males: $65.404 + 7.707 - 0.159$ (weight in kg) $- 0.843$ (time in minutes) Females: $65.404 - 0.159$ (weight in kg) $- 0.843$ (time in minutes) $r = .86$; SEE $= 3.37$	109	Larsen et al. 2002
	Healthy adults (18-29)	Males: $88.02 + 3.716 - 0.1656$ (weight in kg) $- 2.767$ (time in minutes) Females: $88.02 - 0.1656$ (weight in kg) $- 2.767$ (time in minutes) $r = .90$; SEE $= 2.8$	109	George et al. 1993a
2-mile (3,200 m) run	Healthy females (20-37)	$72.9 - 1.77$ (time in minutes); $r = .89$	109	Mello, Murphy, and Vogel 1988
	Healthy males (20-51)	$99.7 - 3.35$ (time in minutes); $r = .91$; SEE $= 3.31$	109	Mello, Murphy, and Vogel 1988
	Female runners (31.1 ± 5.7)	$90.7 - 3.24$ (time in minutes) $+ 0.04$ (time in minutes^2) $r = .94-.96$; SEE $= 2.78-3.58$	109	Weltman et al. 1990
	Male runners (31.1 ± 8.3)	$118.4 - 4.770$ (time in minutes) $r = .73$; SEE $= 4.51$	109	Weltman et al. 1987
3-mile (5K) competition	Trained male runners (27.5 ± 10.3)	$3.1747 \times (0.9139$ (run velocity in km · hr^{-1}) $r = .98$; SEE $= 2.3\%$ *Note:* Run velocity $= 300$ / time in minutes.	109	Tokmakidis et al. 1987
6-mile (10K) competition	Trained male runners (27.5 ± 10.3)	$4.7226 \times (0.8698$ (run velocity in km · hr^{-1}) $r = .88$; SEE $= 4.8\%$ *Note:* Run velocity $= 600$ / time in minutes.	109	Tokmakidis et al. 1987
Marathon (42K) competition	Trained male runners (27.5 ± 10.3)	$6.9021 \times (0.8246$ (run velocity in km · hr^{-1}) $r = .85$; SEE $= 5.6\%$ *Note:* Run velocity $= 2531.7$ / time in minutes.	109	Tokmakidis et al. 1987

Note: A kp is equivalent to a kg of force.

TABLE 5.2 Submaximal Exercise Tests Used to Predict Aerobic Power ($\dot{V}O_2max$)

MODE: TREADMILL

Test protocol	Population (age)	Regression equations ($\dot{V}O_2max = mL \cdot kg^{-1} \cdot min^{-1}$: *r* value; SEE)	Textbook page	Resource
Walking	Healthy adults (20-59)	Males: 15.1 + 21.8 (mph) – 0.327 (HR) – 0.263 (mph × age) + 0.00504 (HR × age) + 5.98 Females: 15.1 + 21.8 (mph) – 0.327 (HR) – 0.263 (mph × age) + 0.00504 (HR × age) *r* = .91; SEE = 3.72 *Note:* Speed in mph, HR immediately postexercise.	112	Ebbeling et al. 1991
Jogging	Healthy adults (18-29)	Males: 54.07 + 7.062 – 0.193 (weight) + 4.47 (mph) – 0.1453 (HR) Females: 54.07 – 0.193 (weight) + 4.47 (mph) – 0.1453 (HR) *r* = .88; SEE = 3.1 *Note:* Weight in kg, speed in mph, HR immediately postexercise.	113	George et al. 1993b
	Healthy adults (18-40)	Males: 58.687 + 7.520 + 4.334 (mph) – 0.211 (weight) – 0.148 (HR) – 0.107 (age) Females: 58.687 + 4.334 (mph) – 0.211 (weight) – 0.148 (HR) – 0.107 (age) *r* = .91; SEE = 2.52 *Note:* Speed in mph, weight in kg, speed in mph, HR immediately postexercise.	113	Vehrs et al. 2007
Walk/jog/run	Healthy adults (18-65)	Males: 30.04 + 6.37 – 0.243 (age) – 0.122 (weight) + 3.2 (mph) + 0.391 (PFA) + 0.669 (PA) Females: 30.04 – 0.243 (age) – 0.122 (weight) + 3.2 (mph) + 0.391 (PFA) + 0.669 (PA) *r* = .94; SEE = 3.09 *Note:* Weight in kg, speed in mph, table 5.4 question responses for PFA and PA[1].	114	George et al. 2009

MODE: CYCLE ERGOMETER

Test protocol	Population (age)	Regression equations ($\dot{V}O_2max = L \cdot min^{-1}$ except YMCA; *r* value; SEE)	Textbook page	Resource
YMCA	Male and female triathletes (19-41)	Equation offers maximal workload (WL) without traditional graphing process: WL2 + [(WL2 – WL1) / (HR2 – HR1)] × (age-predicted HR_{max} – HR2) *Note:* Two stages with HR between 110 and 150 bpm and match WL in kg · min^{-1}. [(Maximal WL in kg · min^{-1} × 1.8) + (weight × 7)] / weight *Note:* Body weight in kg, kg · min^{-1} is bike resistance in kp × 300. *r* = .546; SEE = 14% *Note:* General population error about 10-15% due to age-predicted HR_{max}.	117	Golding, Myers, and Sinning 1989; Dabney and Butler 2006

MODE: CYCLE ERGOMETER (CONTINUED)				
Åstrand	Trained adults (20-30) and healthy males (18-33)	Determine aerobic power using nomogram and age correction factor in figure 5.1. $r = .83\text{-}0.90$; SEE = 5.6-5.7 *Note:* kg · min^{-1} is bike resistance in kp × 300, HR immediately postexercise.	117	Åstrand and Rhyming 1954; Cink and Thomas 1981
Modified Åstrand	Trained adults (20-70)	Determine aerobic power using nomogram in figure 5.1; then use equation: Males: 0.348 (nomogram L · min^{-1}) − 0.035 (age) + 3.011 $r = .86$; SEE = 0.359 L · min^{-1} Females: 0.302 (nomogram L · min^{-1}) − 0.019 (age) + 1.593 $r = .97$; SEE = 0.199 L · min^{-1} *Note:* kg · min^{-1} is bike resistance in kp × 300, HR immediately postexercise.	118	Siconolfi et al. 1982

MODE: DISTANCE FIELD TESTS				
Test protocol	**Population (age)**	**Regression equations ($\dot{V}O_2max = mL \cdot kg^{-1} \cdot min^{-1}$ unless noted; *r* value; SEE)**	**Textbook page**	**Resource**
Quarter-mile walk	College students (18-29)	Males: 88.768 + 8.892 − 0.0957 (weight) − 1.4537 (time) − 0.1194 (HR) Females: 88.768 − 0.0957 (weight) − 1.4537 (time) − 0.1194 (HR) $r = .84$; SEE = 4.03 *Note:* Weight in pounds, 4 × minute time, HR immediately postexercise.	118–119	Greenhalgh, George, and Hager 2001
	College students (18-29)	Males: 132.853 + 6.315 − 0.3877 (age) − 0.1692 (weight) − 3.2649 (time) − 0.1565 (HR) Females: 132.853 − 0.3877 (age) − 0.1692 (weight) − 3.2649 (time) − 0.1565 (HR) $r = .81$; SEE = 4.33 *Note:* Weight in pounds, 4 × minute time, HR immediately postexercise.	118–119	Greenhalgh, George, and Hager 2001
Half-mile walk	Obese females	53.23 − 1.98 (time in minutes) − 0.32 (BMI) − 0.08 (age); $r = 0.76$; SEE = 2.89 *Note:* Refer to chapter 2 for BMI calculation procedures (best accuracy $\leq$ 28 kg · m²)	118–119	Donnelly et al. 1992

(continued)

TABLE 5.2 *(Continued)*

		MODE: DISTANCE FIELD TESTS (CONTINUED)		
Mile walk	High school students (14-18)	Males: 88.768 + 8.892 − 0.0957 (weight) − 1.4537 (time) − 0.1194 (HR) Females: 88.768 − 0.0957 (weight) − 1.4537 (time) − 0.1194 (HR) *r* = .84; SEE = 4.5 *Note:* Weight in pounds, time in minutes, HR immediately postexercise.	118–119	McSwegin et al. 1998
	College students (18-29)	Males: 88.768 + 8.892 − 0.0957 (weight) − 1.4537 (time) − 0.1194 (HR) Females: 88.768 − 0.0957 (weight) − 1.4537 (time) − 0.1194 (HR) *r* = .85; SEE = 7.93 *Note:* Weight in pounds, time in minutes, HR immediately postexercise.	118–119	Dolgener et al. 1994
	College students (18-29)	Males: 88.768 + 8.892 − 0.0957 (weight) − 1.4537 (time) − 0.1194 (HR) Females: 88.768 − 0.0957 (weight) − 1.4537 (time) − 0.1194 (HR) *r* = .85; SEE = 3.93 *Note:* Weight in pounds, time in minutes, HR immediately postexercise.	118–119	Greenhalgh, George, and Hager 2001
Rockport mile walk	High school students (14-18)	Males: 132.853 + 6.315 − 0.3877 (age) − 0.1692 (weight) − 3.2649 (time) − 0.1565 (HR) Females: 132.853 − 0.3877 (age) − 0.1692 (weight) − 3.2649 (time) − 0.1565 (HR) *r* = .80; SEE = 4.99 *Note:* Weight in pounds, time in minutes, HR immediately postexercise.	118–119	McSwegin et al. 1998
	College students (18-29)	Males: 132.853 + 6.315 − 0.3877 (age) − 0.1692 (weight) − 3.2649 (time) − 0.1565 (HR) Females: 132.853 − 0.3877 (age) − 0.1692 (weight) − 3.2649 (time) − 0.1565 (HR) *r* = .84; SEE = 4.03 *Note:* Weight in pounds, time in minutes, HR immediately postexercise.	118–119	Greenhalgh, George, and Hager 2001
	Healthy adults (30-69)	Males: 132.853 + 6.315 − 0.3877 (age) − 0.1692 (weight) − 3.2649 (time) − 0.1565 (HR) Females: 132.853 − 0.3877 (age) − 0.1692 (weight) − 3.2649 (time) − 0.1565 (HR) *r* = .88; SEE = 5 *Note:* Weight in pounds, time in minutes, HR immediately postexercise.	118–119	Kline et al. 1987

1.25-mile (2K) walk	Healthy obese and inactive adults (25-65)	Males: 189.6 – 5.32 (time) – 0.22 (HR) – 0.32 (age) – 0.24 (weight) r = .81; SEE = 6.2 *Note:* Time in minutes, HR immediately postexercise, weight in kg.	118–119	Oja et al. 1991
		Females: 121.4 – 2.81 (time) – 0.12 (HR) – 0.16 (age) – 0.24 (weight) r = .87; SEE = 4.5 *Note:* Time in minutes, HR immediately postexercise, weight in kg.	118–119	Oja et al. 1991
Mile jog	Healthy adults (18-29)	Males: 100.5 + 8.344 – 0.1636 (weight) – 1.438 (time) – 0.1928 (HR) Females: 100.5 – 0.1636 (weight) – 1.438 (time) – 0.1928 (HR) r = .87; SEE = 3.1 *Note:* Weight in kg, time in minutes, HR immediately postexercise.	118–119	George et al. 1993a

Note: PFA is perceived functional ability; PA is physical activity.

TABLE 5.3 Regression Equation Data Collection Variables

Collected data variables	Units	Conversions
Age	year	
Height	in., cm, m	in. × 2.54 = cm / 100 = m
Weight	lb, kg	lbs / 2.2 = kg
Time	sec, min	sec / 60 = min
Distance	yard, m, km, mile	yard × 0.9144 = m / 1,000 = km km × 0.62137119224 = mile
Speed (velocity)	mph, m · sec⁻¹, km · hr⁻¹	mph × 0.44704 = m · sec⁻¹ × 3.6 = km · hr⁻¹
Workload	kg · min⁻¹, watts	kg · min⁻¹ / 6 = watts
Survey	PFA and PA survey answers (table 5.4)	
Body dimensions	Sum of skinfolds, BMI	
Heart rate	bpm	
Aerobic power	mL · km⁻¹, L · km⁻¹, mL · kg⁻¹ · km⁻¹, MET	mL · km⁻¹ × 1,000 = L · km⁻¹ L · km⁻¹ × 1,000 / weight in kg = mL · kg⁻¹ · km⁻¹ mL · kg⁻¹ · km⁻¹ / 3.5 = MET

will be discussed with the assumption that the fitness professional has the time to perform the test and the athlete is willing to provide a maximal effort.

Confirming a maximal effort is essential for improving estimates of aerobic power. Without sophisticated analyzers to identify gas and lactate levels at the completion of a maximal exercise test, heart rate measurements are expected to be above 70% of heart rate reserve or above 85% of age-predicted (220 − age) heart rate maximum (American College of Sports Medicine 2010). Although these maximal heart rate criteria provide objectivity with relative ease, large errors of 10 to 12 bpm at all ages are cause for concern when using the age-predicted value as a reason for test termination or as a basis for maximal effort (American College of Sports Medicine 2000).

The age-predicted maximal heart rate concerns arise from overestimated younger adult and underestimated older adult values (Gellish et al. 2007). To reduce the concern of estimating maximal heart rate, the equation $HR_{max} = 207 − (0.7 \times age)$ is recommended for everyone between the ages of 30 and 75 to reduce estimation errors by 5 to 8 bpm (American College of Sports Medicine 2010; Gellish et al. 2007). Furthermore, examiners should attempt to verify age-predicted maximal heart rate calculations by observing signs of fatigue and performance technique deficiencies when athletes request to stop a maximal effort test (Pettersen, Fredrikson, and Ingjer 2001). Heart rate tests are discussed in more detail in chapter 3.

When interpreting the results of a maximal effort test, critical assumptions must be addressed. Without calibrated equipment, examiners must rely on the previously mentioned relationship between oxygen consumption and heart rate, meaning that they are assuming that the heart rate increases linearly with the workload up to maximal effort. Based on this assumption, the accuracy of the prediction equation will be limited to specific populations as long as the correlations are strong with low standard errors. Nevertheless, the best alternatives to using gas measurements (i.e., oxygen and carbon dioxide) to measure aerobic power are the maximal exercise testing methods identified in table 5.1 (Balke and Ware 1959; Bruce, Kusumi, and Hosmer 1973; George 1996; Spackman et al. 2001; Storer, Davis, and Caiozzo 1990).

Laboratory Maximal Treadmill Tests

The treadmill and the bicycle ergometer are the most popular modes for exercise testing in the United States and Europe (Maeder et al. 2005). The treadmill appears to elicit higher maximal oxygen consumption values than the bicycle ergometer (Hambrecht et al. 1992; Maeder et al. 2005; Myers et al. 1991; Wicks et al. 1978). Higher maximal heart rates have also been observed on the treadmill compared to the bicycle ergometer (Buchfuhrer et al. 1983; Hambrecht et al. 1992; Wicks et al. 1978), but other studies have found that both modes elicit comparable heart rates (Maeder et al. 2005; Myers et al. 1991). Nonetheless, the treadmill is expected to generate the highest aerobic power relative to other exercise modes regardless of the protocol.

The Bruce and Balke–Ware treadmill protocols are most commonly used in clinical and laboratory settings because of their high levels of predictive accuracy and low rates of estimation errors (American College of Sports Medicine 2010; refer to table 5.1 for comparisons). Furthermore, exercise time to exhaustion during the Bruce and Balke protocols was determined to be a simple indication of cardiorespiratory functions and physical fitness capabilities (Balke and Ware 1959; Bruce, Kusumi, and Hosmer 1973). Bruce, Kusumi, and Hosmer (1973) even differentiated between sedentary and physically active lifestyles based on regular participation in jogging, running games, or activities with equivalent exertion levels.

Today, the common practice when testing young and physically active people is to use large increases in speed and grade (i.e., 2 to 3 METs), such as during the Bruce protocol. With older, chronically diseased, or decon-ditioned people, smaller increments (≤ 1 MET per stage) are used, such as during the Balke protocol (American College of Sports Medicine 2010). Although the workload increments are smaller for the Balke protocol, for some subjects (e.g., chronically diseased people), the speed may still be too fast (i.e., 3.1 miles per hour at 0% grade) and challenging (i.e., 20 mL $\cdot$ kg^{-1} $\cdot$ min^{-1}) within the first five minutes of testing.

Modified versions of the Bruce protocol do exist. For instance, one or two preliminary stages (i.e., 1.7 miles per hour at 0% grade and 5% grade) have been added when working with very deconditioned people or cardiac patients. Conversely, the initial stage can be eliminated when testing well-conditioned athletes. However, these modifications are appropriate only when using gas analyzers because the developed regression equations are based on time to completion.

General Guidelines for Laboratory Maximal Treadmill Tests

Once the most appropriate and accurate population-specific equation is chosen (see table 5.1), examiners can use the following steps for data collection:

1. Collect age, height, weight, and resting heart rate measurements.

2. Collect exercise heart rate. The heart rate is taken every minute.

3. Collect recovery heart rate for three to five minutes, and longer if necessary to ensure the safe recovery of the subject.

4. Estimate the subject's $\dot{V}O_2$max using the appropriate population-specific equation identified in table 5.1.

5. Convert absolute (mL $\cdot$ min^{-1}) to relative (mL $\cdot$ kg^{-1} $\cdot$ min^{-1}) $\dot{V}O_2$max by dividing mL $\cdot$ min^{-1} by the subject's body weight in kilograms.

6. Determine the subject's aerobic power by classifying the estimated $\dot{V}O_2$max based on table 5.7 (p. 119).

Note: Throughout the test, the subject should be monitored and questioned for signs (e.g., wheezing, blue or pale skin color) and symptoms (e.g., leg cramps, dizziness, chest pain) indicating the need to terminate the test. In addition, the examiner should make sure to collect the heart rate upon completion of the test along with the reason for termination.

BRUCE PROTOCOL

The examiner collects heart rate every minute of the test, but uses the total number of minutes of the test for calculation.

1. Minutes 0-3: The subject walks at 1.7 miles per hour (2.7 km $\cdot$ hr^{-1}) at a grade of 10%.

2. Minutes 3-6: The subject walks at 2.5 miles per hour (4 km $\cdot$ hr^{-1}) at a grade of 12%.

3. Minutes 6-9: The subject jogs at 3.4 miles per hour (5.5 km $\cdot$ hr^{-1}) at a grade of 14%.

4. Minutes 9-12: The subject jogs at 4.2 miles per hour (6.8 km $\cdot$ hr^{-1}) at a grade of 16%.

5. Minutes 12-15: The subject jogs at 5.0 miles per hour (8 km $\cdot$ hr^{-1}) at a grade of 18%.

6. Minutes 15-18: The subject jogs at 5.5 miles per hour (8.9 km $\cdot$ hr^{-1}) at a grade of 20%.

7. Minutes 18-21: The subject jogs at 6.0 miles per hour (9.7 km $\cdot$ hr^{-1}) at a grade of 22%.

BALKE PROTOCOL (MALES)

The examiner collects heart rate every minute of the test, but uses the total number of minutes of the test for calculation.

1. Minutes 0-1: The subject walks at 3.3 miles per hour (5.3 km $\cdot$ hr^{-1}) at 0% grade.

2. After one minute: Increase 1% grade each minute until volitional fatigue or maximal effort (exertion).

BALKE PROTOCOL (FEMALES)

The examiner collects heart rate every minute of the test, but uses the total number of minutes of the test for calculation.

1. Minutes 0–3: The subject walks at 3 miles per hour (4.8 km · hr^{-1}) at 0% grade.
2. After three minutes: Increase 2.5% grade every three minutes until volitional fatigue or maximal effort (exertion).

Laboratory Maximal Cycle Ergometer Tests

Laboratory cycle ergometer exercise tests are also useful for determining cardiorespiratory endurance. However, subject unfamiliarity with stationary cycling combined with premature fatiguing during maximal efforts results in lower aerobic power values than those generated with treadmill testing (5 to 25% less; American College of Sports Medicine 2010). Those who train in cycling may benefit more from this form of exercise testing. Furthermore, the stationary bike may be more appropriate when balance and joint injuries are a concern, because it offers a non-weight-bearing mode of exercise with stability.

Two popular bicycle ergometer protocols (Storer-Davis and Andersen) differ in workload increments. The American College of Sports Medicine (2010) suggests using small increases in workload (i.e., ≤0.25 kp) for deconditioned and elderly people, which matches the Storer-Davis protocol. The Andersen protocol uses slightly higher increases in workload with the likelihood of fatigue occurring 5 to 10 minutes following the start of 0.5 kp increments. Interestingly, Jung, Nieman, and Kernodle (2001) found that the Andersen protocol had greater error than the Storer-Davis protocol. It should be noted that these equation comparisons were based on testing with the Storer-Davis protocol, whereas the Andersen equation was developed according to its relevant protocol. Nonetheless, both protocols appear to have very low aerobic power prediction errors when compared with the Bruce and Balke treadmill protocols, making them valid and reliable alternatives.

General Guidelines for Laboratory Maximal Cycle Ergometer Tests

Once the most appropriate and accurate population-specific equation is chosen (see table 5.1), examiners should use the following steps for data collection:

1. Collect age, height, weight, resting heart rate, and blood pressure (optional) measurements.

2. Collect exercise heart rate, blood pressure (optional), and rating of perceived exertion (RPE) measurements. The heart rate is taken every minute, whereas the blood pressure and RPE are taken during the last minute of every three-minute stage.

3. Collect recovery heart rate and blood pressure (optional) for three to five minutes, and longer if necessary to ensure the safe recovery of the subject.

4. Estimate the subject's $\dot{V}O_2$max using the appropriate population-specific equation identified in table 5.1.

5. Determine the subject's aerobic power by classifying the estimated $\dot{V}O_2$max based on table 5.7 (p. 119).

Note: The subject should be closely monitored and questioned for signs (e.g., wheezing, blue or pale skin color) and symptoms (e.g., leg cramps, dizziness, chest pain) requiring test termination throughout the test, particularly during running, when excessive arm movements can produce interfering noises that result in unreliable blood pressure measurements (Maeder et al. 2005). All measurements should be collected immediately at the conclusion of the test along with the reason for terminating the test.

STORER-DAVIS PROTOCOL

The examiner should collect heart rate every minute of the test, but use the maximal workload of the test for calculation.

1. Minutes 0-4: The subject pedals at 60 rpm against 0 kp.

2. After four minutes: The subject pedals at 60 rpm and increase 0.25 kp (15 watts) each minute until volitional fatigue.

ANDERSEN PROTOCOL (MALES)

The examiner should collect heart rate every minute of the test, but use the maximal workload of the test for calculation.

1. Minutes 0-7: The subject pedals at 70 rpm against 1.5 kp.

2. After seven minutes: The subject pedals at 70 rpm and increase 0.5 kp (35 watts) every two minutes until volitional fatigue.

ANDERSEN PROTOCOL (FEMALES)

The examiner collects heart rate every minute of the test, but uses the maximal workload of the test for calculation.

1. Minutes 0-7: The subject pedals at 70 rpm against 1.0 kp.
2. After seven minutes: The subject pedals at 70 rpm and increase 0.5 kp (35 watts) every two minutes until volitional fatigue.

5K CYCLE RIDE

Beyond the adolescent and general populations, adult trained cyclists might consider the 5K cycle ergometer ride, which requires timing how long it takes to pedal that distance (Buono et al. 1996). Although the cyclist performs at a self-regulated pace, the objective is to pedal 5K as fast as possible against a resistance calculated by dividing body weight in kilograms by 20 and multiplying the value by 0.5 kp.

1. Determine how long it takes the subject to ride 5K.
2. Minutes 0-2: The subject pedals at a self-selected pace against 1.0 kp.
3. Minutes 2-3: The subject pedals at a self-selected pace against resistance based on body weight (0.5 kp per 20 kg of body weight).
4. Minutes 3-5: The subject rests.
5. After five minutes: The subject pedals at a self-selected pace and resume resistance based on body mass until completion of the 5K ride.

Maximal Field Tests

Maximal field tests offer practical exercise settings outside the laboratory. Field tests are usually much easier to administer than laboratory tests, which require more sophisticated equipment and technical expertise. Instead of relying on laboratory measurements, maximal field tests provide aerobic power estimates based on performance distance or time. As a result of training specificity, athletes improve their distances and times in environments that are practical for field testing.

Timed Maximal Field Tests

There are many maximal running field tests ranging from 5 to 20 minutes. These timed field tests require that the subject be highly motivated to run, bike, or swim as far as possible within a designated time. Because the time limit is the basis of these tests, the main requirement is to monitor how far the subject travels. The examiner must be sure to observe the subject during the entire time limit so that the distance can be determined accurately. For instance, if the selected test requires the subject to travel as far as possible in 12 minutes, a track or pool would permit continuous observation while the subject was running, cycling, or swimming.

Cooper (1968) introduced the 12-minute run to assess aerobic power among male U.S. Air Force officers. Even though the prediction equation was based on the performance of officers between 17 and 52 years of age, most of them were younger than 25; the greatest accuracy was seen in those exceeding 1.4 miles (2.3 km) in distance (Cooper 1968). In another study, Cooper's run test slightly overestimated aerobic power among trained subjects between 17 and 54 years of age, but Wyndham and others (1971) recommended against the use of this protocol with sedentary people in their 40s and 50s. The 5-minute run may be a viable alternative for 18- to 46-year-olds of various fitness levels because it appears to provide an accurate assessment of cardiorespiratory endurance (Berthon et al. 1997b; Dabonneville et al. 2003).

MacNaughton and others (1990) tested competitively active high school students' aerobic power to compare 5- and 15-minute run tests to the Bruce protocol. Obviously, the Bruce protocol provided the most accurate aerobic power measurement, but the next best predictor of aerobic power was the 15-minute run, whereas the 5-minute run provided only satisfactory esti-mates (MacNaughton et al. 1990). Coincidentally, aerobic power estimates made from the 15-minute run demonstrated similar correlation values to those of the 20-minute run, which included a relatively low reported standard error. This suggests that longer durations may be more beneficial for high school students (Murray et al. 1993). However, motivation and local muscular fatigue and discomfort have prompted the recommendation of limiting maximal aerobic power tests to 8 to 10 minutes for youth and untrained people (Massicotte, Gauthier, and Markon 1985).

All the time trial field tests discussed previously estimate aerobic power based on performance distance, but running economy may also need to be taken into consideration to address training efficiency. For instance, most fitness professionals would expect performance to improve with training specificity. However, Cooper (1968) found that repeated 12-minute run testing resulted in minimal training effects. Therefore, Berthon and others (1997a) suggest determining running speed at $\dot{V}O_2max$ to evaluate running economy. The significance of this suggestion is evidenced by the inability to estimate aerobic power as accurately as running speed for runners and athletes (Berthon et al. 1997a), whereas both components of running economy are estimated accurately among the general population (Berthon et al. 1997b). Overall, a 5-minute run appears to be too short for the accurate estimation of running speed (Berthon et al. 1997a; 1997b).

Other maximal field test options that address training specificity are timed swimming and road cycling. Cooper (1982) developed a 12-minute swim and a 12-minute road cycling test. Road cycling distances are best measured using an odometer and pedaling on a flat terrain with winds less than 10 miles per hour (16 km/h). Swimming distances (with any stroke) are best determined by knowing the pool dimensions. Although there are a few equations that estimate aerobic power for swimming, the relatively low correlations and standard errors associated with the estimates indicate a greater value in recording the traveled distance without calculating aerobic power. The same recommendation of recording distance measurements applies to road cycling as well. Although nothing has been published in the literature, these testing strategies could also be used with other endurance activities such as cross-country skiing. Regardless of the endurance event, changes in distances over a training period would be the basis for identifying training effectiveness on swimming, road cycling, and skiing performance.

Distance Maximal Field Tests

Rather than base aerobic power estimates on the duration of a field test, some fitness professionals select a maximal protocol reliant on distance. Regardless of the mode (e.g., walking or running), the objective is to complete a specified distance within the shortest time period.

Several equations that predict aerobic power have been developed for maximal running tests ranging from one mile to marathon distances (see table 5.1). These distances reflect the suggestion that runners must run farther than a mile to estimate cardiorespiratory fitness with the greatest accuracy (Fernhall et al. 1996). During the development of running prediction equations for aerobic capacity, data suggested that at least 600 yards are ideal for healthy populations, but a mile or farther is preferable (Cureton et al. 1995; Disch, Frankiewicz, and Jackson 1975). Based on the specificity principle, common sense suggests that using specific road race distances in tests of competitive runners will result in greater accuracy. Furthermore, Tokmakidis and others (1987) suggested that aerobic power estimation accuracy may be improved by using two running performances under the same conditions (i.e., health status, environment, course). Because of the high-intensity nature of running field tests, sedentary people and those with cardiovascular or musculoskeletal risks should not be assessed using this all-out run approach (American College of Sports Medicine 2010).

General Guidelines for Maximal Distance and Timed Field Tests

Once the most appropriate and accurate population-specific equation is chosen (table 5.1), examiners can use the following steps for data collection:

1. Collect age, height, weight, and resting heart rate measurements. Tricep and subscapular skinfold measurements are required when using the regression equation for the mile run to assess youth

between 10 and 18 years of age (Buono et al 1991). Chapter 2 describes the procedures for determining these skinfold measurements.

2. Have the subject perform a general warm-up using the mode of exercise being tested.

3. Have the subject perform the activity within the specified time limit or distance.

4. Record the distance for a timed protocol or the duration for a distance protocol. Because aerobic power estimation accuracy is questionable with cycling and swimming field tests, performance distances also provides a satisfactory basis for monitoring training progress. Although the swimming and road cycling performance distances are sufficient for assessment purposes, unconfirmed interpretation tables are available (Cooper 1982).

5. Estimate the subject's $\dot{V}O_2$max using the appropriate population-specific equation identified in table 5.1.

6. Convert metabolic equivalent (MET) to relative (mL · kg^{-1} · min^{-1}) $\dot{V}O_2$max by multiplying MET by 3.5.

7. Determine the subject's aerobic power by classifying the estimated $\dot{V}O_2$max based on table 5.7 (p. 119).

Submaximal Exercise Testing Methods

Estimating aerobic power with submaximal exercise testing methods is time efficient. Because most submaximal tests are completed within 6 to 12 minutes with minimal exertion, the risk of medical complications is low. Unfortunately, extrapolating exercise prescriptions is difficult because the testing is performed at submaximal workloads. Only the heart rate responses observed during the submaximal testing session can be incorporated into the exercise prescriptions confidently. Given that the observed heart rates are only within the assessed intensities, any higher heart rates must be assumed based on an estimated maximal heart rate (220 – age). Despite the disadvantages of submaximal exercise testing, the multitude of protocols available provides strong evidence that this form of testing is advantageous to fitness professionals. This section addresses the numerous testing options, including the treadmill, cycle ergometer, and field tests identified in table 5.2 (pp. 98–101).

Laboratory Submaximal Treadmill Tests

Once the most appropriate and accurate population-specific submaximal treadmill equation is chosen, examiners should refer to the following protocol steps for data collection.

TABLE 5.4   Perceived Functional Ability (PFA) and Physical Activity (PA) Questions

Question	Scale
Perceived Functional Ability (26-point scale based on total of both questions)	
1. How fast could you cover a distance of 1 mile and NOT become breathless or overly fatigued. Be realistic.	1 – I could walk the entire distance at a slow pace (18 minutes per mile or more) 2 – I could walk the entire distance at a slow pace (17 minutes per mile) 3 – I could walk the entire distance at a medium pace (16 minutes per mile) 4 – I could walk the entire distance at a medium pace (15 minutes per mile) 5 – I could walk the entire distance at a fast pace (14 minutes per mile) 6 – I could walk the entire distance at a fast pace (13 minutes per mile) 7 – I could jog the entire distance at a slow pace (12 minutes per mile) 8 – I could jog the entire distance at a slow pace (11 minutes per mile) 9 – I could jog the entire distance at a medium pace (10 minutes per mile) 10 – I could jog the entire distance at a medium pace (9 minutes per mile) 11 – I could jog the entire distance at a fast pace (8 minutes per mile) 12 – I could jog the entire distance at a fast pace (7.5 minutes per mile) 13 – I could run the entire distance at a fast pace (7 minutes per mile or less)
2. How fast could you cover a distance of 3 miles and NOT become breathless or overly fatigued. Be realistic.	1 – I could walk the entire distance at a slow pace (18 minutes per mile or more) 2 – I could walk the entire distance at a slow pace (17 minutes per mile) 3 – I could walk the entire distance at a medium pace (16 minutes per mile) 4 – I could walk the entire distance at a medium pace (15 minutes per mile) 5 – I could walk the entire distance at a fast pace (14 minutes per mile) 6 – I could walk the entire distance at a fast pace (13 minutes per mile) 7 – I could jog the entire distance at a slow pace (12 minutes per mile) 8 – I could jog the entire distance at a slow pace (11 minutes per mile) 9 – I could jog the entire distance at a medium pace (10 minutes per mile) 10 – I could jog the entire distance at a medium pace (9 minutes per mile) 11 – I could jog the entire distance at a fast pace (8 minutes per mile) 12 – I could jog the entire distance at a fast pace (7.5 minutes per mile) 13 – I could run the entire distance at a fast pace (7 minutes per mile or less)
Physical Activity (10-point scale)	
Select the number that best describes your overall level of physical activity for the previous 6 months.	0 – Avoid walking exertion (e.g., always use elevator, drive when possible instead of walking) 1 – Light activity: walk for pleasure, routinely use stairs, occasionally exercise sufficiently to cause heavy breathing or perspiration 2 – Moderate activity: 10-60 minutes per week of moderate activity (e.g., golf, horseback riding, calisthenics, table tennis, bowling, weightlifting, yard work, cleaning house, walking for exercise) 3 – Moderate activity: over 1 hour per week of moderate activity as described above 4 – Vigorous activity: run less than 1 mile per week or spend less than 30 minutes per week in comparable activity (e.g., running or jogging, lap swimming, cycling, rowing, aerobics, skipping rope, running in place, soccer, basketball, tennis, racquetball, or handball) 5 – Vigorous activity: run 1-5 miles per week or spend 30-60 minutes per week in comparable physical activity as described above 6 – Vigorous activity: run 5-10 miles or spend 1-3 hours per week in comparable physical activity as described above 7 – Vigorous activity: run 10-15 miles or spend 3-6 hours per week in comparable physical activity as described above 8 – Vigorous activity: run 15-20 miles or spend 6-7 hours per week in comparable physical activity as described above 9 – Vigorous activity: run 20-25 miles or spend 7-8 hours per week in comparable physical activity as described above 10 – Vigorous activity: run over 25 miles or spend over 8 hours per week in comparable physical activity as described above

Reprinted, by permission, from J.D. George, W.J. Stone, and L.N. Burkett, 1997, "Non-exercise $\dot{V}O_2$max estimation for physically active college students," *Medicine and Science in Sports and Exercise* 29:415-423.

General Guidelines for Submaximal Treadmill Tests

Once the most appropriate and accurate population-specific equation is chosen (see table 5.2), examiners should use the following steps for data collection:

1. Collect age, height, weight, and resting heart rate. If administering the walk/jog/run protocol, have the subject complete the perceived functional ability and physical activity questions in table 5.4.

2. Collect exercise heart rate. The heart rate is taken every minute, but the steady state heart rate collected immediately at the conclusion of the test is used for calculation purposes.

3. Collect recovery heart rate and blood pressure (optional) for three to five minutes, and longer if necessary to ensure the safe recovery of the subject.

4. Estimate the subject's $\dot{V}O_2$max using the appropriate population-specific equation identified in table 5.2.

5. Determine the subject's aerobic power by classifying the estimated $\dot{V}O_2$max based on table 5.7 (p. 119).

Single-Stage Submaximal Treadmill Protocols

Walking and jogging single-stage submaximal treadmill protocols are convenient and practical. Unfit or older people appear to get the best aerobic power estimates using the walking submaximal treadmill protocol (Ebbeling et al. 1991; Vehrs et al. 2007). Conversely, the jogging submaximal treadmill test is more appropriate for the relatively fit ($\geq$35.9 mL · kg^{-1} · min^{-1}) between 18 and 29 years of age (George et al. 1993b). In 2007, Vehrs and others added age to the aerobic power prediction equation because they found that accuracy was improved among relatively fit ($\geq$33.4 mL · kg^{-1} · min^{-1}) people older than 29. Following are guidelines for performing submaximal treadmill tests; specific protocols appear immediately afterward.

SUBMAXIMAL TREADMILL WALKING TEST PROTOCOL

1. Minutes 0–4: The subject walks at 0% grade and determines a comfortable speed between 2 and 4.5 miles per hour (3.2 and 7.2 km · hr^{-1}) that elicits 50 to 70% of the age-predicted (220 – age) maximal heart rate.

2. Minutes 4–8: Increase to 5% grade and maintain speed during the first four minutes. The four- to eight-minute pace should elicit 50 to 70% of the age-predicted maximal heart rate (use post-HR in equation).

SUBMAXIMAL TREADMILL JOGGING TEST PROTOCOL (MALES)

1. Minutes 0–2: The subject jogs at 0% grade and determines a comfortable speed between 4.3 and 7.5 miles per hour (7 and 12 km · hr⁻¹).

2. Minutes 2–5: The subject maintains the jogging speed established during the first two minutes. The two- to five-minute pace should not exceed 85% of the age-predicted maximal heart rate (use post-HR in equation).

SUBMAXIMAL TREADMILL JOGGING TEST PROTOCOL (FEMALES)

1. Minutes 0–2: The subject jogs at 0% grade and determines a comfortable speed between 4.3 and 6.5 miles per hour (7 and 10.5 km · hr⁻¹).

2. Minutes 2–5: The subject maintains the jogging speed established during the first two minutes. The two- to five-minute pace should not exceed 85% of the age-predicted maximal heart rate (use post-HR in equation).

Multistage Submaximal Treadmill Protocols

Although a multistage submaximal treadmill protocol may last longer than the single-stage walking and jogging treadmill protocols, George and others (2009) developed a walk/jog/run protocol that offers an opportunity to educate athletes. In addition to performing the exercise test, subjects answer the perceived functional ability and physical activity questions in table 5.4.

The multistage submaximal treadmill exercise protocol ends at the completion of the stage in which 70 to 90% of the age-predicted (220 – age) maximal heart rate is achieved during walking for the lower fitness level, jogging for the average fitness level, and running for the higher fitness level. Furthermore, subjects classify themselves as walkers, joggers, or runners with the perceived functional ability questions, which helps with the selection of training exercises. The subject's previous six-month physical activity rating then permits the fitness professional to discuss realistic training habits.

Athletes' responses on the perceived functional ability and physical activity questionnaire (table 5.4) are incorporated into the multistage treadmill equation in table 5.2 to estimate aerobic power. When subjects' performances on the treadmill are different from their perceptions of their capabilities, the fitness professional has an opportunity to discuss the relationships between training and physiological responses. This empowers the subject while helping the fitness professional design a cardiorespiratory training program based on realistic goals. Overall, the walk/jog/run submaximal treadmill protocol relates the subject's perceptions to personal exercise performance, enabling the fitness professional to teach about choosing safe exercise modes and training at effective intensities to achieve realistic goals (George et al. 2009).

SUBMAXIMAL WALK/JOG/RUN PROTOCOL

1. Minutes 0–4: The subject walks at 0% grade and determines a comfortable speed between 3 and 4 miles per hour (4.8 and 6.4 km · hr^{-1}) within the initial 20 seconds. (End the test at this stage if the subject is within 70 to 90% of the age-predicted [220 – age] maximal heart rate and use the treadmill speed in the equation.)

2. Minutes 4–8: The subject jogs at 0% grade and determines a comfortable speed between 4.1 and 6 miles per hour (6.6 and 9.7 km · hr^{-1}) within the initial 20 seconds. (End the test at this stage if the subject is within 70 to 90% of the age-predicted [220 – age] maximal heart rate and use the treadmill speed in the equation.)

3. Minutes 8–12: The subject runs at 0% grade and determines a comfortable speed above 6 miles per hour (9.7km · hr^{-1}) within the initial 20 seconds. (The final stage should elicit 70 to 90% of the age-predicted [220–age] maximal heart rate and use the treadmill speed in the equation.)

Laboratory Submaximal Cycle Ergometer Tests

Although both maximal and submaximal laboratory cycle ergometer tests raise concerns about training specificity, submaximal tests may have a greater standard error in predicting aerobic power than maximal tests do. Therefore, special attention needs to be paid to the protocol's pedal cadence and the position of the legs during the downstroke. When the lower extremity is straightened at the bottom of the pedaling revolution, the knee angle should be at 5° of flexion for the greatest muscle efficiency (American College of Sports Medicine 2010). Achieving this knee angle requires an adjustment to the proper seat height beforehand.

A review of the research on Åstrand and YMCA submaximal bike tests highlights the aerobic power estimation concerns with these protocols. In 1954, Åstrand and Ryhming developed a nomogram to estimate aerobic power from a six-minute single-stage protocol for well-trained males and females. After exploring various workloads, they discovered that the greatest accuracy occurred at 900 kg · min^{-1} (150 watts) for females and 1,200 kg · min^{-1} (200 watts) for males. Figure 5.1 provides the current Åstrand nomogram that has been modified with an age correction factor (Åstrand 1960). To differentiate fitness levels among males, Cink and Thomas (1981) found that the Åstrand age correction factor must be used to improve the accuracy of the test.

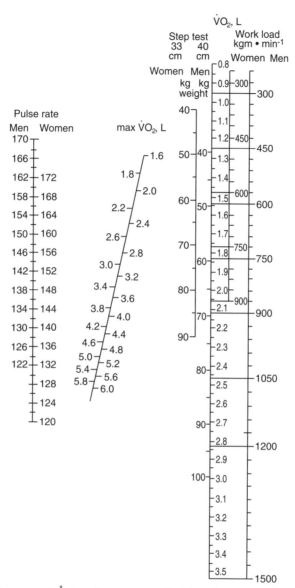

FIGURE 5.1 The current Åstrand nomogram that has been modified with an age correction factor.

Reprinted, by permission, from I. Åstrand, 1960, "Aerobic capacity in men and women with special reference to age," *Acta Physiologica Scandinavica* 49 (Suppl. 169): 51.

Golding, Myers, and Sinning (1989) introduced the multistage YMCA submaximal bike test, which also provides an opportunity to adjust workloads to accommodate various fitness levels. When both submaximal protocols were compared, the YMCA protocol ($r = .73$) was more accurate in estimating aerobic power than the Åstrand protocol was ($r = .56$) among physically active people (Kovaleski et al. 2005). A comparison of the YMCA submaximal bike test and the Bruce protocol revealed that the YMCA test

TABLE 5.5   YMCA Submaximal Bike Test Resistances

Stage 1 HR	Stage 2 load
>100 bpm	1 kp (50 watts)
90-100 bpm	1.5 kp (75 watts)
80-89 bpm	2.0 kp (100 watts)
<80 bpm	2.5 kp (125 watts)

TABLE 5.6   Åstrand Submaximal Bike Test Resistances

Training status	Test load
Untrained	1.5 kp (75 watts)
Moderately trained	2 kp (100 watts)
Well trained	3 kp (150 watts)

underestimated aerobic power values by 14% (Dabney and Butler 2006). These findings indicate that these submaximal bike tests should be limited to trained females and physically active males.

Alternatives are available to fitness professionals working with untrained people. Siconolfi and others (1982) modified the Åstrand submaximal bike test and developed a regression equation based on the nomogram and age for inactive men and women. Another accommodation was to adjust the traditional pedal rate of 50 rpm even though it was well within the recommended pedaling frequency range of 40 to 70 rpm for optimal economy (Åstrand and Rodahl 1986). Sharkey (1988) suggested that pedaling against high resistance at 50 rpm is not easy for untrained people; they perform better at 60 to 70 rpm.

General Guidelines for Submaximal Cycle Ergometer Tests

Once the most appropriate and accurate population-specific submaximal cycle ergometer equation is chosen (see table 5.2), examiners should use the following protocol steps for data collection:

1. Collect age, height, weight, and resting heart rate measurements.
2. Collect exercise heart rate. The heart rate is taken every minute, but the steady state heart rate collected immediately at the conclusion of each stage (YMCA protocol) or at the end of the test is used for calculation purposes.
3. Collect recovery heart rate for three to five minutes, and longer if necessary to ensure the safe recovery of the subject.

4. Estimate the subject's $\dot{V}O_2$max using the appropriate population-specific equation identified in table 5.2.

5. Convert absolute (L · min^{-1}) to relative (mL · kg^{-1} · min^{-1}) $\dot{V}O_2$max by dividing L · min^{-1} by the subject's body weight in kilograms and multiplying the value by 1,000.

6. Determine the subject's aerobic power by classifying the estimated $\dot{V}O_2$max based on table 5.7 (p. 119).

YMCA SUBMAXIMAL BIKE TEST

1. Warm-up: The subject pedals at 50 rpm against 0 kp.

2. Stage 1: The subject pedals at 50 rpm against 0.5 kp (25 watts) and continues the stage for three minutes or longer to achieve steady state HR.

3. Stage 2: The subject pedals at 50 rpm for three minutes at modified resistance based on table 5.5.

4. Additional stages (if necessary): If the steady state HR is not between 110 and 150 bpm for stage 1 and stage 2, the subject continues pedaling at 50 rpm and increases 0.5 kp (25 watts) every three minutes or longer to achieve steady state HR. While the speed is maintained at 50 rpm, the resistance will continue to be increased 0.5 kp (25 watts) for as many stages as necessary to achieve a steady state HR within 110 to 150 bpm for two stages. When within 110 to 150 bpm, the two stages' corresponding heart rates and workloads are then used to determine aerobic power based on the YMCA bike test equation found in table 5.2.

ÅSTRAND SUBMAXIMAL BIKE TEST (MALES)

1. Minutes 0–3: The subject pedals at 50 rpm against 0 kp.

2. Test: Apply resistance according to table 5.6, and have the subject pedal at 50 rpm for six minutes or longer to achieve steady state HR within the 130 to 170 bpm range.

3. Additional stage (if necessary): If the test HR is less than 130 bpm, the subject pedals at 50 rpm and increases 1 to 2 kp (50–100 watts) for an additional six minutes or longer to achieve steady state HR between 130 and 170 bpm. When the subject is within the 130 to 170 bpm range, the immediate postexercise HR and final workload are used in the nomogram.

ÅSTRAND SUBMAXIMAL BIKE TEST (TRAINED FEMALES)

1. Minutes 0–3: The subject pedals at 50 rpm against 0 kp.
2. Test: The subject pedals at 50 rpm against 2 to 3 kp (100–150 watts) for six minutes or longer to achieve steady state within a range of 125 to 170 bpm. When the subject is within the 125 to 170 bpm range, the immediate postexercise HR and final workload are used in the nomogram.

Submaximal Field Tests

Once the most appropriate and accurate population-specific submaximal field test equation is chosen, fitness professionals use the following protocol steps for data collection:

General Guidelines for Submaximal Field Tests

Once the most appropriate and accurate population-specific submaximal field test equation is chosen (see table 5.2), examiners should use the following protocol steps for data collection:

1. Collect age, height, weight, and resting heart rate measurements.
2. Have the subject perform a general warm-up using the specific mode of exercise being tested.
3. Have the subject perform the activity within the protocol-specified distance.
4. Record the duration for a distance protocol and collect postexercise heart rate immediately upon completion of the test if necessary.
5. Estimate the subject's $\dot{V}O_2$max using the appropriate population-specific equation identified in table 5.2.
6. Determine the subject's aerobic power by classifying the estimated $\dot{V}O_2$max based on table 5.7 (p. 119).

Quarter-mile to 2-kilometer (1.25 miles) submaximal walking distances are possible protocol selections for people of all ages, but low-fit people and those whose training regimen consists of walking appear to be the best suited for this mode of field testing. For instance, elderly people and those with physical limitations (e.g., overweight, obese, mentally impaired, cardiopulmonary patients) tend to be assessed using walking tests (Larsen et al. 2002; McSwegin et al. 1998). Conversely, underestimations in aerobic power are common with highly trained people performing these submaximal walking protocols because the cardiorespiratory system is inadequately

TABLE 5.7 Aerobic Power Classifications

Age group	Low	Fair	Average	Good	High	Athletic	Olympic
Women							
20–29	<28	29–34	35–43	44–48	49–53	54–59	60+
30–39	<27	28–33	34–41	42–47	48–52	53–58	59+
40–49	<25	26–31	32–40	41–45	46–50	51–56	57+
50–65	<21	22–28	29–36	37–41	42–45	46–49	50+
Men							
20–29	<38	39–43	44–51	52–56	57–62	63–69	70+
30–39	<34	35–39	40–47	48–51	52–57	58–64	65+
40–49	<30	31–35	36–43	44–47	48–53	54–60	61+
50–59	<25	26–31	32–39	40–43	44–48	49–55	56+
60–69	<21	22–26	27–35	36–39	40–44	45–49	50+

Note: $\dot{V}O_2$max is expressed in tables as milliliters of oxygen per kilogram of body weight per minute.

Adapted, by permission, from I. Åstrand, 1960, "Aerobic capacity in men and women with special reference to age," *Acta Physiologica Scandinavica* 49 (Suppl. 169): 1–92.

challenged (Kline et al. 1987). Anyone who cannot achieve a heart rate above 110 bpm when walking briskly would be considered highly trained (George, Fellingham, and Fisher 1998).

Another approach that goes beyond determining the duration of a submaximal field test is measuring the final heart rate after walking or jogging a mile (1.6 km) (Dolgener et al. 1994; George et al. 1993a; Kline et al. 1987). Note that the mile jog must take longer than eight minutes for males and nine minutes for females, and subjects must maintain a heart rate below 180 bpm for the test to qualify as submaximal (George et al. 1993a).

Regression Equation Calculations

In addition to being skilled at collecting data, fitness professionals also must understand the order of operations to perform regression equation calculations. A common technique for remembering the order of operations is the abbreviation PEMDAS, which stands for Parentheses, Exponents, Multiplication and Division, and Addition and Subtraction. The phrase *Please Excuse My Dear Aunt Sally* is helpful for remembering the order of the letters. When performing calculations, the order of operations refers to a ranking order: (1) parentheses, (2) exponents, (3) multiplication and division working from left to right, and (4) addition and subtraction working from left to right. As an example, we explore the process of determining aerobic power after selecting the submaximal treadmill walk/jog/run protocol and regression equation. Consider the following four-step process:

1. Heart rate is taken during the submaximal treadmill walk/jog/run protocol. A heart rate monitor or electrocardiograph would facilitate the process because of the difficulty of palpating a moving arm during exercise. The purpose of monitoring the heart rate is to determine when a steady state is achieved. The heart rate steady state is the plateau at which the heart rate and rate of oxygen consumption tend to remain relatively stable at a given workload. The examiner can verify steady state, which is optimal for any submaximal test, by determining that the heart rate on the monitor or electrocardiogram is within 6 bpm of each other (American College of Sports Medicine 2010) during the final two minutes of the walking, jogging, and running protocol stages. Even if a steady state is not achieved at the end of the protocol stage, the subject progresses from walking to jogging to running every four minutes until the heart rate falls between 70 and 90% of the age-predicted (220 – age) maximum, which establishes the treadmill speed that will be used in the regression equation. In addition to performing the exercise test, the subject answers perceived functional ability and physical activity questions (table 5.4). The age and weight of the subject must also be known. Here are some results from the submaximal treadmill walk/jog/run protocol to perform the regression equation calculations:

> Age = 40 years
>
> Weight (wgt) = 70 kg
>
> Running treadmill speed (miles per hour) = 7 miles per hour
>
> Perceived functional ability (PFA) = 24
>
> Physical activity (PA) = 8

2. Aerobic power calculations require using the preceding information in the following regression equation for males:

> Aerobic power = 30.04 + 6.37 – 0.243 (age) – 0.122 (wt) + 3.2 (mph) + 0.391 (PFA) + 0.669 (PA)
>
> Aerobic power = 30.04 + 6.37 – 0.243 (40) – 0.122 (70) + 3.2 (7) + 0.391 (24) + 0.669 (8)
>
> Aerobic power = 30.04 + 6.37 – 9.72 – 8.54 + 22.4 + 9.384 + 5.352
>
> Aerobic power = 55.3 mL $\cdot$ kg^{-1} $\cdot$ min^{-1}

3. Aerobic power interpretations are based on the cardiorespiratory fitness levels presented in table 5.7. Within the table, the aerobic power is expressed relative to body weight (mL $\cdot$ kg^{-1} $\cdot$ min^{-1}), which means that 55 mL $\cdot$ kg^{-1} $\cdot$ min^{-1} is classified as athletic. Be aware that absolute (L $\cdot$ km^{-1} or mL $\cdot$ min^{-1}) and metabolic (MET) values need to be converted to relative body weight to use the table. In addition, although classifying the subject may be a goal, the ultimate goal should be to use the aerobic power estimations to improve cardiorespiratory fitness with appropriate exercise prescription strategies.

4. Exercise prescription for developing aerobic power is based on assessments. Whether fitness professionals are determining a baseline or training cardiorespiratory fitness level, interpretation of the aerobic power value will enable them to monitor training specificity. Specificity refers to the principle that the body adapts according to the stimuli it is exposed to during exercise. For example, swimmers train in the water and become very efficient at swimming, but this does not mean they will be good at running or cycling. Nonetheless, as a result of endurance training specificity, aerobic power is expected to improve 5 to 30% regardless of the mode (American College of Sports Medicine 2006). Therefore, a well-selected aerobic power protocol should permit the fitness professionals to monitor and adjust an athlete's training program to accomplish realistic goals based on ongoing assessment results.

Owing to the large variety of cardiorespiratory endurance tests available, fitness professionals must be knowledgeable about them and capable of selecting the best test for assessing an athlete's aerobic power. Proper test selection depends on understanding the physiological and biomechanical principles of a sport or activity while applying the evidence-based research to the athlete's capabilities. Therefore, the maximal (table 5.1) and submaximal (table 5.2) tests presented in this chapter have been organized into SMARTS charts to explore the science and art of exercise selection.

SMARTS stands for Specificity, Mode, Application, Research, and Training Status (see tables 5.8 and 5.9). First, the fitness professional must know the specific metabolic demands of the sport or activity—that is, whether it is predominantly aerobic or anaerobic physiologically. Maximal tests might be more appropriate for sports or activities emphasizing aerobic metabolism, whereas submaximal tests might be best suited for athletes primarily dealing with anaerobic training. Obviously, sports or activities that alternate between aerobic and anaerobic metabolic demands may use either maximal or submaximal tests.

Second, the fitness professional must select an exercise mode that best matches the athlete's training or competitive activity. For instance, a cycle ergometer test might be appropriate for an American football lineman because the athlete must be able to sustain or overcome forces against resistance during an entire game.

Third, the fitness professional must determine whether an aerobic power test would provide applicable information. Referring to the previous example, by determining the aerobic power of the athlete, the coach would have a basis for deciding future training strategies along with duration recommendations for keeping the football lineman in the game without a break.

Professional Applications

(continued)

(continued)

TABLE 5.8 SMARTS Chart for Maximal Exercise Test Selection

SPECIFICITY ↔ MODE				ARTS OF EXERCISE PRESCRIPTION		
Treadmill	**Cycle ergometer**	**Timed field test**	**Distance field test**			
Arizona State University protocol Bruce protocol Balke protocol Modified Bruce protocol	Storer protocol Andersen protocol 5 km cycle ride	Cooper's 12-minute run 15-minute run 20-minute run 5-minute run Cooper's 12-minute swim	Marathon competition 6-mile competition 3-mile competition 2-mile run 1.5-mile run Mile run	Application	Strong ↑ ↓ ↓ Weak	Advanced ↑ ↓ Training Status ↓ Beginner

With Research between Strong and Weak, Training Status between Advanced and Beginner.

TABLE 5.9 SMARTS Chart for Submaximal Exercise Test Selection

SPECIFICITY ↔ MODE			ARTS OF EXERCISE PRESCRIPTION		
Treadmill	**Cycle ergometer**	**Distance field test**			
Jogging protocol Walk/jog/run protocol Walking protocol	YMCA protocol Modified Åstrand protocol Åstrand protocol	Mile jog Rockport mile walk Mile walk 1.25-mile walk Quarter-mile walk Half-mile walk	Application	Strong ↑ ↓ Research ↓ Weak	Advanced ↑ ↓ Training Status ↓ Beginner

Fourth, the fitness professional should refer to the research for population-specific correlations and standard errors to ensure that the selection is evidence based. Because the anaerobic football lineman would be performing a submaximal cycle ergometer test, research appears to favor the YMCA protocol over the Åstrand protocol.

Fifth, the fitness professional must take into account the athlete's training status. Even though the YMCA protocol may be more accurate in estimating aerobic power, the traditional or modified Åstrand protocol might be more appropriate if the football lineman is untrained after a long off-season.

Fitness professionals should keep in mind that these are only examples of how to use the SMARTS charts; no one method is best for assessing all football linemen or any other types of athletes. Nonetheless, specificity, mode, application, research, and training status all play valuable roles in the selection of an appropriate aerobic power test.

Once they have chosen the aerobic power test, fitness professionals must determine the data variables they need to collect. Based on the variables, any skills that need to be developed should be addressed prior to the testing session. Otherwise, undeveloped skills may require the selection of an alternative testing option. Fitness professionals should practice the skills prior to the testing session regardless of their proficiency, especially if time has elapsed since they last performed the test on an athlete.

After collecting the data and calculating the aerobic power estimate, fitness professionals have a foundational cardiorespiratory fitness level for prescribing an individualized training program. This will result in realistic training goals that may maintain or improve the athlete's aerobic power. In addition, fitness professionals should remember that improvements in aerobic power require sustained activities near or above anaerobic threshold; these assessments are presented in the next chapter.

SUMMARY

- The proper selection and administration of a protocol are essential because they affect the accuracy of the results of the cardiorespiratory fitness test. Tests are chosen based on equipment availability, technical expertise, and available time, and they should be population specific while providing the least amount of error in estimating aerobic power. If multiple cardiorespiratory fitness tests are applicable to an athlete, the fitness professional may be able to reduce the standard error by comparing two or more options.

- Knowledge of the athlete's training program exercises prior to testing will allow the fitness professional to make adaptations to address the specificity of the exercise, which will facilitate the selection of an appropriate cardiorespiratory assessment protocol. Regardless, interpreting aerobic power for cardiorespiratory fitness will be based on careful considerations that ensure the test protocol accurately identifies training adaptations and exercise program effectiveness.

Lactate Threshold

Dave Morris, PhD

Lactate is a metabolite that can be produced by the breakdown of glucose or glycogen during the process of glycolysis. Although numerous cells and tissues use glycolysis and produce lactate, the biggest producer during exercise is skeletal muscle, which relies on the glycolytic pathway to provide energy for contractions.

Historically, lactate has been thought of as a waste product of carbohydrate metabolism. In actuality, some amount of the lactate that is produced by the working muscle can be retained by that muscle and used as an energy metabolite. The remaining lactate that is not burned in the working muscle diffuses into the blood where its levels can be measured by a variety of techniques. One such measurement strategy, the lactate threshold test, involves having a subject perform an exercise bout that features progressively higher rates of work. At regular time intervals during the test, blood samples are drawn and analyzed for lactate concentration.

Through the use of the lactate threshold test, researchers have discovered that during low-intensity exercise, blood lactate remains at fairly low and stable levels. However, as exercise becomes more intense, blood lactate levels eventually begin to rise suddenly and continue to rise exponentially as exercise intensity increases. This sudden and distinct rise in blood lactate levels is commonly referred to as lactate threshold.

Because of lactate's role in exercise metabolism, scientists have studied its response to exercise to gain insight into the nuances of bioenergetics. Lactate's link to energy provision during exercise has sparked interest from coaches and athletes looking to design and execute better training programs.

Thanks to Becky Shafer, MS, for her assistance in preparing this chapter.

Energy Pathways and Lactate Metabolism

Properly designing, administering, and interpreting a lactate threshold test requires a comprehensive knowledge of energy pathways and lactate metabolism. As mentioned, lactate can be produced when glycolysis is used to supply energy to the working muscle.

The activation of glycolysis does not always mean that lactate production or blood lactate accumulation will occur in significant amounts. During low- to moderate-intensity exercise (below a rating of perceived exertion of approximately 12 to 13 on the Borg scale), the oxidative energy pathway can provide adequate energy to meet the needs of the working muscle. As exercise intensity increases, the energy demand can begin to overwhelm the capacity of the oxidative energy pathways, forcing the body to rely more heavily on glycolysis to supply adequate energy to fuel muscular contractions. During these times of high energy demand, and high rates of glycolysis, considerable lactate production and accumulation can occur.

Glycolysis is a metabolic pathway that can be activated very quickly. It occurs in the cytosol of the muscle cell and consumes glucose-6-phosphate, using this substrate to produce four molecules that are essential for energy metabolism: adenosine triphosphate (ATP), NADH + H$^+$, pyruvate, and lactate.

The importance of ATP to exercise metabolism is elementary, because the energy held in the phosphate bonds of this molecule provide the free energy needed for performing muscular contractions. Chemical reactions must take place to break these bonds in order for the energy to be released. Once the energy is released, it can be harnessed and utilized for muscular contractions. Because glycolysis can produce ATP very quickly, the body calls on it to provide substantial amounts of ATP during brief exercise bouts (30 seconds to 1 minute). Additionally, glycolysis becomes very active during extended high-intensity bouts of exercise when ATP demand is greater than can be met by oxidative phosphorylation.

Glycolytic ATP formation occurs at two points: the phosphoglycerate kinase and pyruvate kinase reactions. Two molecules of ATP are produced from each reaction, and two or three molecules are produced from glycolysis for each glucose-6-phosphate molecule that is consumed. The discrepancy in the net ATP yield depends on the source of the glucose-6-phosphate that is being used. If blood glucose is being used to form glucose-6-phosphate, two ATP molecules must be invested, one at the hexokinase reaction and one at the phosphofructokinase reaction, for glycolysis to be completed. Therefore, two ATP molecules are harvested when blood glucose is used as the source for glucose-6-phosphate. If muscle glycogen is the source of the glucose-6-phosphate, the hexokinase reaction is skipped, requiring the investment of one less ATP molecule and a higher net ATP yield.

NADH + H$^+$ is formed from nicotinamide adenine dinucleotide, or NAD, at the glyceraldehyde-3-phosphate dehydrogenase reaction. As noted in figure

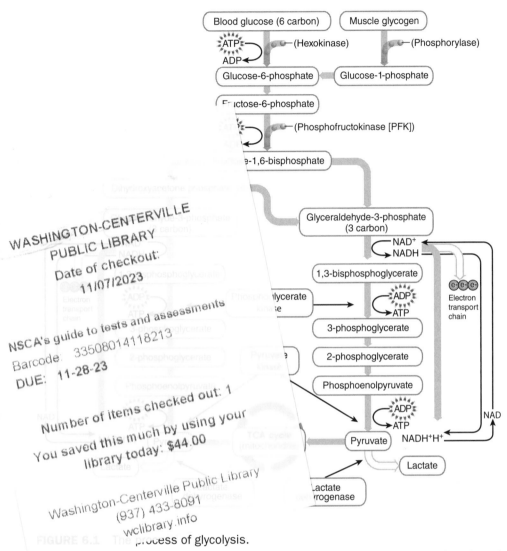

FIGURE 6.1   The process of glycolysis.

Adapted, by permission, from National Strength and Conditioning Association, 2008, Bioenergetics of exercise and training, by J. T. Cramer. In *Essentials of strength training and conditioning*, 3rd ed., edited by T.R. Baechle and R.W. Earle (Champaign, IL: Human Kinetics), 25.

6.1, this oxidation-reduction reaction transfers a hydrogen from glyceraldehyde-3-phosphate to NAD, forming NADH. The associated hydrogen of the NADH + H⁺ comes from a free hydrogen ion in the cytosol. Its association to NADH is due to the attraction of the positively charged hydrogen ion to a negatively charged electron on the nicotinamide molecule.

There are two important aspects of glycolytic NADH + H⁺ production to exercise metabolism. First, the NADH + H⁺ formed during glycolysis can donate its hydrogens to NAD and FAD (flavin adenine dinucleotide) in the mitochondria to form mitochondrial NADH + H⁺ and $FADH_2$. These newly formed mitochondrial NADH + H⁺ or FADH$_2$ are then used in the electron transport chain to regenerate large amounts of ATP. Second, the formation of NADH + H+ at the glyceraldehyde-3-phosphate dehydrogenase allows for the formation of 1,3 bisphosphoglycerate, whose phosphate groups are subsequently used to regenerate ATP at the phosphoglycerate kinase and pyruvate kinase reactions.

The formation of pyruvate occurs in one of the two possible final reactions of glycolysis. Once formed in the muscle cell, pyruvate typically has two fates: conversion to lactate, which will be discussed later in the chapter, or transfer into the mitochondria where it can be consumed by the tricarboxylic acid (TCA) cycle. Once in the mitochondria, pyruvate combines with coenzyme A to form acetyl coA. This process involves a series of reactions that also produces NADH + H⁺, which, like the NADH + H⁺ produced by glycolysis, can be used by the electron transport chain to regenerate ATP. The newly created acetyl coA enters the TCA cycle where it is used to produce ATP, NADH + H⁺, and FADH$_2$; the latter two molecules are used to regenerate ATP in the electron transport chain.

The final ATP tally from one molecule of glucose being consumed through glycolysis, the TCA cycle, and the electron transport chain is approximately 36 to 39 ATP. This number will vary slightly depending on the source of glucose-6-phosphate, the method of transferring the NADH + H⁺ made in the cytosol to the mitochondria, and the efficiency of the coupling of oxidation and phosphorylation in the electron transport chain.

A second fate of pyruvate is its conversion to lactate. Lactate is formed from pyruvate by the donation of hydrogen ions from the NADH + H⁺ created by the glyceraldehyde-3-phosphate dehydrogenase reaction. Once formed in the muscle cell, lactate has two immediate fates. Under some circumstances, this lactate can be converted back into pyruvate and used as a fuel in the oxidative pathways. Lactate that is not used to reform pyruvate is transported out of the muscle to other tissues and used for a variety of purposes. In contrast to pyruvate, lactate itself cannot be consumed by the TCA cycle; thus, lactate that is not used to reform pyruvate cannot be immediately used to further contribute to ATP production. Lactate that appears in the blood therefore represents an ATP yield from glucose-6-phosphate that is limited to the two or three ATP molecules that are produced during glycolysis.

With its superior ATP yield, the consumption of pyruvate by the TCA cycle is obviously the preferred method of pyruvate metabolism during steady state exercise. However, the mitochondria are limited in their ability to produce ATP from pyruvate; and as exercise intensity increases, increased ATP demands must be met, somewhat, by an increase in the rate of glycolysis. However, glycolysis has its own self-limiting mechanism that tempers its ability to produce ATP.

Glycolysis must have adequate levels of NAD to produce NADH + H⁺ at the glyceraldehyde-3-phosphate reaction. Despite the usefulness of NADH

+ HNADH + H$^+$ in ATP regeneration in the electron transport chain, large-scale production of NADH + H+ by glycolysis can lead to a drop in NAD levels in the cytosol. During moderate-intensity exercise, the mitochondria are able to maintain stable levels of NAD in the cytosol by consuming the hydrogens from NADH + H$^+$. However, increases in the rate of glycolysis during heavy exercise can produce NADH + H+ in amounts large enough to overwhelm the consumption capacity of the mitochondria, leading to a buildup of NADH + HNADH + H$^+$ and a drop in the levels of NAD. If the levels of NAD continue to decline, the glyceraldehyde-3-phosphate dehydrogenase (G3PDH) reaction will slow as a result of a lack of NAD. The reduction in the G3PDH reaction will result in lowered rates of glycolysis and glycolytic ATP production and fatigue in the exercising person.

During high-intensity exercise, the formation of lactate plays key roles in exercise metabolism, ATP production, and the maintenance of exercising work rates. The conversion of pyruvate to lactate consumes the hydrogen ions associated with NADH + HNADH + H$^+$, which has two benefits: the regeneration of NAD, which allows glycolysis and glycolytic ATP production to continue at high rates, and the maintenance of relatively neutral pH during exercise (for a comprehensive review, see Robergs, Ghiasvand, and Parker 2004). These benefits of lactate formation are in stark contrast to the traditional beliefs that lactate formation promotes acidosis and fatigue during high-intensity exercise. On the contrary, the formation of lactate actually helps to sustain high-intensity exercise by reducing acidosis and maintaining adequate supplies of NAD.

The production of large amounts of lactate does, however, indicate that the body is using its last line of defense to maintain glycolytic ATP production and exercise intensity. Once this point is reached, further increases in work rates will eventually overwhelm the capacity of lactate production, resulting in acidosis, a drop in NAD levels, and fatigue. Thus, although lactate accumulation and fatigue during exercise are highly correlated, lactate should not be considered a cause of fatigue.

Although lactate is generally associated with high-intensity exercise, some amounts are always being produced regardless of exercising work rates. As exercise intensity increases, accumulation of NADH + HNADH + H$^+$ and pyruvate can cause large increases in the rate of lactate production. Once formed in the working muscle, lactate that is not metabolized locally is transported through the cell membrane and into the blood where it can be delivered to, and consumed by, a variety of tissues.

The lactate dehydrogenase reaction that forms lactate from pyruvate is reversible and allows a variety of tissues including cardiac and nonworking skeletal muscle to use the arriving lactate as a source of pyruvate for the TCA cycle. This process allows these tissues to provide substrate for oxidative metabolism without using their glycogen stores or importing glucose from the blood. Lactate can also be absorbed by the liver where, through the process of gluconeogenesis, it can be converted back into glucose and released into the bloodstream for the working muscle to use. This transport of lactate from the working muscle to the liver, its conversion into glucose, and its redistribution to the working muscle is a process known as the Cori cycle.

Regardless of the fate of lactate, its levels in the blood are a product of lactate production versus lactate consumption. At relatively low to moderate exercise intensities, lactate consumption equals lactate production, resulting in blood lactate levels that are relatively low and consistent. As exercise intensities continue to rise, however, increased rates of glycolysis eventually result in lactate production rates that overwhelm the lactate consumption rate. If high-intensity exercise continues, this inequity ultimately causes an increase in blood lactate concentrations—the lactate threshold (see figure 6.2).

Sport Performance and Lactate Threshold

The objective of a lactate threshold test is to identify the exercise intensity at which the body relies heavily on glycolysis and, consequently, produces excessive amounts of lactate to meet energy demand. Because a lactate threshold test focuses on the ability to use aerobic energy pathways, it is used almost exclusively for endurance athletes such as marathon runners and long-distance cyclists. It identifies the work rate at which the athlete starts to rely more heavily on the inefficient catabolism of the body's limited carbohydrate stores. An athlete with a relatively high lactate threshold is better able to preserve carbohydrate stores when working at high intensities.

Performing a Lactate Threshold Test

During a lactate threshold test, subjects exercise at progressively higher work rates until they are at or near exhaustion. Blood samples are taken at regular time intervals throughout the test and analyzed for lactate concentration. The test begins at a relatively low work rate and progresses slowly so that blood lactate levels remain at, or near, resting levels throughout the early stages of the test. The work rate increases such that a lactate threshold is reached after approximately 12 to 20 minutes of exercise. This strategy of gradually increasing the workload from a low-intensity starting point establishes an exercising baseline level of blood lactate that is useful in identifying the point at which blood lactate accumulation begins.

A variety of exercising modes can be used to perform a lactate threshold test; treadmill running and cycling ergometry are two of the most popular. Although practically any exercise mode is suitable for testing non-endurance-trained athletes, endurance-trained athletes should be tested using the type of exercise that most closely resembles their competitive events. This strategy allows the athlete to perform the test using a familiar mode

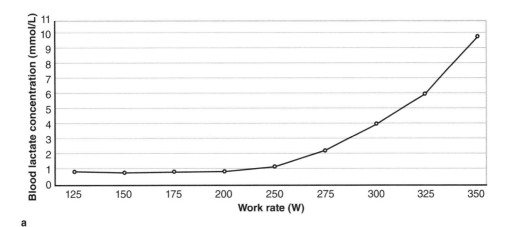

a

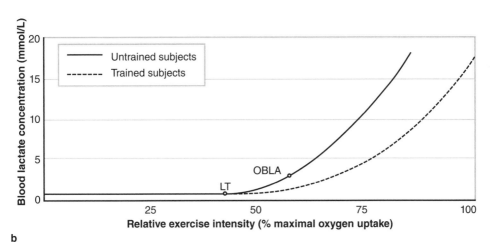

b

FIGURE 6.2 At relatively low to moderate exercise intensities, lactate consumption equals lactate production, resulting in blood lactate levels that are relatively low and consistent. As exercise intensities continue to rise, however, increased rates of glycolysis eventually result in lactate production rates that overwhelm the lactate consumption rate.

of exercise and provides data that are useful in both the design and the assessment of a training program.

Pretest Considerations

Prior to the start of a lactate threshold test, the subject should perform an adequate warm-up of approximately 10 to 15 minutes beginning at a low work rate and progressing to a terminal intensity that is similar to the starting work rate for the lactate threshold test. The warm-up serves two purposes:

- The oxidative energy pathways need several minutes to reach optimal operating capacity. Early in exercise, the body relies heavily on glycolysis to meet ATP demand, resulting in high levels of lactate production. This increased rate of lactate production could lead to blood lactate levels in the initial stages of the test that may not accurately reflect the blood lactate production and consumption dynamics when mitochondria are functioning at their optimal levels.

- People who have never had a lactate threshold test may be apprehensive or nervous before the test begins. These feelings may result in a rise in circulating levels of epinephrine, which can cause increased rates of glycolysis and lactate production. In fact, epinephrine is such a potent stimulator of lactate production that anxious, but otherwise resting, subjects can exhibit blood lactate levels similar to those undergoing intense exercise. These uncharacteristically high levels of blood lactate can make it more difficult to determine the point at which lactate production begins to accelerate as a result of increases in work rate, leading to an inaccurate assessment of lactate threshold. By performing a warm-up prior to the start of the lactate threshold test, subjects can reduce anxiousness and their rates of lactate production, leading to more accurate lactate levels during the early portion of the test.

Starting work rates and the progression of the work rates over the course of the test are dictated by the ability of the subject. Care should be taken when establishing these values to ensure that the subject reaches lactate threshold within approximately 12 to 20 minutes. A test that starts at too high of a work rate or progresses too quickly may not allow the subject to establish an exercising baseline, making identification of the lactate threshold difficult or impossible. A test that starts too low or progresses too slowly wastes both time and materials. Current training paces and previous lactate threshold results can be useful in determining proper starting work rates. If the subject has no prior exercise experience, it is best to err on the conservative side; otherwise, the examiner runs the risk of having to repeat the test because the starting work rate exceeded the subject's lactate threshold work rate or the examiner did not allow for the establishment of an exercise baseline.

Administering the Test

Once the test begins, the progression of the work rate can be accomplished by continuously increasing the work rate over time, which is commonly known as a ramp protocol. The step protocol involves increasing the work rate by a specified amount at consistent intervals, usually every three to four minutes. Ramp protocols can be popular for some types of research applications, but step protocols are generally more useful when evaluating athletes because they determine more precisely the power output or pace that actually elicits the lactate threshold. In a step protocol, work rates typically increase at each stage by approximately 5 to 15% of the starting work rate for the test, whereas the ramp protocol uses similar increases in work rates over a period of three or four minutes (see figure 6.3). Well-conditioned cyclists start at 125 to 150 watts with 20-watt increases every three or four minutes; well-conditioned runners may begin the test at a speed of 8 miles per hour (13 km/h) and increase the pace by 0.5 miles per hour (0.8 km/h) every three or four minutes.

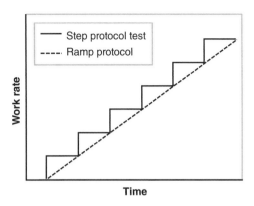

FIGURE 6.3 Ramp versus step protocol work rate increments.

Throughout the lactate threshold test, blood samples are drawn at regular time intervals and analyzed for lactate concentration. If a ramp protocol is used, blood is typically drawn at varied time intervals. Early in the test, blood samples are usually drawn every three or four minutes. As the subject nears lactate threshold, sampling occurs more frequently, usually every 30 seconds to 1 minute. The more frequent blood samples taken near the lactate threshold allow for a more accurate determination of the occurrence of the lactate threshold. Because the work rates remain stable during each stage of a step protocol, the blood is drawn at constant time intervals, generally during the final 30 seconds of each stage.

Taking blood samples too early in the stage may result in lactate readings that do not accurately reflect the lactate production rate for a particular workload. This is because the energy pathways must be given time to increase their rate of operation in response to higher work rates. Furthermore, once glycolytic rates and lactate production rates stabilize in response to the new workload, the lactate must be given time to migrate to the blood and become evenly distributed throughout the bloodstream. Only at that point will lactate levels accurately reflect the levels of lactate production.

Blood samples can be obtained from numerous sites on the body; the three most popular are the fingertips, earlobes, and an antecubital vein. Fingertip and earlobe samples are typically obtained by making a small puncture wound in the skin through which small (approximately 50 µL) samples can be obtained for analysis. Fingertip and earlobe sampling has gained popularity in recent years because it is minimally invasive and modern lactate analyzers require only very small (25 to 50 µL) volumes for analysis. Certain methods of blood lactate analysis, such as spectrophotometry, require larger samples than can be obtained from the earlobe or fingertip. In these cases, blood is typically drawn from an antecubital vein using a catheter or venipuncture technique.

The blood sampling site may be dictated by the equipment available, but is otherwise up to the technician and subject. It should be noted that blood lactate levels can vary by 50% or more depending on the sampling site

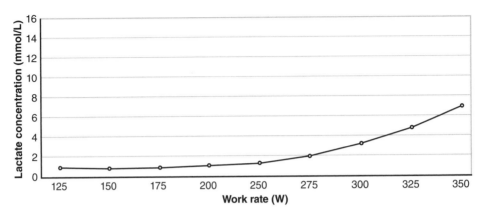

FIGURE 6.4 Lactate threshold results from a subject who exhibited a gradual rise in blood lactate levels; in this case, no definitive lactate threshold could be determined using the visual inspection method.

(El-Sayed, George, and Dyson 1993); thus, once a sampling site is chosen, it should be used consistently throughout the test.

Once the blood sample is obtained, it should be analyzed with a lactate analyzer immediately. If this is not possible, the sample should be placed in a lysing agent to destroy the red blood cells as quickly as possible because they produce lactate as part of their normal metabolism. If left intact, red blood cells will continue to produce lactate after the blood sample has been obtained resulting in blood lactate levels that are not reflective of lactate production by the working muscle.

Test Termination and Data Analyses

The lactate threshold test continues until the subject reaches exhaustion, or until a clear and continued rise in blood lactate concentration is observed. Once blood lactate data have been obtained, lactate threshold is determined by plotting the lactate values against their respective work rates. As shown in figure 6.2, blood lactates at lower work rates are typically maintained at fairly low and consistent levels. This maintenance of consistent lactate concentration in the face of increasing work rates is commonly referred to as a baseline, or as baseline lactate values.

As work rates exceed a certain level, blood lactate levels begin to exhibit substantial increases as work rates increase. This inflection point in blood lactate concentration is considered by many to be the lactate threshold, which can often be identified by visually inspecting the plotted lactate values for changes in lactate concentrations in response to increases in work rate (Davis et al. 2007).

Unfortunately, lactate plots may not always exhibit a clear and decisive threshold such as the one shown in figure 6.2. Figure 6.4 illustrates data from a subject who exhibited a gradual rise in blood lactate levels; in this

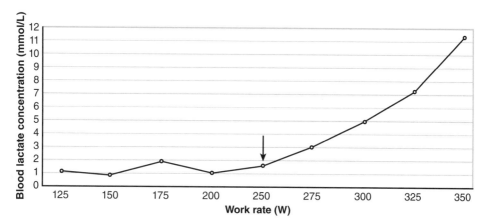

FIGURE 6.5 Lactate threshold results from a subject whose blood lactate values stayed relatively low and stable through 250 watts, but at a work rate of 275 watts, the lactate value increased by greater than 1.0 mmol · L⁻¹.

case, no definitive lactate threshold could be determined using the visual inspection method. Because such cases occur with regularity, many exercise physiologists advocate the use of more objective methods of determining lactate threshold. These methods include the 0.5 mmol · L⁻¹ criteria, the 1.0 mmol · L⁻¹ criteria, the extrapolation method, and the D-max method.

0.5 and 1.0 mmol · L⁻¹ Criteria

The 0.5 (Zoladz, Rademaker, and Sargeant 1995) and 1.0 mmol · L⁻¹ (Thoden 1991) criteria use similar methods for identifying lactate threshold, but differ in the magnitude of the change required to qualify as a threshold. With these methods, blood lactate concentrations are plotted against their respective work rates. The lactate threshold is then identified as the highest work rate that does not result in a 0.5 or 1.0 mmol · L⁻¹ increase in blood lactate concentration in response to at least two consecutive increases in work rate. The requirement of two consecutive increases in blood lactate reduces the possibility of erroneously identifying a lactate threshold from irregular lactate responses to low exercising work rates.

In figure 6.5, the blood lactate values stayed relatively low and stable through 250 watts. At a work rate of 275 watts, the lactate value increased by greater than 1.0 mmol · L⁻¹. This 1.0 mmol · L⁻¹ increase was again seen between the 275- and 300-watt outputs, which meets the requirement of a 1.0 mmol · L⁻¹ increase in blood lactate concentration in response to at least two consecutive increases in work rate.

A major limitation of the visual inspection and 0.5 and 1.0 mmol · L⁻¹ methods of determining lactate threshold is that the accuracy of the threshold measurement is somewhat dictated by the work rate increments of the stages. For instance, in figure 6.2, the lactate threshold is clearly 250 watts.

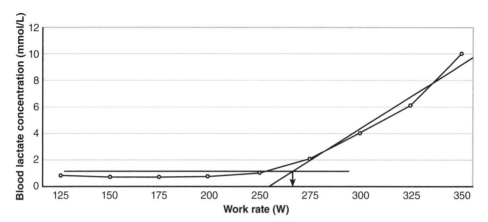

FIGURE 6.6   Regression lines. A vertical line is passed through the point of intersection and extrapolated downward until it intersects with the x-axis. The point of intersection on the x-axis marks the work rate at which lactate threshold supposedly occurs.

However, because lactate levels were measured only at 250 watts and 275 watts, we can only be certain that blood lactate was not accumulating at 250 watts, but was accumulating at 275 watts. Thus, we cannot be certain of the precise work rate that causes blood lactate to accumulate, only that it is somewhere between just above 250 watts and 275 watts.

Regression Analyses

In an attempt to make more precise assessments of the work rates that induce lactate threshold, some exercise physiologists advocate using regression analyses to analyze blood lactate data. To perform this procedure, the lactate curve is divided into two parts: baseline, which includes all of those lactate values up to the point at which blood lactate levels begin to rise, and the exponential portion of the curve, which includes all values from this inflection point until the termination of the test. Separate regression analyses are performed on each portion of the curve to generate lines of best fit for the respective portions. Once established, the regression lines are extrapolated until they intersect. A vertical line is passed through the point of intersection and extrapolated downward until it intersects with the x-axis. The point of intersection on the x-axis marks the work rate at which lactate threshold supposedly occurs (see figure 6.6).

A criticism of the extrapolation method is that lactate threshold is influenced by the rate at which blood lactate concentrations increase following the exhibition of a lactate inflection point. Consider two athletes whose lactate profiles are presented in figure 6.7, *a* and *b*. Athlete A's blood lactate accumulated at a much quicker rate after the exhibition of a lactate inflection point than did athlete B's. Note that by virtue of the interaction of the two regression lines, athlete A has a higher lactate threshold than athlete B, even though their lactate inflection points occurred at the same work rate.

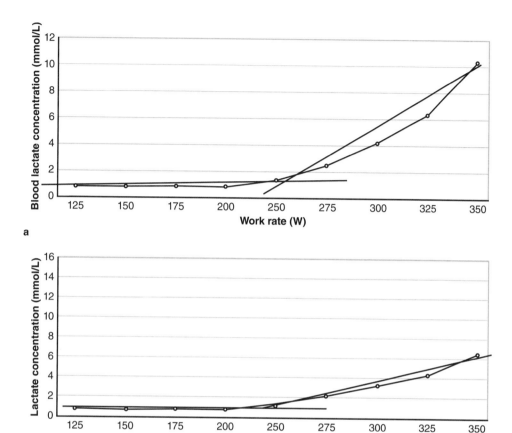

FIGURE 6.7 Comparing the interaction of the two regression lines, athlete A has a higher lactate threshold than athlete B, even though their lactate inflection points occurred at the same work rate.

Factors that dictate this rate of increase in blood lactate levels following the exhibition of an inflection point, such as the activity of the lactate dehydrogenase enzyme, muscle fiber composition, and blood volume, may have nothing to do with the work rate that actually results in the accumulation of blood lactate. Thus, determination of the lactate threshold by the extrapolation method may be unjustifiably influenced by factors that do not result in an initial increase in blood lactate levels.

D-Max Method

To perform the D-max method of lactate analysis, the subject must exercise to volitional exhaustion during the lactate threshold test (Cheng et al. 1992). The resulting data are plotted using a third-order curvilinear regression. Next, a straight line is drawn connecting the first and last lactate values. A second line is drawn perpendicularly from the first line to the point on the plotted lactate value that is farthest from the first line. From the point of

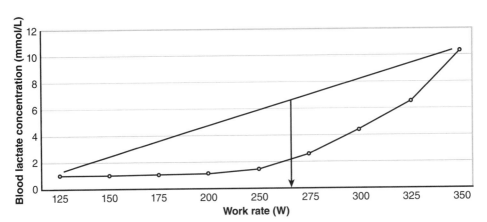

FIGURE 6.8 The work rate that elicits lactate threshold is at the point at which the second line intersects with the x-axis.

intersection of the second line and the plotted lactate values, a third, vertical line is drawn downward until it intersects with the x-axis. The work rate that elicits lactate threshold is said to be at the point at which the third line intersects with the x-axis (see figure 6.8).

Although the D-max method suffers from the same criticism as the extrapolation method, a high degree of repeatability has been reported for this approach (Zhou and Weston 1997). Furthermore, in a comparison of 10K running pace to pace at lactate threshold determined by a number of methods, the D-max method predicted competitive running performance with the greatest degree of accuracy (Nicholson and Sleivert 2001), demonstrating the method's usefulness for evaluating competitive athletes.

Maximal Lactate Steady State

Although lactate threshold is probably the most commonly used lactate measurement test, the maximal lactate steady state test (MLSS) is sometimes used to predict maximal sustainable work rates in exercising people. This test monitors blood lactate levels during extended periods of consistent exercise intensity seeking to identify the highest workload at which blood lactate levels remain stable (Beneke 2003).

The maximal lactate steady state concept was born from criticism that, although lactate threshold marks the point of increased blood lactate accumulation, it may not identify the highest work rate a person can maintain without continued increases in lactate production when this intensity is maintained over an extended period of time. Increases in lactate production and blood lactate levels are sometimes mistakenly considered to be an indication that the body is unable to maintain homeostasis in the glycolytic pathway. In fact, lactate production assists in the maintenance of proper rates

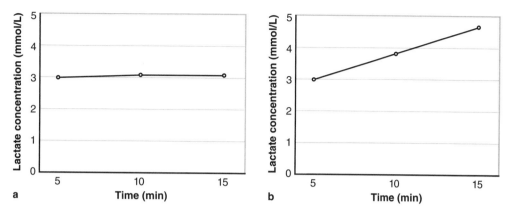

FIGURE 6.9 Lactate values from two consecutive stages of an MLSS test; *(a)* at 250 watts and *(b)* at 260 watts.

of ATP production by maintaining adequate levels of NAD for glycolysis.

Some have demonstrated that work rates in excess of those that result in lactate threshold can be maintained with consistent, albeit elevated, levels of lactate production in many people (Morris and Shafer 2010). Proponents of MLSS argue that, even though the lactate levels in response to a given workload are higher than exercising baseline, their consistent levels over time indicate that homeostasis within glycolysis is occurring and exercise intensity can be maintained for an extended period of time. Thus, the MLSS test monitors the blood lactate response to a specific work rate over an extended period of time.

Determination of MLSS involves a series of tests and may take several days to complete. Initially, the subject should perform a lactate threshold test as described earlier in this chapter. From this data, the work rate that elicits lactate threshold is identified. The subject then performs a series of discontinuous exercise stages separated by several minutes or hours of rest. The durations of the stages vary considerably by protocol and usually range from 9 to 30 minutes (Beneke 2003). The work rates are held at a constant level within each stage while blood is drawn at regular time intervals and analyzed for lactate levels. If the subject maintains consistent blood lactate levels throughout a stage, a rest period is provided and the procedure is repeated at a slightly higher work rate. This strategy continues until significant increases in blood lactate levels are observed within a single stage. MLSS is defined as the highest work rate that does not result in an increase in blood lactate concentration exceeding the criteria for steady state lactate levels.

Figure 6.9 illustrates lactate values from two consecutive stages of an MLSS test. At 250 watts (see figure 6.9a), the subject was able to maintain a consistent blood lactate level throughout the duration of the stage. During the next stage, when the work rate was increased to 260 watts, the lactate values did not remain at a consistent level and increased over the duration of the stage (see figure 6.9*b*). From these data, we can determine that MLSS is 250 watts for this subject.

The duration of the stages and rest periods, the progression in work rates between stages, and the criteria for a rise in blood lactate vary considerably depending on the mode of exercise and the specific protocol. For instance, in protocols using 30-minute stages, blood lactate levels may be measured every 5 minutes and lactate increases may be limited to no more than 1.0 mmol · L^{-1} between the 10th and 30th minutes of exercise (Beneke 2003); whereas others may limit increases to no more than 0.5 mmol · L^{-1} between the 20th and 30th minutes (Urhausen et al. 1993). Shorter protocol, such as 9 minutes, may measure blood lactate every 3 minutes and limit blood lactate increase to no more than 1.0 mmol · L^{-1} between the 3rd and 9th minutes (Morris, Kearney, and Burke 2000).

Rest periods between stages may vary between 30 minutes for the shorter staged protocols and 24 hours for the protocols using 30-minute stages. When evaluating athletes for training purposes, the shorter protocols are more appropriate because athletes typically do not have time to devote to the multiple days of testing required for the longer MLSS protocols. However, more accurate determinations of MLSS may be obtained from longer protocols, which may make them more appealing to researchers.

The work rate for the initial stage is usually slightly above the work rate at lactate threshold. Work rate progressions can be arbitrarily set or calculated as a percentage of the work rate for the initial stage. For rowing and cycling protocols, common increments are 5 to 10 watts, whereas runners may increase by 0.2 to 0.3 miles per hour (0.3 to 0.5 km/h) per stage.

Using Lactate Threshold Data

Information provided by a lactate threshold test has a number of purposes. By understanding the role that lactate plays in exercise metabolism, the exercise physiologist can use the information from lactate threshold tests to predict proper racing and training paces, and assess the fitness of a subject or the efficacy of the training program. Although lactate production does not contribute to acidosis and lactate itself does not appear to cause fatigue, blood lactate accumulation does indicate that the body is relying on substantial contributions from anaerobic glycolysis to meet exercising energy requirements. Knowing the exercise intensity at which this occurs is valuable for two reasons: When glucose and glycogen are metabolized to lactate, only two or three ATP molecules are generated per molecule of carbohydrate consumed compared to the 36 to 39 ATP molecules that are generated when pyruvate is produced and consumed through oxidative phosphorylation. Thus, the advent of lactate threshold signals that the body is consuming glucose and glycogen at an increased rate in respect to ATP production, which, ultimately, can lead to premature carbohydrate depletion and exhaustion. Therefore, athletes who partake in events that challenge their glycogen storage capacity should take into consideration the need to preserve carbohydrate stores when planning their pacing strategies.

Increases in blood lactate concentrations also indicate that the subject's ATP consumption rate is beginning to exceed the ability to provide ATP through the oxidative pathway. The increase in blood lactate levels seen at this transitional intensity indicates that the body has to rely on glycolysis to provide adequate ATP supplies for the exercising muscle. Though lactate production does not result in acidosis and has a questionable role in causing fatigue, the accumulation of lactate in the blood indicates that maximal sustainable rates of exercise and ATP production are close at hand (Morris and Shafer 2010).

The relationship between lactate threshold and the rate of consumption of carbohydrate stores, and correlations between lactate threshold and maximal sustainable work rate, make lactate threshold a good predictor of endurance exercise performance. Previous studies (Foxdal et al. 1994; Tanaka 1990) have demonstrated close agreements between running paces at lactate threshold and average paces during competitive running events in distances ranging from 10,000 meters to the marathon. In studies using cycling ergometry, power outputs that elicited lactate threshold were similar to average power outputs during time trials ranging from 60 to 90 minutes (Bentley et al. 2001; Bishop, Jenkins, and Mackinnon 1998). However, in time trials ranging from 25 to 35 minutes, subjects typically maintain significantly higher power outputs than those that elicited lactate threshold (Bentley et al. 2001; Kenefick et al. 2002). Despite these discrepancies, correlations between power outputs at lactate threshold and average power outputs during the shorter time trials remained remarkably high, suggesting that performance in these events can be predicted from lactate threshold data with reasonable accuracy.

As in many physiological and anatomical systems, the mechanisms that influence lactate threshold are responsive to exercise training. Properly designed training programs can increase the capacity of the oxidative pathway by increasing oxygen delivery to the working muscle (Schmidt et al. 1988), mitochondrial numbers (Holloszy and Coyle 1984), and oxidative enzyme levels (Henriksson and Reitman 1976). These improvements in oxidative capacity increase the muscle's ability to produce ATP, consume pyruvate, and regenerate NAD resulting in a reduced reliance on lactate production and an increase in work rates that are required to elicit lactate threshold.

Unlike maximal oxygen consumption, which can be significantly influenced by genetic factors (Bouchard et al. 1986), the exhibition of lactate threshold when expressed as a percentage of maximal oxygen consumption is primarily influenced by the level of conditioning (Henritze et al. 1985). This sensitivity to exercise training makes lactate threshold useful for assessing aerobic fitness and the efficacy of training programs. Well-trained

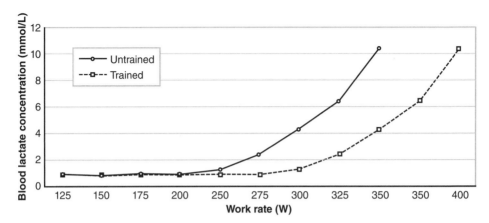

FIGURE 6.10   The lactate threshold training effect.

endurance athletes tend to exhibit lactate threshold when exercising at 80% or more of their maximal oxygen consumption, whereas untrained people experience lactate threshold at substantially lower intensities (Joyner and Coyle 2008). Continued training at or above the work rate that elicits lactate threshold also results in increases in the power outputs that cause increased rates of lactate production and accumulation (Henritze et al. 1985). Therefore, the efficacy of a training program can be assessed by measuring lactate threshold prior to, and following, program implementation. A rightward shift, as seen in figure 6.10, suggests that the training program has been successful in increasing the work rate that elicits lactate threshold and maximal sustainable work rates.

The ability of lactate threshold to respond to training and predict competitive performance also makes it useful in prescribing proper training intensities. Scientific evidence supports the overload principle of training (Weltman et al. 1992), which suggests that the most effective way to improve physiological capacity is to train at an intensity that exceeds current ability. Thus, effective training strategies involve assessing athletes' current performance capacities and using work intervals that exceed their current maximal sustainable work rates. Undoubtedly, the most accurate way of measuring an athlete's performance capacity in a particular event is to measure performance during that event. Unfortunately, lengthy endurance events such as the marathon are physically taxing, which makes performing them simply to test performance capacity impractical. However, the relatively short and low-stress nature of a lactate threshold test makes it ideal for frequently assessing an athlete's ability.

Tim is a competitive distance runner who has recently set a goal of running his first marathon. He has a history of strong performances in 10K road races and wants to run a fast time in his first marathon. Tim recognizes the concept of progressive overload and knows that to improve his ability in the marathon, he must train at a pace that is faster than the speed he could maintain for the entire 26.2 miles. However, if he trains at a pace that is too fast, he won't be able to do the volume of training that is required to perform well in his upcoming competition. He is very aware of his abilities at the 10K distance, but the marathon is roughly four times longer than the 10K, and he knows that he cannot maintain this pace for the entire marathon.

Tim visits an exercise physiologist, who is also a distance runner, for advice. The exercise physiologist agrees that Tim's competitive pace for the 10K is far faster than what he could maintain for the entire marathon. The exercise physiologist is aware of research demonstrating that pace at lactate threshold is typically very similar to the pace that can be maintained for a marathon and suggests that Tim undergo a lactate threshold test.

The exercise physiologist chooses a step protocol because it will identify the running pace that elicits lactate threshold more accurately than a ramp protocol. Stages for the test will be three minutes long to stabilize blood lactate levels in response to each new workload. The pace of each stage will increase by one-half mile per hour to determine the pace that results in lactate threshold.

The starting pace must be one that will allow Tim to complete four or five stages before blood lactate levels begin to rise. This will establish a baseline from which to identify lactate threshold. Tim has recently competed in a 10K run, finishing in 36:00, which roughly translates into a six-minute mile, or a pace of about 10 miles per hour. Well-conditioned endurance runners can maintain a pace for a 10K race that is slightly faster than their pace at lactate threshold. Thus, 9.5 miles per hour is a good estimation for a pace that will elicit lactate threshold. To start the test at a speed that will put Tim at 9.5 miles per hour within four stages, the exercise physiologist multiplies the number of stages (four) by the rate of increase in speed for each stage (0.5 mph). The resulting figure of 2 miles per hour is then subtracted from the suspected lactate threshold speed of 9.5 miles per hour to give a starting speed of 7.5 miles per hour.

Prior to starting the test, Tim warms up for 12 minutes. The warm-up begins at a relatively slow speed of five miles per hour and remains here for the first two minutes of the warm-up. At the two-minute mark, the speed is increased by 0.5 miles per hour and is increased by this amount every two minutes for the remainder of the warm-up. This progression will have Tim running at the starting pace for the lactate threshold test (7.5 mph) for the final two minutes of the warm-up.

(continued)

(continued)

This approach accomplishes three things:

- It allows Tim's body to adjust to the metabolic demands of the starting work rate of the lactate threshold test.
- It allows Tim to experience the starting speed for the test and reduce his apprehension going into the test.
- It gives Tim the chance to experience the pacing progressions for each stage of the lactate threshold test.

Once he has finished the warm-up, Tim steps off of the treadmill. He and the exercise physiologist have four to five minutes to make final preparations for the test. For Tim, this may include using the restroom, stretching, or double-knotting his shoelaces to make sure they do not come untied and interrupt the test once it has started. The exercise physiologist takes this time to double-check that all of the necessary equipment is at hand and properly calibrated.

To begin the test, the exercise physiologist starts the treadmill and sets the starting speed of 7.5 miles per hour. Tim then steps on the treadmill belt, and the exercise physiologist starts the stopwatch. After three minutes of running, Tim straddles the treadmill belt and the exercise physiologist uses a needle to make a small puncture in Tim's finger. A small blood sample is taken from the wound and introduced immediately to the lactate analyzer. The exercise physiologist then places a small piece of gauze on Tim's wound before the treadmill speed is increased by 0.5 miles per hour, and Tim returns to running on the treadmill. This procedure is repeated until an obvious and sustained increase in blood lactate levels is observed over the course of several stages.

Upon termination of the test, the exercise physiologist plots the lactate values against their respective running paces and sees an obvious inflection point at a speed of 9.5 miles per hour. This pace is likely the highest average pace that Tim could maintain for a marathon. Because his objective is to improve his ability before the competition, Tim should use 9.5 miles per hour as a minimum pace for his long training runs, and paces in excess of 10 miles per hour for interval workouts.

With proper training, Tim's lactate threshold will increase, which will increase his minimum training pace. Measureable improvements can be expected within about four to six weeks, necessitating a subsequent retest of Tim's lactate threshold. These regular reassessments will be useful in assessing the efficacy of the training program and in reestablishing proper training paces as Tim's ability improves.

SUMMARY

- The lactate threshold test is used to evaluate endurance exercise capacity.

- Lactate threshold is typically marked by a sharp increase in blood lactate concentration in response to rising work rate.

- Changes in blood lactate levels in response to changing work rates provide insight into an athlete's ability to efficiently catabolize carbohydrate for energy.

- The lactate threshold can be indicative of an athlete's maximal sustainable work rate and, thus, can be used to predict exercise performance and prescribe training intensity.

- Lactate threshold is responsive to endurance exercise training and can therefore be used to evaluate the efficacy of a training program.

7

Muscular Strength

Gavin L. Moir, PhD

Muscular strength has long been identified as an important component in sport performance and health (e.g., Dorchester 1944; Murray and Karpovich 1956; Paschall 1954; Sampon 1895). For this reason, tests used to identify both prognostic and diagnostic information regarding muscular strength are of great value to the strength and conditioning professional. The ability to test muscular strength has significant applications when working with athletes. For example, tests of muscular strength have been suggested as a way to monitor the responses to a training program (Stone, Stone, and Sands 2007; Zatsiorsky 1995), determine the training loads to use during resistance training programs (Baechle, Earle, and Wathen 2008; Bompa and Haff 2009), and monitor rehabilitation following injury (Flanagan, Galvin, and Harrison 2008; Meller et al. 2007). Muscular strength tests also help identify talent in sports such as rugby and soccer (Pienaar, Spamer, and Steyn 1998; Reilly, Bangsbo, and Franks 2000).

In addition to sport performance applications, tests of muscular strength have been used in clinical settings to determine the risk for falls in older subjects (Perry et al. 2007; Wyszomierski, Chambers, and Cham 2009) and to highlight the functional consequences of sarcopenia (Vandervoort and Symons 1997). Additionally, muscular strength has been positively correlated to bone mineral density in older people (Iki et al. 2006; Miller et al. 2009). Clearly, the selection of appropriate tests of muscular strength is a pertinent issue for researchers and practitioners alike.

The purpose of this chapter is to outline appropriate methods for testing muscular strength, particularly maximal muscular strength. The reliability and validity of the tests will be highlighted when possible. We begin, however, by defining muscular strength, which requires a brief discussion of the mechanical and physiological factors that have been shown to influence the expression of muscular strength.

Definition of Muscular Strength

Muscular strength is often equated with muscular force (Siff 2000; Stone, Stone, and Sands 2007; Zatsiorsky 1995) and can be defined as the ability of a muscle or group of muscles to produce a force against an external resistance. From this definition, the expression of muscular strength lies along a continuum from zero (no force generated) to maximal force production (maximal muscular strength). A force is an agent that changes, or tends to change, the motion of an external resistance. (Note that because muscles produce "pulling," or tensile forces, as a result of actomyosin cycling, many refer to the tension developed by a muscle as opposed to the force. However, the term *force* will be used in this chapter for the sake of continuity.) The rearrangement of Newton's second law of motion defines the relationship between an applied force (F) and the mass (m) and acceleration (a) of the external resistance.

$$F = ma$$

where
F = applied force, measured in newtons (N),
m = mass of the external resistance, measured in kilograms (kg), and
a = acceleration of the external resistance, measured in meters per second^2 (m · s^{-2}).

Thus, the magnitude of a force can be determined by the acceleration of an external resistance. Forces, however, take time to change the motion of an external resistance, and so the product of force and time, called the impulse of the force, is often calculated in mechanics:

$$\text{Impulse} = Ft$$

where
Impulse is measured in newton-seconds (Ns),
F = applied force (N), and
t = time, measured in seconds (s).

The importance of the impulse of a force becomes apparent with the relationship between impulse and linear momentum (which can be derived from an equation of motion):

$$Ft = mv_f - mv_i$$

where
Ft = impulse of the applied force (Ns),
mv_f = final linear momentum of an external resistance, measured in kilograms-meters per second (kg/m · s^{-1}), and
mv_i = initial linear momentum of an external resistance, measured in kilograms-meters per second (kg/m · s^{-1}).

From this relationship, the impulse of an applied force acts to change the momentum of an external resistance. Given that linear momentum is the product of mass and linear velocity, and that the mass of external resistances encountered in sporting and clinical situations will remain constant throughout the time of force application, the impulse–momentum relationship defined earlier tells us that to change the linear velocity of an external resistance, we have to apply an impulse—a force that acts over a certain time period.

In the majority of sporting situations and activities of daily living we are required to change the velocity of an external resistance, which may be the mass of our own or someone else's body, or the mass of an object or implement. The impulse–momentum relationship tells us that we can increase the change in motion experienced by an external resistance by increasing the magnitude of the average force applied, increasing the time that the force is applied, or increasing both of these variables. Therefore, the impulse of a force is important from both a mechanical and a practical perspective.

Relating muscular strength to the ability of a muscle or group of muscles to produce a force highlights the importance of muscular strength in sport and clinical settings. Defining muscular strength in terms of the force capabilities of the muscles is also informative because the mechanical and physiological factors that influence force production in skeletal muscle have been determined. As a result, these factors can be considered when establishing the utility of muscular strength tests.

Factors Affecting Muscular Force Production

The factors that affect force production in skeletal muscle include contraction type, muscle architecture, muscle fiber type, contractile history, and neural influences. This section addresses these factors as well as joint torque. It concludes with a definition of maximal muscular strength.

Contraction Type

A muscle can develop force under either static conditions (muscle length remains constant) or dynamic conditions (muscle length changes). When the force is developed and muscle length remains constant, the muscle is said to be performing an isometric contraction. Under dynamic conditions, the muscle can contract eccentrically (i.e., force is developed as the muscle lengthens) or concentrically (i.e., force is developed as the muscle shortens). Recently, muscle physiologists have asserted that the terms *eccentric* and *concentric* are inappropriate and misleading (Faulkner 2003); however, the terms are still widely used in coaching circles, and will be used here.

A special case of a dynamic muscle contraction is an isokinetic contraction. Here, force is developed with the muscle acting either eccentrically

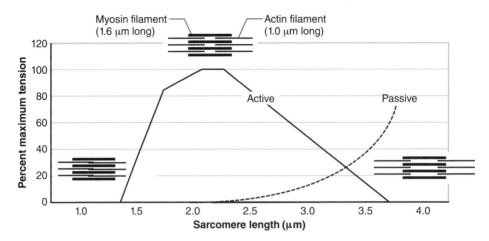

FIGURE 7.1 The force–length relationship. The passive portion of the curve comes from the force exerted by passive structures, such as titin, as the fiber is lengthened.

Reprinted, by permission, from R.L. Lieber, 2002, *Skeletal Muscle Structure, Function and Plasticity. The Physiological Basis of Rehabilitation* (Baltimore, MD: Lippincott Williams & Wilkins), 62.

or concentrically, but the velocity of the contraction apparently remains constant. This type of contraction will be covered in greater depth later in the chapter (see the section Isokinetic Strength Testing).

It should be noted that although the type of contraction performed by a muscle may be obvious *in vitro*, the distinction is not always clear *in vivo*. For example, previous researchers have shown that muscle behavior does not necessarily correspond to joint movement because of the presence of extensible tendons operating in series with the muscle (Reeves and Narici 2003). Specifically, when a joint is accelerated into extension and the muscles crossing the joint are assumed to be operating eccentrically, an isometric contraction may be performed while the tendon is stretched. Such issues may affect the external validity of a test of muscular strength.

It has been established that the force developed by a muscle while operating isometrically depends upon muscle length (Rassier, MacIntosh, and Herzog 1999). This *force–length relationship* (see figure 7.1) is essentially due to changes in the overlap of the myofilaments (shallow ascending limb, plateau, and descending limb) and the thick filaments abutting the Z-disks (steep ascending limb). The practical significance of this relationship is that the expression of muscular strength will vary with muscle length, which in turn will vary with the joint angle selected during the specific test of strength.

Although the force–length relationship can be used to describe the force developed under isometric conditions, this relationship cannot be used to describe the behavior of muscle contracting dynamically. Rather, the *force–velocity relationship* describes the force developed by a muscle when contracting eccentrically or concentrically (see figure 7.2). The precipitous drop in

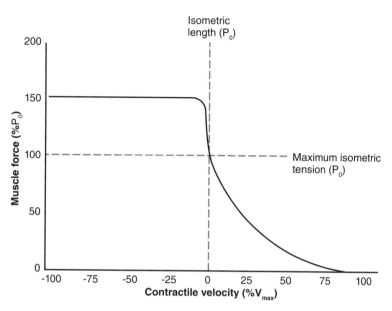

FIGURE 7.2 The force–velocity relationship.

Reprinted, by permission, from R.L. Lieber, 2002, *Skeletal Muscle Structure, Function and Plasticity. The Physiological Basis of Rehabilitation* (Baltimore, MD: Lippincott Williams & Wilkins), 55.

force development as the shortening velocity increases can be explained in terms of chemical reaction rates associated with actomyosin cycling as described by the cross-bridge theory of muscle contraction (Lieber 2002). The rise in force associated with eccentric muscle contractions cannot readily be explained by the original cross-bridge theory; some authors propose sarcomere inhomogeneities as an explanation (Harry et al. 1990; Morgan 1990).

It should be noted that the force–velocity relationship depicted in figure 7.2 represents the relationship generated from a series of experiments performed on an isolated whole muscle in which the muscle was allowed to contract against various loads (strictly, it is the load–velocity relationship). *In vivo* measurements of the relationship using isokinetic dynamometry do not always conform strictly to this idealized relationship; eccentric forces are no greater than isometric forces (Dudley et al. 1990). These differences are probably due to inhibitory reflexes that are initiated when the contractions are performed *in vivo*.

What is apparent from the research is that the force associated with eccentric contractions exceeds that for concentric contractions when the measurements are recorded *in vitro* as well as *in vivo* (Drury et al. 2006; Harry et al. 1990). Although fitness professionals often measure concentric capabilities *in vivo*, measuring eccentric forces is difficult without the use of specialized equipment (e.g., isokinetic dynamometers, force platforms). This is significant given the importance of eccentric forces during many movements (LaStayo et al. 2003). Issues of eccentric force measurement are addressed in the discussion of specific tests later in this chapter.

Researchers have demonstrated that the force developed during a concentric contraction can be enhanced when it is preceded by an eccentric contraction (Finni, Ikegawa, and Komi 2001). This sequencing of concentric and eccentric muscle contractions is termed the *stretch-shortening cycle* (SSC) and has been shown to enhance concentric force development through mechanisms including elastic energy contributions, reflex activation, and architectural changes (Komi 2003). Because the SSC is a naturally occurring sequence of muscle contractions used in sporting and daily activities, its inclusion in a test of muscular strength will influence the validity of the test.

Muscle Architecture

The architectural characteristics that can affect the expression of muscular strength are the cross-sectional area of the muscle and the pennation angle.

Cross-Sectional Area

The cross-sectional area (CSA) of a muscle is related to the number of sarcomeres in parallel. Because this number affects the muscle's ability to develop force, greater CSA is associated with greater force production (McComas 1996). Thus, hypertrophy of a muscle is a way to increase force capabilities. Despite the importance of CSA to the force capabilities of a muscle, the relationship is not applicable to pennate muscles where the muscle fibers operate at an angle to the line of action of the muscle (e.g., rectus femoris). In such situations, the physiological cross-sectional area should be calculated (Leiber 2002), whereby the angle between the orientation of the fascicles and the line of action of the muscular force, the pennation angle, is considered.

Pennation Angle

The pennation angle, defined as the angle between the orientation of the fascicles and the line of action of muscular force, can have a significant effect on muscular force—a greater pennation angle indicates greater force capabilities (Ichinose et al. 1998) with more fibers packed into a given volume of muscle. Researchers have reported significant positive correlations between muscle thickness and pennation angles (Ichinose et al. 1998; Kawakami, Abe, and Fukunaga 1993), suggesting that increases in pennation angle may contribute to muscle hypertrophy. Because the pennation angle of a muscle can change depending on the joint angle (Kawakami et al. 2000), the force capability of a muscle will likely be affected by the joint angle selected in a given strength test.

Muscle Fiber Type

Skeletal muscle is composed of fibers that differ in terms of their contractile properties. The heterogeneity in the contractile properties is partly dependent on the myosin heavy chain (MHC) isoforms present. The type of MHC isoform (of which Types I, IIa, and IIx are found in human skeletal muscle) is used to classify muscle fiber types (Baldwin and Haddad 2001). Research with muscle fibers *in vitro* has revealed that MHC Type IIx fibers have greater specific tension than MHC Type I fibers (Stienen et al. 1996). *In vivo* recordings in humans tend to substantiate these findings; researchers have found positive correlations between MHC Type II percentage and muscular strength (Aagaard and Andersen 1998). Conversely, Type I fibers have a greater oxidative capacity and therefore have greater endurance capabilities (Bottinelli and Reggiani 2000).

Contractile History

Prior muscular contractions can have a significant effect on the ability of a muscle to develop force through fatigue and postactivation potentiation mechanisms.

Fatigue

Fatigue can be defined as a reversible decline in muscle performance associated with muscle activity and is marked by a progressive reduction in the force developed by a muscle (Allen, Lamb, and Westerblad 2008). The reduction in force may not be as pronounced during submaximal contractions as it is during maximal contractions, during which fatigue manifests as an inability to maintain the activity at the required intensity (Allen, Lamb, and Westerblad 2008). Muscle fibers expressing a high proportion of MHC Type I are better able to resist fatigue during repeated contractions (Bottinelli and Reggiani 2000). Although the mechanisms behind fatigue are complex and specific to the task (MacIntosh, Gardiner, and McComas 2006), it is clear that the completion of prior muscular contractions can have a significant effect on the expression of muscular strength.

It is important to note that fatigue is not just an acute phenomenon that occurs immediately following muscular contractions, dissipating rapidly to restore muscle function; the depression in force following muscular contractions could last days, especially when the movements involve the SSC (Nicol, Avela, and Komi 2006; Stewart et al. 2008). Therefore, both the short- and long-term effects of prior muscular contractions on muscular force should be considered when measuring muscular strength.

Postactivation Potentiation

Research has shown that performing maximal or near-maximal muscular contractions can produce short-term increases in the maximal force produced by the stimulated muscles in a phenomenon known as postactivation potentiation (PAP) (Hodgson, Docherty, and Robbins 2005). The mechanical specificity between the exercise used to induce PAP and the performance exercise appears to confer a substantial influence on the efficacy of the PAP effect (Hodgson et al. 2005). Although the mechanisms responsible for the PAP effect are not completely clear (Robbins 2005), PAP represents a method to potentially increase the expression of muscular strength in the short-term.

Neural Influences on Muscular Strength

Up to this point, consideration has only been given to the mechanical variables associated with isolated skeletal muscle or groups of muscles and how force production is affected. However, during muscular efforts by the intact motor system, the central nervous system has a profound effect on the expression of muscular strength. Increasing the number of motor units recruited during a voluntary contraction can increase the magnitude of muscular force, while increasing the rate at which the motor neurons discharge action potentials (rate coding) will have a similar effect (Duchateau, Semmler, and Enoka 2006). The force at which the voluntary recruitment of motor units is complete differs among muscles (Moritz et al. 2005; Oya, Riek, and Creswell 2009).

An understanding of neural influences on the expression of strength has led to the development of methods to augment muscular strength. For example, the superimposition of an electrical stimulus during a maximal voluntary muscular contraction has been shown to increase the magnitude of the force developed (Paillard et al. 2005). This has led some authors to distinguish between voluntary muscular strength and absolute (superimposed stimulation) muscular strength (Zatsiorsky 1995). Although such superimposition methods have been used to test the strength of isolated muscles or the activity of muscles acting across a single joint, their utility with complex, multijoint movements such as those experienced in sport and daily activities has been questioned on both practical and safety grounds (Stone, Stone, and Sands 2007).

As previously stated, the expression of muscular strength in a given test is likely to result from the interaction of the force developed by groups of muscles. A simplified representation of a joint served by an antagonistic pair of muscles shows that the force associated with the contraction of the agonist is influenced by the activity of the antagonist. Therefore, the net force developed during a given movement depends on the degree of coactivation between the antagonistic pair of muscles acting across a joint. Researchers have shown that athletes exhibit less coactivation during muscular strength tests than sedentary people do (Amiridis et al. 1996), which may partly explain the greater strength values recorded for well-trained subjects.

Finally, the activation of motor units during a task has been shown to be affected by the orientation of the body segments (Brown, Kautz, and Dairaghi 1996; Person 1974) and the direction of force applied during a given movement (Ter Haar Romney, van der Gon, and Gielen 1982; 1984). This implies that the expression of muscular strength is influenced by posture.

Joint Torque

Although the aforementioned neuromechanical properties determine force production in skeletal muscle, during movements of the human body, the motion of body segments is the result of torques acting at joints as opposed to muscular

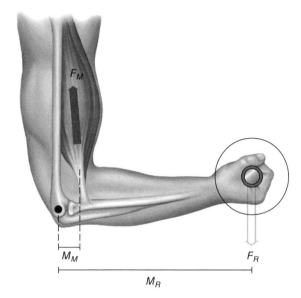

FIGURE 7.3 Schematic representation of a muscular torque acting at a joint.

Reprinted, with permission, from National Strength and Conditioning Association, 2008, Biomechanics of resistance training, by E. Harman. In *Essentials of Strength Training and Conditioning*, 3rd ed., edited by T.R. Baechle and R.W. Earle (Champaign, IL: Human Kinetics), 70.

forces alone. (In a strictly mechanical sense, a torque involves pure rotation and so the correct mechanical terminology refers to the moment of a force, or simply the moment, acting at a joint [Chapman 2008]. However, the term *torque* will be used in this chapter.) A torque is the rotational effect of a force acting on a body that is constrained to rotate about a fixed axis. It is calculated as the product of a force and the perpendicular distance between the line of action of the force and the axis of rotation:

$$\tau = Fd$$

where
τ = muscular torque, measured in newton-meters (N·m),
F = muscular force (N), and
d = the perpendicular distance between the line of action of the force and the axis of rotation, measured in meters (m).

Figure 7.3 shows the schematic representation of a muscle torque ($F_M \times M_M$) and an opposing torque associated with a resistance held in the hand ($F_R \times M_R$).

The perpendicular distance between the line of action of the force and the axis of rotations is known as the moment arm of the muscular force.

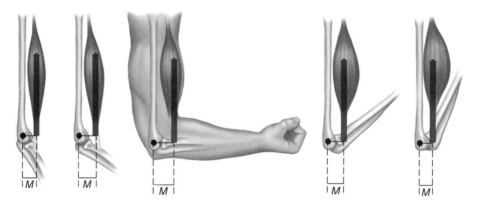

FIGURE 7.4   Changes in the moment arm associated with the muscular torque as the joint is accelerated through a range of motion.

Reprinted, with permission, from National Strength and Conditioning Association, 2008, Biomechanics of resistance training, by E. Harman. In *Essentials of Strength Training and Conditioning*, 3rd ed., edited by T.R. Baechle and R.W. Earle (Champaign, IL: Human Kinetics), 71.

From the equation of muscular torque, it is clear that alterations in muscular force or alterations in the moment arm can affect the torque produced. It is important to note that the moment arm associated with the muscular force will change as the joint is accelerated through a range of motion (see figure 7.4).

The torque measured at a joint in mechanical analyses of movements is the net torque exerted around the axis of rotation, the main cause of which is assumed to be the activity of the muscle groups crossing the joint. The contributions of other structures (i.e., ligaments, joint capsule) are considered minimal, as are the contributions from muscles that may be active but do not cross the joint of interest (see Zajac and Gordon, 1989, for a discussion of the complexity of determining the influence of active musculature on joint torques during multijoint movements). In some tests of muscular strength, joints are isolated so that the torque can be assumed to result from the active musculature crossing the joint (see the section Isokinetic Strength Testing). Such tests may not be valid for the assessment of multijoint movements that typically occur in sport and daily activities.

Dynamic muscle contractions are often referred to as isotonic, meaning that the tension developed by the muscle remains constant during the contraction (Lieber 2002). Although this may be true in isolated muscle preparations, it is unlikely to be true for muscular contractions taking place *in vivo* because of the concomitant moment arm changes. Therefore, the term *isoinertial* has been suggested to describe the *in vivo* muscle actions when performing dynamic contractions against loads of constant mass (Abernethy, Wilson, and Logan 1995). This term is used in this chapter.

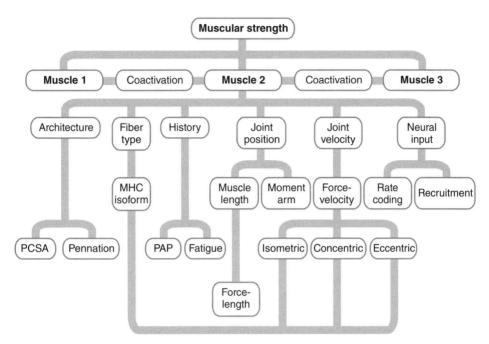

FIGURE 7.5 Mechanical factors affecting the expression of muscular strength in a given test. MHC = myosin heavy chain isoform; PCSA = physiological cross-sectional area; PAP = postactivation potentiation.

Adapted from V. Baltzopoulos, and N.P. Gleeson. 1996. Skeletal muscle function. In *Kinanthropometry and Exercise Physiology Laboratory Manual: Tests, Procedures and Data*, edited by R. Eston and T. Reilly, 7-35. London, UK: Routledge.

It is important to recognize that joint motion *in vivo* rarely results from the torque produced by a single muscle. Rather, a number of muscles operate simultaneously, each of which has unique mechanical characteristics (e.g., fiber type, architecture, moment arms). Therefore, the expression of strength in a given test will result from the interaction of mechanical properties associated with groups of activated muscles (see figure 7.5).

Muscular Strength Defined

From the knowledge of the many mechanical and physiological factors that contribute to the force developed by a muscle, our definition of muscular strength can now be refined to the ability of a muscle or group of muscles to voluntarily produce a force or torque against an external resistance under specific conditions defined by muscle action, movement velocity, and posture. *Maximal muscular strength* is then the ability to voluntarily produce a maximal force or torque under specific conditions defined by muscle action, movement velocity, and posture.

Sport Performance and Muscular Strength

The first step when developing a training program for any athlete is to perform a needs analysis to evaluate the important physical characteristics of both the sport and the athlete (Baechle, Earle, and Wathen 2008). Physical tests should be used to determine areas of weakness relative to the specific demands of the sport. This will allow the development of an appropriate training program. As the athlete progresses, the effectiveness of the training program should be evaluated using physical tests. The expression of maximal muscular strength has been shown to be important in many sports including baseball, basketball, American football, rugby, soccer, and sprint running (Baker and Newton 2006; Bartlett, Storey, and Simons 1989; Cometti et al. 2001; Fry and Kraemer, 1991; Latin, Berg, and Baechle 1994; Meckel et al. 1995). Clearly, tests of maximal muscular strength would help strength and conditioning professionals develop and monitor training programs for athletes in these sports.

Performances in many sports are limited by the time athletes have to develop force. For example, foot contact times of 220 milliseconds or less have been reported for the long jump and high jump (Dapena and Chung 1988; Luhtanen and Komi 1979), and contact times of 120 milliseconds or less have been reported during sprint running (Kuitunen, Komi, and Kyrolainen 2002). Because tests of maximal muscular strength are often unconstrained by time, some authors have suggested that such tests are not indicative of the mechanical capabilities of the muscle (Green 1992; Komi 1984; Tidow 1990). As a result, tests in which force production is limited by time (rate of force development) have been recommended (these tests are discussed in chapter 9).

Because maximal muscular strength appears to be strongly related to the ability to develop force quickly, strong people are able to generate force rapidly even when the external load they are moving is relatively light (Moss et al. 1997). Indeed, Schmidtbleicher (1992) postulated that maximal strength was the foundation on which muscular power is developed. Therefore, a mesocycle in which maximal strength is increased precedes a mesocycle emphasizing muscular power in the development of a periodized training program (Bompa and Haff 2009; Stone, Stone, and Sands 2007). Measures of maximal muscular strength can also be used to determine the training loads used during these mesocycles. This again highlights the importance of maximal muscular strength tests for strength and conditioning professionals.

Methods of Measurement

Although many of the factors affecting the expression of muscular strength cannot be controlled by the fitness professional interested in assessing muscular strength, many can. Therefore, before selecting a specific test of muscular strength, the fitness professional must consider several issues including the specificity of the test, the warm-up protocol, and the timing and order of muscular strength tests.

Specificity of Muscular Strength

From the preceding discussion of the mechanical and physiological factors affecting muscular strength, it should be apparent that the expression of muscular strength is specific to the test employed. Using tests of muscular strength that are mechanically dissimilar to the performance of interest can compromise the external and predictive validity of the data gathered. For example, differences between training and testing exercises in terms of the type of muscle contraction used (Abernethy and Jürimäe 1996; Rutherford and Jones 1986), open- versus closed-kinetic chain movements (Augustsson et al. 1998; Carroll et al. 1998), and bilateral versus unilateral movements (Häkkinen et al. 1996; Häkkinen and Komi 1983) have been shown to influence the magnitude of the gains in muscular strength accrued following a period of resistance training. Therefore, fitness professionals should consider the movement characteristics of any strength test used; the movements should be similar to the performance of interest with respect to the following mechanical factors (Siff 2000; Stone, Stone, and Sands 2007):

Movement Patterns

- *Complexity of movement.* This involves such factors as single versus multijoint movements.

- *Postural factors.* The posture adopted in a given movement dictates the activation of the muscles responsible for force production.

- *Range of motion and regions of accentuated force production.* During typical movements, the range of motion at a joint will change as will the associated muscular forces and torques. Such information can be gathered from a biomechanical analysis of the movement.

- *Muscle actions.* This concerns the performance of concentric, eccentric, or isometric muscle contractions. As mentioned previously, such information is not always intuitive and may not be identifiable from observing the joint motion associated with the movement.

Force Magnitude (Peak and Mean Force)
Force magnitude refers to joint torques as well as ground reaction forces (GRF) during the movement. This information is garnered from biomechanical analyses.

Rate of Force Development (Peak and Mean Force)
Rate of force development refers to the rate at which a joint torque or the GRF is developed.

Acceleration and Velocity Parameters

Usually, in sporting and everyday movements, both velocity and acceleration characteristics change throughout the movement. Velocity is defined as the rate at which the position of a body changes per unit of time, whereas acceleration refers to the rate at which the velocity changes per unit of time. Given Newton's second law of motion ($a = F / m$), the greatest accelerations are observed when the net forces acting on the body are largest. However, the greatest velocities will not coincide with the largest accelerations and, therefore, the largest net forces (unless the person is moving in a dense fluid such as water).

Ballistic Versus Nonballistic Movements

Ballistic movements are those in which motion results from an initial impulse from a muscular contraction, followed by the relaxation of the muscle. The motion of the body continues as a result of the momentum that it possesses from the initial impulse (this is the impulse-momentum relationship). This is in contrast to nonballistic movements, in which muscular contraction is constant throughout the movement. These categories of movements involve different mechanisms of nervous control.

Consideration of these mechanical variables will increase the likelihood of selecting a valid test of the muscular strength. Researchers have raised the concern that the relationships among the dependent variables associated with strength tests (e.g., maximal external load lifted, maximal force generated) and performance variables are rarely actually assessed (Abernethy, Wilson, and Logan 1995; Murphy and Wilson 1997). These relationships are discussed in relation to each test covered in this chapter where appropriate.

The type of equipment used for muscular strength tests has significant implications. For example, some tests of muscular strength can be performed using either machine weights, in which the movement is constrained to follow a fixed path, or free weights, in which the movement is relatively unconstrained. However, a test performed with machine weights will not necessarily produce the same outcome as the same test performed with free weights. Cotterman, Darby, and Skelly (2005) reported that the values recorded for measures of maximal muscular strength were different during both the squat and bench press movements when the exercises were performed in a Smith machine compared to when they were performed with free weights. Testing muscular strength with different types of equipment introduces significant systematic bias into the data and therefore severely compromises the reliability of the measures as well as the external validity.

Warm-Up Considerations

A warm-up is often performed prior to exercise to optimize performance and reduce the risk of injury (Bishop 2003, *a* and *b*; Shellock and Prentice 1985). As stated previously, the force capabilities of a muscle can be affected by the completion of previous contractions, resulting in either a decrease in force (fatigue) or an increase in force (PAP). Indeed, both fatigue and PAP are proposed to exist at opposite ends of a continuum of skeletal muscle contraction (Rassier 2000). Therefore, exercises performed as part of an active warm-up could significantly alter the expression of muscular strength during the test.

An increase in the temperature of the working muscles has been reported following both passive (e.g., external heating) and active (e.g., engaging in specific exercises) warm-up activities (Bishop 2003, *a* and *b*). However, the effects of increased temperature on measures of maximal muscular strength are unclear with increases in maximal isometric torque reported by some authors (Bergh and Ekblom 1979), whereas others have reported no change (de Ruiter et al. 1999).

Static stretches are often included in the warm-up routines of athletes. Researchers have reported a reduction in force during maximal voluntary contractions following an acute bout of static stretches (Behm, Button, and Butt 2001; Kokkonen, Nelson, and Cornwell 1998), leading some to propose that static stretches be excluded from warm-up routines prior to strength and power performances (Young and Behm 2002). However, Rubini, Costa, and Gomes (2007) recently noted methodological issues with many of the static stretching studies, concluding that an interference with muscular strength is usually observed following a stretching protocol in which many exercises are held for relatively long durations, which runs counter to common practice. Therefore, including static stretches in a warm-up routine prior to muscular strength testing may be permissible, as long as the total stretch duration is not excessive (four sets of exercises for each muscle group with 10-30 seconds stretch duration is recommended) and that the exercises are performed consistently during subsequent testing sessions.

Clearly, the warm-up performed prior to a strength test can have a significant influence on the expression of muscular strength, and so the examiner should give the warm-up due consideration. However, the most important factor associated with the warm-up would appear to be the consistency of the exercises incorporated; any alteration in the exercises performed will compromise the validity and reliability of the test. Jeffreys (2008) outlined the following warm-up protocols:

- *General warm-up.* Five to 10 minutes of low-intensity activity aimed at increasing heart rate, blood flow, deep muscle temperature, and respiration rate.

- *Specific warm-up.* Eight to 12 minutes of performing dynamic stretches incorporating movements that work through the range of motion required in the subsequent performance. This period is followed by gradually increasing the intensity of the movement-specific dynamic exercises.

Timing and Order of Tests

Researchers have reported that the expression of strength under both isometric and isokinetic conditions is affected by the time of day the tests are taken, with greater strength values being recorded in the early evening (Guette, Gondin, and Martin 2005; Nicolas et al. 2005). Although the mechanisms behind this diurnal effect are unclear, the implication is that examiners need to consider the time of day when administering strength tests and to ensure consistency when administering the test during future sessions.

A test of muscular strength may be one of a number of tests performed on a person. In this case, the fitness professional needs to consider where to place the muscular strength test in the battery. This consideration is important given the effect that contractile history can have on the expression of muscular strength. Harman (2008) proposed the following order for tests in a battery based on energy system requirements and the skill or coordination demands of the tests:

Nonfatiguing tests (anthropometric measurements)

Agility tests

Maximum power and strength tests

Sprint tests

Muscular endurance tests

Fatiguing anaerobic tests

Aerobic capacity tests

Following this order should maximize the reliability of each test.

Field Tests for Muscular Strength

Field tests do not require the use of specialized laboratory equipment, such as force platforms or dynamometers. Field tests for muscular strength tend to be isoinertial, meaning that subjects lift a load in a specified movement; the magnitude of the load provides a measure of maximal muscular strength. Although many field tests incorporate the SSC, concentric- and eccentric-only measures are also possible.

The maximal load that can be lifted during a low number of repetitions (usually a single repetition or three repetitions) in a specific movement with appropriate technique constitutes a field test for maximal muscular strength. Although the maximal load lifted during the specific test is recorded by the examiner, this value is often expressed relative to the subject's body mass using an allometric method (load lifted / body mass$^{2/3}$), which can account for differences in anthropometric dimensions that could influence the expression of maximal muscular strength (Jaric, Mirkov, and Markovic

2005). Such scaling techniques can enhance the comparisons in maximal muscular strength values among subjects.

Some authors have noted that tests employing three repetitions (3-repetition maximum, or 3RM) are safer and more reliable than those in which the subject lifts a maximal load once (1RM) (Tan 1999). However, 1RM tests have been used with children (Faigenbaum, Milliken, and Wescott 2003) and elderly people (Adams et al. 2000; Rydwik et al. 2007) without any injuries reported. Similarly, 1RM tests have been shown to have acceptable reliability (correlation coefficients ≥.79) in a variety of movements (Braith et al. 1993; Hoeger et al. 1990; Ploutz-Snyder and Giamis 2001; Rydwik et al. 2007). Therefore, only 1RM tests are discussed here—specifically, the bilateral back squat, unilateral back squat, leg press, and bench press (free weights and machine). Only tests that have clear procedures and published reliability data (systematic bias, test–retest correlation, and within-subject variation, where possible) are included. It should be noted that because all of the procedures discussed here require the examiner to make an *a priori* estimation of a load equivalent to the subject's 1RM, errors in the final value are possible.

1RM BILATERAL BACK SQUAT

The 1RM bilateral back squat protocol has been used with recreationally active college-aged men; the 1RM values were achieved within five attempts on average (Moir et al. 2005; 2007). McBride and colleagues (2002) used this protocol successfully with well-trained resistance athletes performing the squat in a Smith-type machine. Adams and colleagues (2000) used a similar protocol to test the 1RM strength of older women (mean age: 51 years) using a squat press machine.

EQUIPMENT

- Standard squat rack (crossbars placed at appropriate height)
- Olympic barbell
- Olympic plates

TECHNIQUE (EARLE AND BAECHLE 2008)

The subject grasps the barbell with a closed, pronated grip slightly wider than shoulder width. The barbell should be placed above the posterior deltoids (high bar position). The feet should be slightly wider than shoulder width and pointing slightly outward when the subject begins the descent. The subject reaches the lowest point in the descent when the top of the thighs are parallel to the ground (see figure 7.6), and the barbell should rise in a continuous motion without assistance. For safety, at least two spotters should stand on either side of the barbell and follow the bar during the descent and the ascent.

PROCEDURE (BAECHLE, EARLE, AND WATHEN 2008)

1. The subject warms up by performing repetitions with a load that allows 5 to 10 repetitions.

2. One-minute rest.

3. Estimate a warm-up load that allows the subject to complete three to five repetitions by adding 30 to 40 pounds (14 to 18 kg), or 10 to 20%, to the load used in step 1.

4. Two-minute rest.

5. Estimate a near-maximal load that will allow the subject to complete two or three repetitions by adding 30 to 40 pounds (14 to 18 kg), or 10 to 20%, to the load used in step 3.

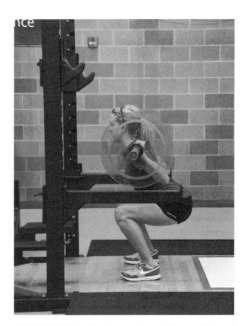

FIGURE 7.6 The lowest position achieved during the 1RM back squat. Note also the high bar position of the barbell.

6. Two- to four-minute rest.

7. The subject performs a 1RM attempt by increasing the load used in step 5 by 30 to 40 pounds (14 to 18 kg), or 10 to 20%.

8. Two- to four-minute rest.

9. If the subject fails the 1RM attempt, decrease the load by removing 15 to 20 pounds (7 to 9 kg), or 5 to 10%, and have the subject perform one repetition.

10. Two- to four-minute rest.

11. Continue increasing or decreasing the load until the subject can complete one repetition with appropriate technique. The subject's 1RM should be achieved within five attempts.

RELIABILITY

Test–retest correlations of between .92 and .99 have been reported for 1RM back squat loads using the procedure outlined here with recreationally active and resistance-trained men (McBride et al. 2002; Sanborn et al. 2000).

VALIDITY

Moderate ($r = .47$) to very large ($r = .85$) correlations between 1RM back squat loads and measures of athletic performance such as sprint running and agility have been reported (Chaouachi et al. 2009; Peterson, Alvar, and Rhea 2006; Requena et al. 2009; Young and Bilby 1993). Also, 1RM back

TABLE 7.1 Percentile Values for the 1RM Back Squat for American Football Players of Various Ages and Playing Levels

% rank	HIGH SCHOOL (14–15 YEARS)		HIGH SCHOOL (16–18 YEARS)		NCAA DIVISION I		NCAA DIVISION III	
	lb	kg	lb	kg	lb	kg	lb	kg
90	385	175	465	211	500	227	470	214
80	344	156	425	193	455	207	425	193
70	325	148	405	184	430	195	405	184
60	305	139	365	166	405	184	385	175
50	295	134	335	152	395	180	365	166
40	275	125	315	143	375	170	365	166
30	255	116	295	134	355	161	335	152
20	236	107	275	125	330	150	315	143
10	205	93	250	114	300	136	283	129
Mean	294	134	348	158	395	180	375	170
SD	73	33	88	40	77	35	75	34
n	170		249		1,074		588	

Data from Hoffman 2006.

squat loads have been shown to discriminate among playing positions within collegiate American football and basketball (Carbuhn et al. 2008; Latin et al. 1994) as well as differentiating playing levels in collegiate American football (Fry and Kraemer 1991). Similarly, 1RM back squat values have been shown to predict playing time in collegiate basketball (Hoffman et al. 1996). Percentile values for the 1RM back squat for American football players of various ages and playing levels are shown in table 7.1.

1RM UNILATERAL BACK SQUAT

Because many sporting and daily activities require unilateral force production by the lower body (e.g., walking, running, kicking), the discussion of a 1RM unilateral squat test is included here.

EQUIPMENT

- Standard squat rack (crossbars placed at appropriate height)
- Olympic barbell
- Olympic plates
- An extra support surface is required to place the foot of the noninvolved leg on during the movement.

TECHNIQUE (MCCURDY ET AL. 2004)

The subject approaches and lifts the barbell as per the 1RM back squat. The top of the foot of the noninvolved leg is placed behind the subject on a supporting surface that is placed at a distance that maintains hip extension of the noninvolved leg. For safety, at least two spotters should stand on either side of the barbell and follow the bar during the descent and the ascent. The subject descends until the angle between the tibia and the femur reaches 90° and then begins the ascent (see figure 7.7).

During the descent, the examiner observes the subject's involved leg and the barbell. A successful lift is determined by an absence of posterior movement of the barbell and concomitant anterior movement of the knee, thus ensuring that the load remains primarily over the involved leg.

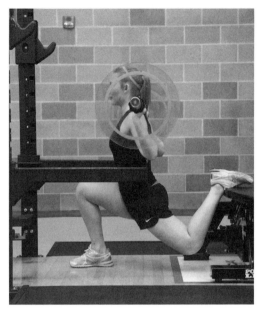

FIGURE 7.7 Unilateral back squat. The subject is at the lowest point of the movement, with a 90° angle at the knee joint.

PROCEDURE (MCCURDY ET AL. 2004)

1. Familiarization sessions are performed to establish appropriate submaximal loads allowing for 5 to 10 repetitions to be completed.

2. The subject performs five minutes of jogging and self-selected stretching exercises.

3. A load is selected such that the subject can achieve 5 to 10 repetitions.

4. One-minute rest.

5. The load is increased by 10 to 20%, and the subject performs five repetitions.

6. Three- to five-minute rest.

7. The load is increased by 20 to 30%, and the subject performs one repetition.

8. If the subject is successful, provide a three- to five-minute rest, increase the load by 10 to 20%, and have the subject attempt another single repetition. If the subject is unsuccessful, provide a three- to five-minute rest, decrease the load by 5 to 10%, and have the subject complete one repetition.

9. Continue increasing or decreasing the load until the subject can complete one repetition with appropriate technique. The subject should achieve 1RM within five attempts.

RELIABILITY

Test–retest correlation coefficients of .98 and .99 have been reported for trained college-aged men and women, respectively, using the outlined procedure (McCurdy et al. 2004). In untrained college-aged men and women, correlation coefficients of .99 and .97, respectively, have been reported (McCurdy et al. 2004).

VALIDITY

There are currently no published data to validate this test.

1RM MACHINE LEG PRESS

Fitness professionals may not wish to have older subjects perform a 1RM test using free weights for safety reasons (Hoffman 2006). The 1RM machine leg press is often used as a measure of maximal lower body muscular strength with older subjects (Foldvari et al. 2000; Henwood, Riek, and Taafe 2008; Marsh et al. 2009).

EQUIPMENT

Various types of machines have been used to test 1RM leg press strength in older subjects. For example, Foldvari and colleagues (2000) used a pneumatic resistance machine (Keiser Sports Health Equipment Inc., Fresno, CA), and Phillips and colleagues (2004) used a plate-loaded machine (Paramount Fitness Corp., Los Angeles, CA). The protocol outlined here is that to be used on a plate-loaded machine.

TECHNIQUE (PHILLIPS ET AL. 2004)

The subject sits in the leg press chair with both feet on the foot-plates and an internal angle of 90° at the knee (see figure 7.8). The subject should not produce excessive lordosis of the lumbar spine during the movement.

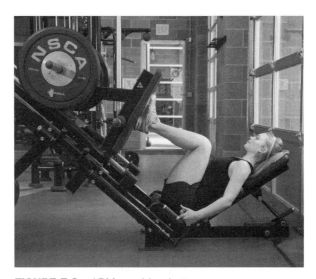

FIGURE 7.8 1RM machine leg press.

TABLE 7.2 Percentile Values for 1RM Leg Press Normalized to Body Mass for the General Population

% rank	20–29 YEARS M	20–29 YEARS F	30–39 YEARS M	30–39 YEARS F	40–49 YEARS M	40–49 YEARS F	50–59 YEARS M	50–59 YEARS F	60+ YEARS M	60+ YEARS F
90	2.27	2.05	2.07	1.73	1.92	1.63	1.80	1.51	1.73	1.40
80	2.13	1.66	1.93	1.50	1.82	1.46	1.71	1.30	1.62	1.25
70	2.05	1.42	1.85	1.47	1.74	1.35	1.64	1.24	1.56	1.18
60	1.97	1.36	1.77	1.32	1.68	1.26	1.58	1.18	1.49	1.15
50	1.91	1.32	1.71	1.26	1.62	1.19	1.52	1.09	1.43	1.08
40	1.83	1.25	1.65	1.21	1.57	1.12	1.46	1.03	1.38	1.04
30	1.74	1.23	1.59	1.16	1.51	1.03	1.39	0.95	1.30	0.98
20	1.63	1.13	1.52	1.09	1.44	0.94	1.32	0.86	1.25	0.94
10	1.51	1.02	1.43	0.94	1.35	0.76	1.22	0.75	1.16	0.84

Reprinted, by permission, from J. Hoffman, 2006, *Norms for fitness, performance, and health* (Champaign, IL: Human Kinetics), 35.

PROCEDURE (PHILLIPS ET AL. 2004)

1. The subject performs a five-minute general warm-up on a stationary recumbent cycle.

2. The subject performs several lifts at low or zero resistance to reestablish familiarity with the movement.

3. Select an initial resistance slightly above that of the familiarization resistance (add 5 to 15 lb, or 2.25 to 6.75 kg).

4. The subject performs one lift with good technique.

5. The subject rates perceived exertion on a rating of perceived exertion (RPE) scale of 6 to 20.

6. The subject rests for one minute if RPE is below 12, and for two minutes if RPE is above 12.

7. Add 5 to 10 pounds (2.25 to 4.50 kg) depending on the RPE, and have the subject repeat step 4.

8. Have the subject repeat the process to momentary muscular fatigue (i.e., the subject cannot continue) or volitional fatigue (i.e., the subject does not wish to continue).

9. Record the maximum load lifted.

RELIABILITY

Phillips and colleagues (2004) reported within-subject variations of 3.4 and 5.6% in older men (mean age: 75.8 years) and women (mean age: 75.2 years), respectively, following a familiarization session.

VALIDITY

Foldvari and colleagues (2000) reported a moderate correlation (r = -.43) between 1RM leg press load and functional status in older women (mean age: 74.8 years). However, on the strength of this relationship, 1RM leg press explains less than 20% of the variance in functional status in older women. Percentile values for the 1RM leg press normalized to body mass (1RM value / body mass) for the general population are shown in table 7.2. Note that the 1RM values are recorded in pounds.

1RM ECCENTRIC MACHINE LEG PRESS

Because of the importance of eccentric muscular strength in performance (LaStayo et al. 2003), Hollander and colleagues (2007) developed a protocol to test eccentric strength during a leg press movement using a modified leg press machine.

EQUIPMENT

A weight stack machine (Master Trainer, Rayne, LA) was modified with levers attached to allow spotters to lift and hold the load prior to the subjects' eccentric attempts (see figure 7.9).

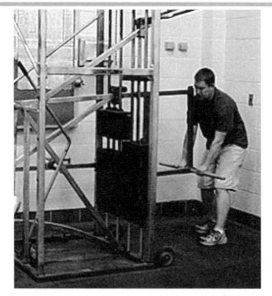

FIGURE 7.9 Modified weight stack machines in the 1RM eccentric leg press.

Reprinted, by permission, from D.B. Hollander et al., 2007, "Maximal eccentric and concentric strength discrepancies between young men and women for dynamic resistance exercise," *Journal of Strength and Conditioning Research* 21: 34-40.

TECHNIQUE (HOLLANDER ET AL. 2007)

The load is held in place by spotters, and the subject is instructed to lower the load in three seconds. The motion of the load during descent is observed to ensure the appropriate cadence.

PROCEDURE (HOLLANDER ET AL. 2007)

1. The subject performs two or three sets of 5 to 10 repetitions with a load that is 40 to 60% of the estimated maximum with three- to five-minute rests between sets.

2. The subject performs one or two sets of five repetitions with a load that is 80% of the estimated maximum with three- to five-minute rests between sets.

3. The subject attempts the estimated 1RM.

4. Following a three- to five-minute rest, the load is increased or decreased depending on whether the subject has succeeded in lifting the estimated 1RM load.

5. The process is repeated until the subject achieves a 1RM load within five lifts.

RELIABILITY

There are currently no published reliability data for this test.

VALIDITY

There are currently no published data to validate this test.

1RM BENCH PRESS (FREE WEIGHTS)

The 1RM bench press protocol has been used with recreationally active college-aged men where the 1RM values were achieved within four attempts on average (Moir et al. 2007). Adams and colleagues (2000) used a similar protocol successfully to test maximal strength in older females (mean age: 51 years).

EQUIPMENT

- Standard flat bench with barbell stands
- Olympic barbell
- Olympic plates

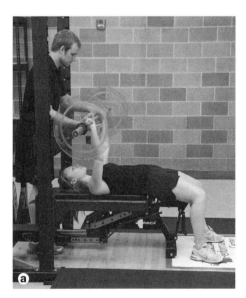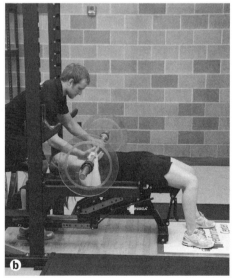

FIGURE 7.10   Starting position and the lowest position achieved during the 1RM bench press.

Photos courtesy of Gavin L. Moir.

TECHNIQUE (EARLE AND BAECHLE 2008)

The subject lies supine on the bench with the head, shoulders, and buttocks in contact with the bench and both feet in contact with the floor (five-point contact). The bar is grasped with a closed, pronated grip slightly wider than shoulder width. The spotter assists the subject in removing the bar to the beginning position, where the bar is held with the elbows extended. For safety, a spotter should stand close to the subject's head holding the bar with a closed, alternated grip, and follow the bar during the descent and the ascent without touching it. Each repetition begins from this position. The bar is lowered to touch the chest at around the level of the nipple and is then raised in a continuous movement until the elbows are fully extended (see figure 7.10). During the movement, the subject should maintain the five contact points and not bounce the bar from the chest at the lowest part of the movement.

PROCEDURE (BAECHLE, EARLE, AND WATHEN 2008)

1. The subject warms up by performing repetitions with a load that allows 5 to 10 repetitions.
2. One-minute rest.
3. Estimate a warm-up load that allows the subject to complete three to five repetitions by adding 10 to 20 pounds (4.5 to 9 kg), or 5 to 10%, to the load used in step 1.
4. Two-minute rest.
5. Estimate a near-maximal load that will allow the subject to complete two or three repetitions by adding 10 to 20 pounds (4.5 to 9 kg), or 5 to 10%, to the load used in step 3.
6. Two- to four-minute rest.
7. Instruct the subject to perform a 1RM attempt by increasing the load used in step 5 by 10 to 20 pounds (4.5 to 9 kg), or 5 to 10%.
8. Two- to four-minute rest.
9. If the subject fails the 1RM attempt, decrease the load by removing 5 to 10 pounds (2.3 to 4.5 kg), or 2.5 to 5%, and have the subject perform one repetition.
10. Two- to four-minute rest.
11. Continue increasing or decreasing the load until the subject can complete one repetition with appropriate technique. The subject's 1RM should be achieved within five attempts.

RELIABILITY

There are no published reliability data for this test.

TABLE 7.3   Percentile Values for the 1RM Back Squat for American Football Players of Various Ages and Playing Levels

% rank	HIGH SCHOOL (14–15 YEARS) lb	HIGH SCHOOL (14–15 YEARS) kg	HIGH SCHOOL (16–18 YEARS) lb	HIGH SCHOOL (16–18 YEARS) kg	NCAA DIVISION I lb	NCAA DIVISION I kg	NCAA DIVISION III lb	NCAA DIVISION III kg
90	243	110	275	125	370	168	365	166
80	210	95	250	114	345	157	325	148
70	195	89	235	107	325	148	307	140
60	185	84	225	102	315	143	295	134
50	170	77	215	98	300	136	280	127
40	165	75	205	93	285	130	273	124
30	155	70	195	89	270	123	255	116
20	145	66	175	80	255	116	245	111
10	125	57	160	73	240	109	225	102
Mean	179	81	214	97	301	137	287	130
SD	45	20	44	20	53	24	57	26
n	214		339		1,189		591	

Reprinted, by permission, from J. Hoffman, 2006, *Norms for fitness, performance, and health* (Champaign, IL: Human Kinetics), 36.

VALIDITY

Bench press tests of maximal muscular strength were able to discriminate among collegiate American football players of differing abilities (Fry and Kraemer 1991), while the 1RM bench press values performed in a Smith-type machine have been shown to differentiate among performance levels in rugby league players (Baker 2001; Baker and Newton 2006). A large correlation ($r = .64$) between 1RM load during the bench press and ball throwing velocity has been reported in handball players (Marques et al. 2007). Normative values for the 1RM bench press are shown in table 7.3.

1RM BENCH PRESS (MACHINE)

Because of possible safety issues, examiners may want to test the maximal upper body strength of older people using weight machines (Humphries et al. 1999; Izquierdo et al. 1999; Smith et al. 2003).

EQUIPMENT

As with the 1RM leg press, various machines have been used to test 1RM bench press strength in older people. For example, Smith and colleagues (2003) used a plate-loaded machine (Global Gym and Fitness Equipment Ltd, Weston, ON), and Izquierdo and colleagues (1999) used a Smith-type machine. The protocol outlined here is for use with a plate-loaded machine.

TECHNIQUE (PHILLIPS ET AL. 2004)

The subject holds the bar with a pronated grip and the elbows placed directly under the bar with the forearms vertical to create a 90° angle at the elbow joint. This configuration determines the grip width for each subject. The feet are placed on either side or on top of the bench, depending on subject preference. The bar should be placed directly over the midchest area. The subject is instructed to keep the back in contact with the bench throughout the lift and to breathe out when lifting the bar and breathe in when lowering the bar.

PROCEDURE (PHILLIPS ET AL. 2004)

1. The subject performs a five-minute general warm-up on a stationary recumbent cycle.
2. The subject performs several lifts at low or zero resistance to reestablish familiarity with the movement.
3. Select an initial resistance slightly above that of the familiarization resistance (add 5 to 15 lb, or 2.23 to 6.8 kg).
4. The subject performs one lift with good technique.
5. The subject rates perceived exertion on an RPE scale of 6 to 20.
6. The subject rests one minute if the RPE is below 12, and two minutes if the RPE is above 12.
7. Add 5 to 10 pounds (2.3 to 4.5 kg) depending on the RPE, and repeat step 4.
8. Have the subject repeat the process to momentary muscular fatigue (i.e., the subject cannot continue) or volitional fatigue (i.e., the subject does not wish to continue).
9. Record the maximum load lifted.

RELIABILITY

Phillips and colleagues (2004) reported within-subject variations of 5.4 and 5.2% in older men (mean age: 75.8 years) and women (mean age: 75.2 years), respectively, in the absence of familiarization sessions.

VALIDITY

The 1RM bench press has been used to differentiate dynamic strength of middle-aged (35 to 46 years) and older (60 to 74 years) men (Izquierdo et al. 1999), as well as middle-aged (45 to 49 years) and older (60 to 64 years) women (Humphries et al. 1999).

Predicting 1RM Values From Multiple Repetitions

Objections to maximal strength testing abound in the literature, including possible injury to untrained or older people as well as prohibitive time demands. Although the validity of some of these objections may be questioned, equations that allow fitness professionals to estimate a subject's 1RM value in a specific test based on multiple repetitions to failure performed with submaximal loads have been developed. In general, the accuracy of these equations tends to diminish as the number of submaximal repetitions performed increases (Kemmler et al. 2006; Mayhew et al. 2004; Reynolds, Gordon, and Robergs 2006). It is important to note that these equations have been developed for specific cohorts performing specific exercises.

An underlying assumption of these prediction equations is that the relationship between maximal strength and the number of repetitions performed at a percentage of 1RM does not change with training. In college-aged men, this assumption appears to hold true for multijoint exercises such as the bench press and leg press, but not for many single-joint exercises such as arm curls and leg extensions (Hoeger et al. 1990; Shimano et al. 2006). As such, the discussion here is broadly divided into equations developed for younger subjects (<40 years) and those developed for older subjects (>40 years) focusing on 1RM values for bench press and squat or leg press exercises.

Prediction Equations for Younger Subjects

Using a combined group of college-aged men and women, LeSuer and colleagues (1997) compared various equations and found the following to produce the most accurate prediction of a 1RM value from <10 repetitions to failure in both the squat and bench press exercises:

$$1RM = 100 \times l[48.8 + 53.8 \times e(-0.75 \times r)]$$

where
l = the load for a given RM range,
e = approximately 2.7181, and
r = the number of repetitions achieved.

This equation overestimated both squat and bench press loads by less than 1%. Kravitz and colleagues (2003) developed the following regression equation to predict 1RM back squat values based on a 10 to 16RM target in male high school powerlifters (15 to 18 years):

$$1RM = 159.9 + (0.103 \times r \times l) + (-11.552 \times r)$$

where
r = the number of repetitions achieved, and
l = the load for a given RM range.

This equation produced errors of approximately 5 kilograms (11 lb) in the estimation of 1RM back squat loads. The same authors developed the following regression equation to predict 1RM bench press values based on a 14 to 18RM target in the same subjects:

$$1RM = 90.66 + (0.085 \times r \times l) + (-5.306 \times r)$$

where
r = the number of repetitions achieved, and
l = the load for a given RM range.

This equation produced errors of less than 3 kilograms (6.6 lb) in the estimation of 1RM bench press loads.

Prediction Equations for Older Subjects

Very few equations to predict 1RM values have been developed for older subjects, particularly men. In a mixed group of older men (mean age: 73.1 years) and women (mean age: 69.1 years), Knutzen, Brilla, and Caine (1999) reported that the following equation provided the most accurate prediction of 1RM bench press load when using 7 to 10RM loads:

$$1RM = 100 \times l / [52.2 + 41.9 \times e(-0.55 \times r)]$$

where
l = the load for a given RM range,
e = approximately 2.7181, and
r = the number of repetitions achieved.

A correlation of .90 was demonstrated between the predicted and actual 1RM loads, although the equation underestimated the load. Using 3-5, 6-10, 11-15, and 16-20 repetition maximum (RM) loads, Kemmler and colleagues (2006) recently developed the following polynomial equation that could be used to predict the 1RM loads in trained postmenopausal women (mean age: 57.4 years) for exercises including the leg press and bench press:

$$1RM = l(0.988 - 0.0000584r^3 + 0.00190r^2 + 0.0104r)$$

where
l = the load for a given RM range, and
r = the number of repetitions achieved.

The 1RM loads using this prediction equation were generally underestimated for both the leg press and the bench press, although the errors were small ($\geq 2.5\%$).

In summary, the prediction equations may have some utility for fitness professionals given the associated accuracy. However, because all of the equations either overestimate or underestimate the actual 1RM value, values of maximal muscular strength should be measured directly.

Laboratory Tests for Maximal Muscular Strength

Laboratory tests require the use of equipment to test maximal muscular strength, usually a force platform (Blazevich, Gill, and Newton 2002; Kawamori et al. 2006) or a force transducer in a custom-designed system (Requena et al. 2009). Laboratory tests for maximal muscular strength generally provide a more objective assessment than field tests do. The discussion here focuses on the use of force platforms in tests for maximal muscular strength.

The use of a force platform allows for a direct measurement of GRF during multijoint, closed-kinetic chain movements. Usually, the vertical component of the GRF is measured in tests of muscular strength. The peak value is a common outcome measure, although measures of the impulse of the force are also possible, but rarely reported. The most common types of force platforms used in kinesiology can be divided into piezoelectric platforms (e.g., Kistler type 9281) and strain-gauge platforms (e.g., Advanced Mechanical Technologies Inc. type BP400600). All force platforms should have high linearity, low hysteresis, low cross-talk, and adequate system sensitivity (see Bartlett, 2007, for details on these variables).

The accuracy of measurements of maximal GRF during tests of maximal muscular strength depends on the system's sensitivity, which in turn depends on the analog-to-digital (A/D) converter used. Ideally, a 12-bit converter should be used to minimize the errors in the measurement of maximal force. However, the type of A/D converter used is absent from the methodologies published. Similarly, rarely are other signal-processing procedures (e.g., filtering of the force trace prior to analysis) reported in the methodologies. Such procedures can have a significant impact on the accuracy of the measurements.

Laboratory tests for muscular strength using force platforms can involve either dynamic or isometric muscular contractions. Both are discussed here.

Dynamic Measures of Maximal Muscular Strength

An advantage of using a force platform during dynamic tests of muscular strength is that eccentric forces can be measured directly. Tests for measuring eccentric forces during the back squat and bench press movements have been published, although only those associated with the back squat have reliability data. The loads used during the movements to record eccentric force vary between absolute loads (or percentages of body mass) and percentages of maximal strength (1RM).

Peak Eccentric Force During a Bilateral Back Squat

In a group of recreationally active college-aged men, Murphy and Wilson (1997) measured peak force during the eccentric phase of a back squat in a modified Smith machine (Plyopower Technologies, Lismore, Australia) positioned over a piezoelectric force platform (Kistler) sampling at 1,000 Hertz. The authors used a load of 200% body mass, and the bar descent was prevented beyond an internal knee angle of 109°. On command, subjects were instructed to resist the accelerating mass as quickly and with as much force as possible. The load was determined from pilot work as the greatest load that could be controlled in an eccentric–concentric action (i.e., the subjects were able to reverse the descent of the bar). Unfortunately, reliability statistics were not reported for peak eccentric force values. However, it was reported that the values did not change significantly following an eight-week resistance training program that elicited improvements in performance measures (sprint running and cycling) as well as increased 1RM back squat loads.

Frohm, Halvorsen, and Thorstensson (2005) measured eccentric force in a group of active men using a hydraulic motor machine that assisted the subjects in raising the load and controlled the velocity to a near-constant value during the eccentric phase. An absolute load of 200 kilograms (441 lb) was used. These authors reported a test–retest correlation coefficient of .81 and a within-subject variation of 9%.

Peak Eccentric Force During a Bench Press

Two studies have tested peak eccentric force during a bench press movement, both using a modified Smith machine placed over a piezoelectric force platform (Murphy, Wilson, and Pryor 1994; Wilson, Murphy, Giorgi 1996). Both used loads relative to the subjects' maximal muscular strength in the bench press. Wilson and colleagues (1996) used a load equivalent to 130% 1RM, and Murphy and colleagues (1994) used loads up to 150% of 1RM. Murphy and colleagues (1994) reported large correlations between eccentric force and a series of upper body performance tests ($r > .78$). However, Wilson and colleagues (1996) reported that eccentric force production did not change following eight weeks of resistance training. Unfortunately, method reliability was not reported in either study.

Isometric Measures of Maximal Muscular Strength

As previously mentioned, an isometric contraction occurs when muscular force is developed but the length of the muscle remains constant. Isometric measures of maximal muscular strength are common in the published literature. In general, these tests have been shown to have high reliability, although the validity of these tests for use with athletic populations has been questioned (see Wilson, 2000, for a review).

The problems with isometric muscular strength tests are attributed mainly to the poor relationships between isometric measures and dynamic performances arising from neural and mechanical differences. There is certainly evidence to support this view. For example, peak isometric force (PIF) in unilateral, single-joint exercise (knee extension) demonstrated only a moderate correlation ($r = -.42$) to sprinting performance in well-trained soccer players (Requena et al. 2009). However, this relationship was only slightly weaker than that between an isoinertial measure of maximal muscular strength and sprint performance ($r = -.47$). Baker, Wilson, and Carlyon (1994) reported that the changes in isometric and dynamic measures of maximal muscular strength were relatively unrelated ($r = .12$ to $.15$) following a 12-week resistance training program using isoinertial exercises with trained men.

Despite these studies' demonstrating the poor relationships between isometric measures and dynamic performance, others have provided contrary findings. For example, large ($r \geq .50$) and very large ($r = .87$) correlations have been reported between PIF during a multijoint movement (midthigh clean pull) and sprint cycling performance in trained cyclists (Stone et al. 2004) as well as vertical jump performance in trained weightlifters (Kawamori et al. 2006). Elsewhere, Stone and colleagues (2003) reported large to very large correlations between isometric peak force in a multijoint movement and athletic performance ($r = .67$ to $.75$). In a clinical setting, PIF during a leg press movement demonstrated a large correlation with functional tests in older women (mean age: 68.8 years), although less than 40% of the variance in the functional tests was explained by PIF (Forte and Macaluso 2008).

Taken together, isometric measures of maximal muscular strength can explain up to almost 80% of the variance in dynamic performance. This is not dissimilar to some of the dynamic tests of muscular strength reviewed here. Isometric tests also have the advantage of being relatively easy to administer in terms of time and require little skill to perform the movements.

General Procedures for Isometric Tests

With isometric testing, the joint angle significantly affects muscular force (see the section Factors Affecting Muscular Force Production); the joint angle used should be the one that elicits peak force (Murphy et al. 1995; Stone et al. 2003). Typically during the isometric tests, the force recordings are taken for at least three seconds with a minimum of one minute of rest between contractions (Bazett-Jones, Winchester, and McBride 2005; Blazevich, Gill, and Newton 2002; Brock Symons et al. 2004; Cheng and Rice 2005; Heinonen et al. 1994). The force trace may then be averaged across a time window (one second), which is likely to reduce the impact of any noise in the signal. At least two trials are recorded, and the trial in which the greatest PIF value was achieved is used in the analysis (Ahtiainen et al. 2005; Bazett-Jones et al. 2005; Blazevich, Gill, and Newton 2002; Brock Symons et al. 2004; Cheng and Rice 2005; Heinonen et al. 1994; Kawamori et al. 2006). When the outcome variable is PIF, the subject should be instructed to contract as hard as possible throughout the test to ensure that force is maximized (Christ et al. 1993).

PEAK ISOMETRIC FORCE DURING BILATERAL SQUATS

EQUIPMENT (BLAZEVICH, GILL, AND NEWTON 2002)

The exercise is performed in a Smith machine, and the vertical force trace is recorded from a piezoelectric force platform (Kistler, Winterthur, Switzerland) sampling at 1,000 Hertz.

TECHNIQUE (BLAZEVICH, GILL, AND NEWTON 2002)

The subject performs a squat with a bar, descending until the internal angle at the knee is 90°. The hip angle is measured in this position. The subject then approaches the bar in the Smith machine and descends from a standing position until the same knee and hip angles are achieved. The bar is then locked at this height to prevent any movement.

PROCEDURE (BLAZEVICH, GILL, AND NEWTON 2002)

1. The subject performs five minutes of moderate-intensity running followed by several warm-up repetitions with free weight squats.

2. The subject performs two warm-up repetitions of the isometric squat in the Smith machine, one at 60% of perceived maximum and the other at 80%.

3. The subject performs three maximal isometric efforts lasting four seconds, separated by three-minute rests.

Newton and colleagues (2002) used a similar protocol with a group of older men (average age: 61 years), in which they measured maximal force using chain-mounted force transducers.

RELIABILITY

A test–retest correlation coefficient of .97 has been reported for this protocol using recreationally active college-aged men (Blazevich, Gill, and Newton 2002).

VALIDITY

Large correlations ($r = .77$) have been reported between peak isometric force using this protocol and 1RM back squat load performed with free weights (Blazevich, Gill, and Newton 2002). However, this still leaves over 40% of the variance in squat performance unexplained.

PEAK ISOMETRIC FORCE DURING MIDTHIGH CLEAN PULLS

EQUIPMENT (KAWAMORI ET AL. 2006)

A custom adjustable squat rack (Sorinex Inc, Irmo, SC) that allows the bar to be fixed at the appropriate height. Force data are collected from a force platform (Advanced Mechanical Technologies Inc., Newton, MA) sampling at 500 Hertz. The subject is strapped to the bar using lifting wraps and athletic tape (see figure 7.11).

TECHNIQUE (KAWAMORI ET AL. 2006)

The height of the bar is determined by the subject's knee and hip angles. These angles are based on those used in the dynamic midthigh pull during training (mean knee angle: 141°; mean hip angle: 124°). The subject approaches the bar and grasps it as though performing the dynamic midthigh pull.

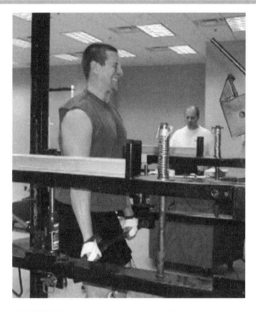

FIGURE 7.11   Isometric midthigh pull test.

Reprinted, by permission, from N. Kawamori et al., 2006, "Peak force and rate of force development during isometric and dynamic mid-thigh clean pulls performed at various intensities," *Journal of Strength and Conditioning Research* 20: 483-491. Journal of strength and conditioning research by National Strength & Conditioning Association (U.S.) Reproduced with permission of LIPPINCOTT WILLIAMS & WILKINS INC in the format Journal via Copyright Clearance Center.

PROCEDURE (KAWAMORI ET AL. 2006)

1. The subject performs a warm-up including dynamic exercises focusing on the muscle groups to be used in testing and five power cleans at 30 to 50% of the current 1RM.

2. The subject adopts the appropriate position under the bar and performs three practice isometric pulls.

3. Following a three-minute rest, the subject performs the first isometric pull as hard and fast as possible.

4. Following another three-minute rest, the subject performs the second and final isometric pull.

RELIABILITY

A test–retest correlation of .97 has been reported with male weightlifters (Kawamori et al. 2006).

VALIDITY

In trained weightlifters, moderate to strong correlations ($r = .55$ to $.82$) have been reported between isometric and dynamic measures of peak force during midthigh pulls, particularly as the load used during dynamic movement increased (Haff et al. 1997; Kawamori et al. 2006). One may expect such a finding given that the increase in load used during the dynamic movements may render them more "quasi-isometric." However, large correlations ($r = .82$ to .87) have been reported between peak force during the isometric midthigh pull and vertical jump performance (Kawamori et al. 2006). Similarly, Stone and colleagues (2003) reported moderate to large correlations ($r = .67$ to .75) between peak force during an isometric midthigh pull and shot put distance in a group of collegiate throwers. Interestingly, the relationships became stronger as the subjects progressed through an eight-week training period focusing on increasing maximal strength and strength-power. However, these correlation values still leave a large proportion of variance in athletic performance unexplained.

PEAK ISOMETRIC FORCE DURING A BENCH PRESS

EQUIPMENT (FALVO ET AL. 2007)

Standard bench and power rack placed over a commercial-grade floor scale containing four load cells (Rice Lake Weighing Systems, Rice Lake, WI) to sample vertical force at 1,000 Hertz.

TECHNIQUE (FALVO ET AL. 2007)

The subject grasps the bar as in the bench press. The height of the bar above the floor is adjusted so that the upper arms are parallel to the floor and the internal angle of the elbow joint is 90°. The bar should be in line with the midsternum. The bar is then fixed in this position (see figure 7.12).

PROCEDURE (FALVO ET AL. 2007)

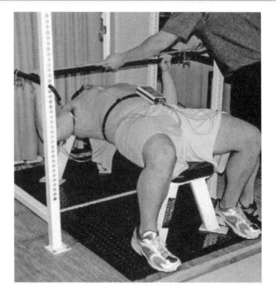

FIGURE 7.12 Isometric bench press test.

Reprinted, by permission, from M.J. Falvo et al., 2007, "Efficacy of prior eccentric exercise in attenuating impaired exercise performance after muscle injury in resistance trained men," *Journal of Strength and Conditioning Research* 21: 1053-1060. Journal of strength and conditioning research by National Strength & Conditioning Association (U.S.) Reproduced with permission of LIPPINCOTT WILLIAMS & WILKINS INC in the format Journal via Copyright Clearance Center.

1. The subject performs two submaximal repetitions at 50 and 75% of perceived maximal effort.

2. The subject performs a maximal isometric effort for three to five seconds with the instruction to contract as hard and as fast as possible.

3. Following a 30-second rest, the subject performs a second maximal isometric effort.

4. The force trace is filtered (fourth-order Butterworth with a 30 Hz cutoff), and the maximal value of peak force obtained from the two trials is recorded.

RELIABILITY

Using college-aged resistance-trained men, Falvo and colleagues (2007) reported a test–retest correlation of .90 and a within-subject variation of 6.6% for PIF.

VALIDITY

Ojanen, Rauhala, and Häkkinen (2007) found that peak isometric force during a bench press exercise was able to differentiate among male throwing athletes (shot put, discus, hammer) of various ages, and between the athletes and age-matched controls. PIF has been shown to be significantly reduced following eccentric contractions performed in the bench press movement (Falvo et al. 2007). Elsewhere, however, PIF during the bench press explained less than 30% of the variance in dynamic upper body performance (Murphy and Wilson 1996).

Isokinetic Strength Testing

Isokinetic means constant velocity, referring specifically to the angular velocity of a joint, which is constrained to rotate at a constant velocity across a range of the movement by a dynamometer (obviously, the velocity cannot be constant across the entire range given that there must be acceleration at the beginning and deceleration at the end of the movement). Isokinetic dynamometers allow rotations about a fixed axis and maintain constant, predetermined joint angular velocity by means of hydraulic (Akron) or electromagnetic (Biodex, Con-Trex, Cybex Norm, IsoMed 2000) mechanisms or a combination of both (Kin-Com).

It is important to recognize that although the joint motion may be constant across a given movement range during isokinetic testing, the shortening velocity of the contracting muscle fibers is unlikely to be (Ichinose et al. 2000). Furthermore, many of the tests involve single-joint, open-kinetic chain movements in which concentric and eccentric actions are performed. However, multijoint, closed-kinetic chain movements are available with certain dynamometers (Müller et al. 2007). Modifications can be made to isokinetic dynamometers to allow the testing of children (Deighan, De Ste Croix, and Armstrong 2003). The present focus is on single-joint rotational measurements performed on isokinetic dynamometers in which the outcome variable of interest is peak torque.

Validity of Isokinetic Measures of Muscular Strength

A criticism of isokinetic testing is that the angular velocities achievable on available dynamometers do not approach those achieved during sporting movements. For example, commercially available dynamometers are capable of achieving angular velocities of up to $555° \cdot s^{-1}$ (Baltzopoulos, 2008). However, angular extension velocities of greater than $1,000° \cdot s^{-1}$ have been reported at the knee joint during sprint running (Kivi, Maraj, and Gervais 2002), and internal shoulder rotation angular velocities in excess of $5,800° \cdot s^{-1}$ have been reported during the baseball pitching motion (Chu et al. 2009).

It would appear, therefore, that the criticisms of isokinetic dynamometry on the grounds of external validity would have some merit. However, low movement speeds are achieved during most tests of maximal muscular strength, and of course, no external movement occurs during isometric tests. Nevertheless, these tests are still widely used with athletes. Moreover, it is important to remember that the purpose of an isokinetic test is to assess the magnitude of the torque at a given velocity rather than the maximal angular velocities achievable in a given movement.

Using sprint running as an example, Johnson and Buckley (2001) reported a peak hip extensor torque of 377 N·m during the foot contact phase at a time when the joint angular velocity was around $400° \cdot s^{-1}$ (a peak hip extension angular velocity in excess of $800° \cdot s^{-1}$ occurred after this peak torque). When testing the peak isokinetic hip extension torque in trained sprinters, Blazevich and Jenkins (2002) reported average values of 302 N·m at a velocity of $60° \cdot s^{-1}$ and 254 N·m at a velocity of $480° \cdot s^{-1}$. Interestingly, these peak torque values increased following a period of resistance training that resulted in an improvement in sprinting speed and to the same extent as an isoinertial measure of muscular strength (1RM back squat).

In baseball pitching, Chu and colleagues (2009) reported peak internal shoulder rotation torques of around 65 N·m and peak internal shoulder rotation angular velocities in excess of $5,800° \cdot s^{-1}$. Carter and colleagues (2007) reported peak isokinetic internal rotation torques of around 60 N · m at an angular velocity of $300° \cdot s^{-1}$ measured on an isokinetic dynamometer. Again, the magnitude of the torque increased following a period of plyometric training that resulted in an improvement in throwing velocity.

It appears that isokinetic dynamometers are unable to produce the angular velocities recorded during sporting movements, but are able to elicit the magnitude of the joint torques observed. As already noted, force/torque magnitude constitutes an important element of specificity of strength tests (albeit with other mechanical variables).

Another criticism of isokinetic tests is that very rarely in sporting and everyday movements does a joint rotate with constant angular velocity. Indeed, this may be a more valid objection to isokinetic testing than the relatively low velocities associated with current dynamometers and is more difficult to defend. Similarly, the posture adopted during isokinetic tests may limit the external validity of the measures obtained. Indeed, peak torque during a single-joint movement (knee extension) at slow ($60° \cdot s^{-1}$), moderate ($180° \cdot s^{-1}$), and high ($270° \cdot s^{-1}$) testing velocities demonstrated only moderate correlations ($r \leq .31$) to sprinting performance in both well-trained and recreationally active subjects (Murphy and Wilson 1997; Requena et al. 2009). The strength of these relationships was below that reported using both dynamic and isometric measures of maximal muscular strength.

Abernethy and Jürimäe (1996) reported that measures of isokinetic peak torque were not immediately sensitive to the increases in muscular strength accrued from isoinertial resistance training methods. The strength gains demonstrated by isokinetic measures were achieved weeks following those observed with isoinertial and even isometric tests of maximal muscular strength.

Despite the studies that bring the validity of isokinetic measures of muscular strength into question, some studies support its validity. For example, internal shoulder rotation peak torque at $210° \cdot s^{-1}$ is significantly related to peak serve velocity ($r = .86$) in collegiate female tennis players (Kraemer et al. 2000), and external shoulder rotation peak torque at 240 and 400° $\cdot s^{-1}$ demonstrated large correlations ($r \geq .76$) with javelin throw distance in trained javelin throwers (Forthomme et al. 2007). Others have reported moderate correlations ($r > .55$) between various isokinetic measures and sprint running performance (Dowson et al. 1998; Nesser et al. 1996). Similarly, peak torque during both concentric and eccentric contractions of the knee extensors has been shown to discriminate among sprinters, rugby players, and sedentary subjects (Dowson et al. 1998).

On a more practical level, the time needed for setting up the dynamometer for each subject and the prohibitive cost of isokinetic dynamometers, as well as the associated space requirements, may render isokinetic dynamometry inappropriate for many fitness professionals. Baltzopoulos (2008) and Wrigley and Strauss (2000) offer a complete discussion of these issues.

Reliability of Isokinetic Measures of Muscular Strength

In general, isokinetic measures of maximal muscular strength (peak torque) have shown acceptable reliability. For example, Maffiuletti and colleagues (2007) have reported test–retest correlation values for concentric peak torque of $\geq.98$ and within-subject variations of $\leq3.3\%$ for velocities between 60 and $180° \cdot s^{-1}$ for the knee flexors and extensors in a group of recreationally active men and women. Peak torque values about the ankle joint tend to be less reliable (Müller et al. 2007).

Peak knee extension torques obtained during both concentric and eccentric contractions have been shown to be reliable (test–retest correlations $\geq.88$) in a group of older (average age: 72 years) women (Brock Symons et al. 2004). Test–retest correlation coefficients of $\geq.72$ (within-subject variation $\leq 15\%$) have been reported for the peak extensor torques at the elbow and knee joints at low ($30° \cdot s^{-1}$) and moderate ($180° \cdot s^{-1}$) velocities in young (average age: 10.1 years) boys using a modified dynamometer (Deighan, De Ste Croix, and Armstrong 2003). The peak flexor torques were slightly less reliable (test–retest correlation $\geq .55$; within-subject variation $\leq 15\%$).

General Procedures for Isokinetic Tests

The general procedures to follow when using isokinetic tests of muscular strength are outlined here. The issues discussed are taken from the reviews by Baltzopoulos (2008) and Wrigley and Strauss (2000).

- *Dynamometer calibration.* An isokinetic dynamometer should be calibrated prior to data collection to ensure the reliability and validity of the measures. The calibration procedure usually involves suspending a range of loads of known mass from the dynamometer arm at low velocities as well as using a goniometer to calibrate angular position.

- *Gravity correction.* Measurement error can be reduced by performing gravity correction prior to each test. Most dynamometers have computerized procedures for gravity correction.

- *Order of test velocities.* The typical testing order used in isokinetic dynamometry is to begin with slow velocities and progress to fast velocities.

- *Positioning of the subject.* The subject should be positioned in such a way that the recorded torque is generated by the musculature crossing the joint of interest. This often means that contralateral limbs and the torso should be stabilized with appropriate harnesses or belts. Similarly, the limb of interest should be secured to the dynamometer arm to avoid any "overshoot" torque recordings or impact injuries. The appropriate joint angles should be adopted, even of those joints that may not appear to be involved in the movement (particularly if the test involves biarticular muscles). An important aspect of isokinetic testing is the alignment of the axis of rotation of the dynamometer arm with that of the joint of interest. Although anatomical axes may be difficult to establish visually (and indeed are likely to move throughout the range of motion), a prominent anatomical landmark is usually used (e.g., the lateral epicondyle of the femur for the knee joint). However, it is important to establish appropriate alignment during submaximal or maximal contractions given the potentially large change in joint position between rest and contraction.

- *Instructions and feedback.* The examiner should explain to the subject the purpose of the test and emphasize that maximal muscular effort should be given throughout the test. Familiarization trials should be provided before the data are collected at each testing velocity. During the test, the examiner should provide verbal instruction and encouragement, as well as visual feedback of joint torque data.

- *Rest intervals.* Rest intervals of 40 to 60 seconds are generally recommended between contractions.

MAXIMAL MUSCULAR STRENGTH OF KNEE FLEXORS AND EXTENSORS

Maximal muscular strength is defined as the peak torque achieved during the contractions at predetermined speeds.

EQUIPMENT (MAFFIULETTI ET AL. 2007)

Con-Trex dynamometer (Con-Trex MJ, CMV AG, Dübendorf, Switzerland) with angular velocities of 60, 120 and 180° · s^{-1} for concentric contractions and a velocity of –60° · s^{-1} for eccentric contractions. The torque values are sampled at 100 Hertz.

TECHNIQUE (MAFFIULETTI ET AL. 2007)

The subject sits in the chair of the dynamometer with an internal angle of 85° at the hip joint. The distal shin pad of the dynamometer arm is attached 2 to 3 centimeters (0.8 to 1.2 in.) proximal to the lateral malleolus of the dominant leg. Straps are also fixed across the subject's chest, pelvis, and midthigh to prevent extraneous movement during the test. The subject places each arm on the contralateral shoulder during each contraction to avoid the involvement of the arms. Alignment between the dynamometer rotational axis and that of the knee joint is checked prior to each test. During the contractions, verbal encouragement and visual feedback (instantaneous joint torque readings) are provided. The range of motion for each contraction is 70°—from 80° to 10° of knee flexion (0° corresponding to full knee extension).

PROCEDURE (MAFFIULETTI ET AL. 2007)

1. The subject performs a warm-up of 20 submaximal (20 to 80% of perceived maximal effort) reciprocal concentric and eccentric contractions at low velocities (15° · s^{-1} for concentric, –15° · s^{-1} for eccentric).

2. The subject performs three continuous, reciprocal extension and flexion contractions with maximal effort at a predetermined angular velocity of 60° · s^{-1}.

TABLE 7.4 Data for Peak Knee Extension and Flexion Torques (N·m) in Athletic Populations

Population	Gender	60° · s⁻¹		180° · s⁻¹		300° · s⁻¹	
		Flexion	Extension	Flexion	Extension	Flexion	Extension
NCAA DI basketball	M	165.4 ± 26.2	178.1 ± 32.9	133.2 ± 21.2	135.3 ± 29.7	101.1 ± 30.7	96.9 ± 34.0
NCAA DI soccer	M	152.0 ± 9.3	240.3 ± 11.1				
NCAA DI wrestling	M	156.9 ± 9.9	256.2 ± 12.1			98.6 ± 7.0	100.8 ± 6.8
NCAA DI volleyball	F	77.8 ± 10.3	153.3 ± 26.2	59.2 ± 9.1	115.8 ± 21.0	48.5 ± 8.1	88.8 ± 19.4

Values are group means ± standard deviations.

Adapted, by permission, from J. Hoffman, 2006, *Norms for fitness, performance, and health* (Champaign, IL: Human Kinetics), 30.

3. The subject rests passively for 60 seconds.

4. Steps 2 and 3 are repeated at angular velocities of 120 and 180° · s⁻¹.

5. The subject performs three alternating isometric contractions for the knee extensors and flexors (60° flexion) with a 60-second passive recovery after each one.

6. The subject performs three maximal eccentric contractions of the knee extensors at an angular velocity of –60° · s⁻¹; contractions are separated by 60 seconds of passive rest.

7. The subject repeats step 6 for the knee flexors.

RELIABILITY

For both concentric and eccentric peak torque values achieved by the knee extensors, Maffiuletti and colleagues (2007) reported test–retest correlations of ≥.99 at angular velocities of 60, 120, 180 and –60° · s⁻¹ in a group of recreationally active men and women. The within-subject variations were 2.8, 1.9 and 1.9% for the concentric contractions at angular velocities of 60, 120, and 180° · s⁻¹, respectively; a value of 3.4% was reported for the eccentric contraction. Very similar test–retest correlations were reported for the knee flexors (≥.99). However, the within-subject variations were slightly greater; values of 3.6, 2.9, and 2.7% were reported for the concentric contractions at angular velocities of 60, 120, and 180° · s⁻¹, respectively.

Table 7.4 provides descriptive data for peak knee flexion and extension torques collected from various athletes using the isokinetic test discussed here.

TABLE 7.5 Practical Summary of Tests of Maximal Muscular Strength

Test	Contraction type	Specific resources	Published validity	Published reliability	Published normative/descriptive data	Ease of administration	Skill requirements
1RM bilateral back squat	SSC Multijoint	Free weights and squat rack	Yes	Yes	Yes	Time consuming Likely to require long recovery	Familiarity with back squat
1RM unilateral back squat	SSC Multijoint	Free weights and squat rack	No	Yes	No	Time consuming Likely to require long recovery	Familiarity with single-leg back squat
1RM machine leg press	Concentric and eccentric Multijoint	Plate-loaded machine	Yes, but poor	Yes	Yes	Time consuming Likely to require long recovery	Limited skill requirements
1RM eccentric machine leg press	Eccentric Multijoint	Modified weight stack machine	No	No	No	Time consuming Likely to require long recovery	Limited skill requirements
1RM bench press (free weights)	SSC Multijoint	Free weights and rack	Yes	No	Yes	Time consuming Likely to require long recovery	Familiarity with bench press
1RM bench press (machine)	Concentric and eccentric Multijoint	Plate-loaded machine	Yes	Yes	No	Time consuming Likely to require long recovery	Limited skill requirements
Peak isometric force during bilateral squats	Isometric Multijoint	Force platform	Yes	Yes	No	Reduced time for administration Limited recovery time following tests	Limited skill requirements
Peak isometric force during midthigh clean pulls	Isometric Multijoint	Force platform	Yes	Yes	No	Reduced time for administration Limited recovery time following tests	Limited skill requirements

Test	Contrac-tion type	Specific resources	Published validity	Pub-lished reliability	Published normative/ descriptive data	Ease of administra-tion	Skill require-ments
Peak iso-metric force during bench press	Isometric Multijoint	Force plat-form	Yes, but poor	Yes	No	Reduced time for adminis-tration Limited recov-ery time fol-lowing tests	Limited skill require-ments
Peak torque during isokinetic knee flexion and exten-sion	Isokinetic Single-joint	Isokinetic dynamom-eter	Yes	Yes	Yes	Time consuming Eccentric tests are likely to require long recovery	Limited skill require-ments

Note. SSC = stretch-shortening cycle

Comparing Muscular Strength Measurement Methods

Table 7.5 summarizes the field and laboratory tests that have been discussed in this chapter and provides a rating of the tests in terms of the type of muscular contraction involved, the resources required, published validity and reliability, published normative data, ease of administration, and potential skill requirements of the subject.

Many tests of maximal muscular strength are available, each with its own benefits and limitations. No one test should be regarded as the gold standard for maximal muscular strength. Rather, the fitness professional should determine the utility of each test based on the subject population, the mechanical specificity between the test and the performance of interest, available equipment, ease of data analysis and interpretation, and time available.

The time available refers not only to that for the specific testing session, but also for the recovery that the subject may require following the test. As mentioned earlier, high-intensity movements involving the SSC can result in fatigue that lasts for days (Nicol et al. 2006). This is an important consideration given that most sporting movements involve the SSC and therefore a test of maximal muscular strength that demonstrates high levels of mechanical specificity is likely to involve this action as well. The significant fatigue following the completion of

(continued)

Professional Applications

(continued)

the test may preclude its regular administration during the athlete's wider training program. This highlights the need to carefully plan the placement of testing sessions within an athlete's long-term training cycle.

When to administer a test during an athlete's training program is also an important consideration. It would appear practical to administer tests at the completion of a mesocycle to establish the effectiveness of the training period. However, researchers have identified possible lag times in the improvements accrued from a period of training—improvements in specific physical capacities such as maximal muscular strength may not be realized immediately following the completion of a specific mesocycle (Siff 2000; Stone, Stone, and Sands 2007).

The timing of improvements elicited by a specific mesocycle of training may be determined in part by the specificity between the test of maximal muscular strength and the training exercises used in the program. This was demonstrated by Abernethy and Jürimäe (1996), who reported that a dynamic isoinertial test of maximal muscular strength was better than either an isometric or an isokinetic test in tracking the changes in strength elicited from a resistance training program comprising isoinertial exercises.

The selection of a nonspecific test of maximal muscular strength may cause the fitness professional to erroneously label a training program as ineffective. Clearly, tests of maximal muscular strength are not interchangeable; once the professional has identified the most appropriate test given the circumstances, only this test should be administered when a measure of maximal muscular strength is required. Failure to use the same test for a specific physical capacity prevents the professional from effectively monitoring the athlete's progress.

For the tests of maximal muscular strength reviewed here, large correlations have been reported between the test scores and performance measures regardless of whether the tests are isoinertial, isometric, or isokinetic. However, authors have called for tests of strength to be validated through the relationships between the changes in the test scores and those of performance measures following an intervention (Abernethy, Wilson, and Logan 1995; Murphy and Wilson 1997). Unfortunately, such analyses are largely absent from the literature. Where the relationships between the tests and performance measures have been reported, dynamic isoinertial tests appear to be better at tracking changes in dynamic performance, as the principle of mechanical specificity would dictate.

Regardless of the type of strength test used, and at what point during the athlete's training program it is administered, the fitness professional must administer the test consistently (e.g., warm-up, instructions during the test, postures adopted during the test, time of day the test is performed). This will ensure the effective recording and monitoring of the athlete's strength.

SUMMARY

- Maximal muscular strength can be defined as the ability of a muscle or group of muscles to produce a maximal force or torque against an external resistance under specific conditions defined by posture, muscle action, and movement velocity.

- The fitness professional should determine the utility of a maximal muscular strength test based on the subject population, the mechanical specificity between the test and the performance of interest, and the equipment and time available.

- Fitness professionals should measure values of maximal muscular strength directly rather than predicting them from multiple repetitions performed with submaximal loads.

- Reliability is crucial for any physical test. The magnitude of a change in muscular strength required for a real change to have occurred following an intervention can be determined from reliability statistics, and sample sizes for future studies can also be computed (Hopkins 2000). As such, the reliability of tests of maximal muscular strength and muscular strength endurance are important for both fitness professionals and researchers. Hopkins (2000) noted the following three important reliability statistics:

  1. Systematic bias (a change in the mean between consecutive test scores)

  2. Within-subject variation

  3. Test–retest correlation (the intraclass correlation as opposed to bivariate statistics should be used)

- Without reliability statistics, a fitness professional cannot make informed decisions about the utility of a strength test for a given subject population. Many of the tests reviewed here have associated test–retest correlations, although many of these are bivariate statistics (Pearson's r), which limits the comparisons of the tests. Few of the tests have systematic bias or within-subject variations reported. This is a substantial omission from the literature and one that should be addressed in future research.

- The fitness professional must administer tests consistently (e.g., warm-up, instructions during the test, postures adopted during the test, time of day the test is performed).

8

Muscular Endurance

Gavin L. Moir, PhD

Chapter 7 introduced muscular strength as an important aspect of both health and athletic performance. The selection of an appropriate test of muscular strength should concern fitness professionals dealing with athletic, clinical, and even general populations. This chapter focuses on tests of muscular endurance.

Tests of muscular endurance are not often administered to athletic populations, certainly in comparison to tests of maximal muscular strength. However, muscular endurance tests commonly appear in the battery of physical tests administered to children, military and law enforcement personnel, and firefighters (Baumgartner et al. 2007; Hoffman 2006); in fact, the outcome scores for many of these tests are used as minimum entry standards. Such tests typically involve large numbers of subjects being tested concurrently, and so they are generally easy to administer and interpret. As a result of the size of these populations, extensive normative data sets are available for many tests of muscular endurance. This chapter outlines the appropriate methods for testing muscular endurance and identifies the associated reliability and validity statistics. We begin, however, by defining muscular endurance.

Definition of Muscular Endurance

Muscular strength is often equated with muscular force and can be defined as the ability of a muscle or group of muscles to produce a force against an external resistance (Siff 2000; Stone, Stone, and Sands 2007; Zatsiorsky 1995). This implies that the expression of muscular strength lies along a continuum from zero (no force generated) to maximal force production (maximal muscular strength). The physiological and mechanical factors influencing the expression of muscular strength are discussed in chapter 7.

These factors included the contraction type (isometric, eccentric, concentric), the architectural characteristics of the muscle fibers (cross-sectional area, pennation angle), the fiber type, and the contractile history (fatigue, postactivation potentiation). From this discussion, maximal muscular strength was defined as the ability to voluntarily produce a maximal force or torque under specific conditions defined by muscle action, movement velocity, and posture. We can now define muscular endurance as the ability to voluntarily produce force or torque repeatedly against submaximal external resistances, or to sustain a required level of submaximal force in a specific posture for as long as possible.

A relationship exists between maximal muscular strength and muscular endurance (Reynolds, Gordon, and Roberts 2006). Indeed, this relationship forms the basis of the prediction equations used to estimate a 1RM value from multiple submaximal lifts performed in a specific test, as highlighted in chapter 7. In general, the outcome of muscular endurance tests in which repetitions are continued to failure with an absolute load are strongly related to maximal muscular strength; stronger people can perform a greater number of repetitions and therefore a greater amount of work (Stone et al. 2006; Zatsiorsky 1995). Conversely, matching the load to the strength of the subject results in similar numbers of repetitions among subjects, regardless of strength.

The definition of muscular endurance presented here relates to the two divergent testing methods that are often used to test muscular endurance. The first method requires the subject to perform as many repetitions as possible against a submaximal load until volitional failure using both eccentric and concentric contractions (e.g., push-ups to failure). The second method requires the subject to maintain a prespecified posture for as long as possible and therefore involves predominantly isometric contractions (e.g., flexed-arm hang). Despite the quantitative and qualitative differences between these two broad methods of evaluating muscular endurance, the defining characteristic of both is the ability of the active musculature to resist fatigue, defined as a reversible decline in muscle performance associated with muscle activity that is marked by a progressive reduction in the force developed by a muscle (Allen, Lamb, and Westerblad 2008).

One issue to be addressed in relation to the definition of muscular endurance is the determination of the submaximal loads during tests in which the number of repetitions achieved before volitional failure is the dependent variable. The selection of submaximal loads can be based on a percentage of body mass (Baumgartner et al. 2002), a percentage of maximal muscular strength (Mazzetti et al. 2000; Rana et al. 2008; Woods, Pate, and Burgess 1992), or an absolute load (Baker and Newton 2006; Mayhew et al. 2004; Vescovi, Murray, and Van Heest 2007). Each of these methods has inherent problems. For example, using a load relative to body mass assumes a linear relationship between body mass and muscular strength and does not accurately account for differences in body composition among subjects. Conversely, basing the load on a percentage of maximal muscular strength requires that the subject initially complete a 1RM test and therefore increases the length of the testing sessions.

Some authors have questioned the validity of relative tests of muscular endurance, suggesting that rarely in sporting or daily activities are loads relative to maximal muscular strength or even body mass encountered (Stone et al. 2006). Absolute loads, where the external load is the same for each subject are more common. However, a problem with using absolute loads to measure muscular endurance is that the load may be too heavy for some subjects, which risks changing the test to one of maximal strength rather than muscular endurance. Indeed, Kraemer and colleagues (2002) recommended that 10 to 25 or more repetitions be required for an exercise emphasizing muscular endurance. These numbers can be used as a guide when using a test of muscular endurance based on repetitions to failure.

Another factor for consideration is that of the cadence of the repetitions performed during a test using repetitions to failure. LaChance and Horto-bagyi (1994) reported that the selection of a cadence can have a significant effect on the number of repetitions performed during strength exercise. However, very few of the published tests of muscular endurance specify a cadence, allowing the subjects to set their own. Failure to specify a cadence could reduce the reliability of the test, whereas selecting one may compro-mise the external validity of the test. Both of these situations can limit the ability of the test to track changes in a person's performance across time.

Other tests of muscular endurance require the subject to maintain a prespecified posture for as long as possible using isometric contractions. At issue is the time the subjects are required to hold the posture for the test to be a measure of muscular endurance. Previously it was noted that, when an external load is being moved repeatedly, a minimum number of repeti-tions is required to qualify a test as a measure of muscular endurance; an equivalent time threshold is difficult to determine for tests in which subjects must maintain a specific posture.

As with all isometric tests of muscular strength, the choice of posture, and therefore joint angle, is important because the length–tension rela-tionship of a muscle has a significant impact on the expression of strength (Rassier, MacIntosh, and Herzog 1999). The issue of the most appropriate posture to adopt during the test also arises. The fitness professional should determine the utility of a specific test in relation to the postures adopted in the performance for which the subject is being trained, as the principle of specificity would dictate. This requires a thorough needs analysis of the performance activity before selecting a test.

Tests of muscular endurance should not be used interchangeably because only moderate correlations have been reported between tests, even when the active musculature involved appears to be similar (Clemons et al. 2004;

Halet et al. 2009; Sherman and Barfield 2006). This reflects the importance of the specificity of the tests and also highlights the need to select the test carefully and to use the same test when tracking muscular endurance over time in the same person, or when comparing the muscular endurance of various people. Failure to use the same test will negate the possibility of effectively monitoring clients' progress.

Field Tests for Muscular Endurance

The majority of field tests of muscular endurance presented in the literature are specific to the abdominal musculature and that of the upper body. The tests discussed here include the bench press, push-up, pull-up, sit-up, and leg press or squat, all of which are performed to failure. The flexed-arm hang, a posture-specific isometric test, is also discussed. The methods for selecting the external resistance used in these tests are discussed where appropriate. Where there are multiple forms of the same test available (e.g., bench press), only those protocols with published reliability and validity data will be discussed in detail.

Bench Press to Failure (Load as a Percentage of Body Mass)

Baumgartner and colleagues (2002) had male and female college-aged men and women perform repetitions to failure on a machine weight bench press. The load for the men was 70% of body mass; the load for the women was 40%. Although no reliability data were reported for the test, the men (average repetitions: 15.2) produced significantly greater repetitions than the women did (average repetitions: 13.6). Although these average values tend to fall within the prescribed repetitions for strength endurance as outlined by Kraemer and colleagues (2002), there was a very large range of repetitions; some subjects were unable to achieve a single repetition with the selected loads. Therefore, the selection of a load equivalent to 70% and 40% of body mass for men and women, respectively, may limit the validity of this test for the general population.

Bench Press to Failure (Load as a Percentage of 1RM)

Mazzetti and colleagues (2000) used repetitions to failure with a load equivalent to 80% of 1RM in moderately trained men employing free weights. The authors reported that the number of repetitions achieved (six to eight) did not change following 12 weeks of resistance training, although significant increases in 1RM values did occur.

Baker (2009) had well-trained rugby league players perform repetitions to failure using a load equivalent to 60% of 1RM; the exercise was performed in a Smith-type machine. The number of repetitions performed was not able to differentiate performance level in rugby league players, despite both the elite and lower-level players achieving more than 20 repetitions on average during the test.

Adams and colleagues (2000) used a free-weight bench press to volitional failure performed with a load equivalent to 50% of 1RM in older females (mean age: 51 years). The subjects in this study were able to achieve more than 20 repetitions on average (range: 10 to 30).

Woods, Pate, and Burgess (1992) tested upper body muscular endurance using repetitions to failure with a load equivalent to 50% of 1RM in pre-pubescent boys and girls (mean age: 10 years). The exercise was performed on a weight machine. The subjects achieved an average of 18.3 repetitions (boys' mean: 19.9; girls' mean: 17.3). Unfortunately, there are no published reliability data for repetitions to volitional failure in the bench press when loads relative to maximal muscular strength are used.

Bench Press to Failure (Absolute Load)

Vescovi, Murray, and Van Heest (2007) used a load of 150 pounds (68 kg) to measure the muscular endurance of well-trained ice hockey players during a free-weight bench press exercise. The subjects were required to lift at a cadence of 50 repetitions per minute during the test, which was terminated when the subject could no longer maintain this cadence. The number of repetitions achieved prior to failure allowed the researchers to differentiate among playing positions: goalkeepers achieved an average of 3.3 repetitions, and defensemen achieved an average of 9.2 repetitions.

Mayhew and colleagues (2004) used a load of 225 pounds (102 kg) in the bench press with NCAA Division II American football players. Although no set cadence was used, the subjects were encouraged to take no more than a 2-second pause between repetitions. A repetition was counted if the bar touched the chest, was not bounced from the chest, and was returned to full elbow extension. The players were able to perform an average of 11.7 repetitions before failure.

Other researchers reported an average of 7.2 repetitions in the same test using a similar subject sample (Chapman, Whitehead, and Binkert 1998). Baker (2009), using the number of repetitions performed with a load of 225 pounds (102 kg), was able to differentiate among rugby league players of differing playing abilities, but players in the lower divisions achieved a low number of repetitions (an average of 5.9).

Given that the recommendation for an exercise to develop muscular endurance is a minimum of 10 repetitions (Kraemer et al. 2002), these absolute loads would appear to be inappropriate for measuring muscular endurance in many athletic subjects. Furthermore, there is no reported reliability for the bench press to failure performed with a load of 225 pounds (102 kg) despite its widespread use, particularly in American football (Chapman, Whitehead, and Binkert 1998; Mayhew et al. 2004).

BENCH PRESS TO FAILURE WITH AN ABSOLUTE LOAD OF 132 POUNDS (60 KG)

Baker and Newton (2006) used a load of 132 pounds (60 kg) during a bench press movement performed using free weights to test the muscular endurance of well-trained rugby league players. The protocol employed by these researchers is discussed here.

TECHNIQUE (EARLE AND BAECHLE 2008)

The subject lies supine on the bench with the head, shoulders, and buttocks in contact with the bench and both feet in contact with the floor (five-point contact). The bar is grasped with a closed, pronated grip slightly wider than shoulder width. The spotter assists the subject in removing the bar to the beginning position, where the bar is held with the elbows extended. Each repetition begins from this position. The bar is lowered to touch the chest at around the level of the nipple, and is then raised in a continuous movement until the elbows are fully extended (see figure 8.1). During the movement, the five contact points should be maintained, and the subject should not bounce the bar from the chest at the lowest part of the movement.

PROCEDURE (BAKER AND NEWTON 2006)

1. In their study, Baker and Newton (2006) had rugby athletes perform the muscular endurance test after completing a 1RM bench press test. However, the fitness professional should determine an appropriate warm-up routine that avoids fatigue.

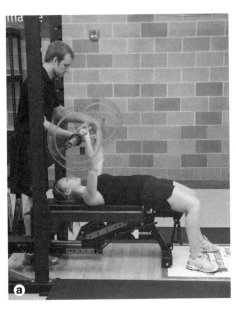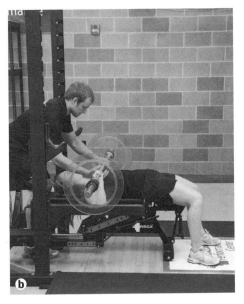

FIGURE 8.1 Starting position and the lowest position achieved during the bench press exercise.

TABLE 8.1 Normative Values for Repetitions Completed in the YMCA Bench Press Test to Failure

% rank	18–25 years		26–35 years		36–45 years		46–55 years		56–65 years		65+ years	
	M	F	M	F	M	F	M	F	M	F	M	F
95	42	42	40	40	34	32	28	30	24	30	20	22
75	30	28	26	25	24	21	20	20	14	16	10	12
50	22	20	20	17	17	13	12	11	8	9	6	6
25	13	12	12	9	10	8	6	5	4	3	2	2
5	2	2	2	1	2	1	1	0	0	0	0	0

Reprinted, by permission, from J. Hoffman, 2006, *Norms for fitness, performance, and health* (Champaign, IL: Human Kinetics), 47; Adapted from *YMCA fitness testing and assessment manual*, 4th ed., 2000, with permission of YMCA of the USA, 101 N. Wacker Drive, Chicago, IL 60606.

2. The barbell is loaded to 132 pounds (60 kg).

3. The subject is required to perform as many repetitions as possible until volitional failure or technique deterioration. No cadence is specified for this test, but the subject is prohibited from resting between repetitions.

RELIABILITY

A test–retest correlation coefficient of .94 has been reported for repetitions to failure with an absolute load of 132 pounds (60 kg) performed with no set cadence in rugby league players (Baker and Newton 2006).

VALIDITY

The number of repetitions achieved in this test was found to differentiate among playing abilities in rugby league players; elite players achieved an average of 35.6 repetitions before test termination, whereas lower-level players achieved an average of 23.8 repetitions (Baker and Newton 2006). These repetitions are closely aligned to those recommended in the literature for muscular endurance (Kraemer et al. 2002). No data are available for athletic females using this test.

The absolute load of 132 pounds (60 kg) may be too heavy for the general population. An alternative would be the YMCA bench press test, which specifies a load of 80 pounds (36.3 kg) for men and 35 pounds (15.9) for women (Hoffman 2006). This test follows a set cadence of 30 repetitions per minute. Table 8.1 shows normative values for repetitions achieved by the general population in the YMCA bench press test to failure.

PUSH-UPS TO FAILURE

PROCEDURE (BAUMGARTNER ET AL. 2002)

1. The subject adopts a prone position on the floor with the hands placed shoulder-width apart, fingers pointing forward, and elbows pointing backward (figure 8.2).

2. From the starting position the subject pushes up to full arm extension with the body straight, such that a straight line can be drawn from the shoulder joint to the ankle joint (this is the up position).

3. The subject then lowers until all of the body from the chest to the thighs makes contact with the floor.

4. The subject then pushes up to full arm extension, keeping the body straight.

5. The subject continues the exercise at a comfortable rate (20 to 30 repetitions per minute) until no more push-ups can be performed with the correct form.

6. A push-up is counted when the subject is in the up position, and no resting is allowed between repetitions.

RELIABILITY

Test–rest correlation coefficients of .95 and .91 have been reported for this test in college-aged men and women, respectively (Baumgartner et al. 2002).

VALIDITY

Williford and colleagues (1999) reported that the number of push-ups before failure (41) was a strong indicator of performance during a specific firefighting task in a group of firefighters. The number of repetitions performed during push-ups to failure at a cadence of 50 repetitions per minute was able to differentiate ice hockey playing positions; goalkeepers achieved 22.7 repetitions and defensemen achieved 26.6 repetitions (Vescovi et al. 2007). Very large correlations ($r = .80$ to .87) between push-ups to failure and bench press to failure have been reported in both college-aged men and women (Baumgartner et al. 2002). In this study the average number of push-up repetitions for the men was 26.4; the average number for the women was 9.5.

Other researchers provided a modification to the push-up for women (see figure 8.3), allowing them to place the knees on the floor with the feet crossed behind (Boland et al. 2009). This allowed the women to achieve more than 20 repetitions on average. The test can be modified for children by having them begin the test in the push-up position and descend until

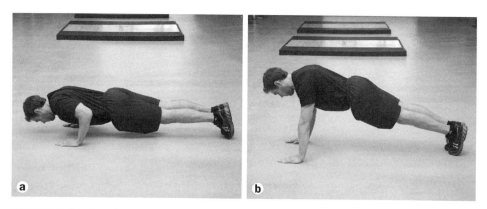

FIGURE 8.2   Starting position and ending position during a push-up.

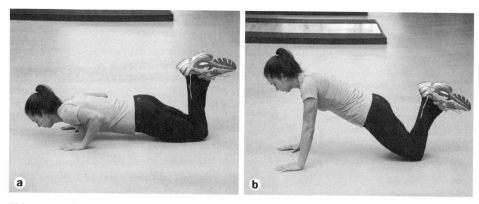

FIGURE 8.3   Starting position and ending position of a modified push-up.

the elbow joint is at 90°, repeating this process at a cadence of 20 push-ups per minute (Saint Romain and Mahar 2001). This modified test has been shown to have a test–retest correlation greater than .97 (Saint Romain and Mahar 2001).

Some examiners use the number of push-ups completed in 60 seconds as a measure of muscular endurance. This measure is used for law enforcement personnel (Hoffman 2006) and has been shown to differentiate among athletes from diverse sports (Rivera, Rivera-Brown, and Frontera 1998). Military personnel are often assessed on the number of push-ups completed in 120 seconds (Hoffman 2006). Normative values for push-ups to failure for various populations are shown in tables 8.2, 8.3, and 8.4.

TABLE 8.2 Normative Values for Push-Ups to Failure in the Adult General Population

% rank	20–29 YEARS		30–39 YEARS		40–49 YEARS		50-59 YEARS		60+ YEARS	
	M	F	M	F	M	F	M	F	M	F
90	57	42	46	36	36	28	30	25	26	17
80	47	36	39	31	30	24	25	21	23	15
70	41	32	34	28	26	20	21	19	21	14
60	37	30	30	24	34	18	19	17	18	12
50	33	26	27	21	21	15	15	13	15	8
40	29	23	24	19	18	13	13	12	10	5
30	26	20	20	15	15	10	10	9	8	3
20	22	17	17	11	11	6	9	6	6	2
10	18	12	13	8	9	2	6	1	4	0

Reprinted, by permission, from J. Hoffman, 2006, *Norms for fitness, performance, and health* (Champaign, IL: Human Kinetics), 45; Adapted from D.C. Nieman, 1999, *Exercise testing & prescription: A health related approach*, 4th ed. (Mountain View, CA: Mayfield Publishing), with permission of The McGraw-Hill Companies.

TABLE 8.3 Normative Values for Push-Ups to Failure in Youth

% rank	AGE (YEARS)											
	6	7	8	9	10	11	12	13	14	15	16	17+
Boys												
90	11	17	19	20	25	30	34	41	41	44	46	56
80	9	13	15	17	21	26	30	35	37	40	41	50
70	7	11	13	15	18	23	25	31	30	35	36	44
60	7	9	11	13	16	19	20	28	25	32	32	41
50	7	8	9	12	14	15	18	24	24	30	30	37
40	5	7	8	10	12	14	15	20	21	27	28	34
30	4	5	7	8	11	10	13	16	18	25	25	30
20	3	4	6	7	10	8	10	12	15	21	23	25
10	2	3	4	5	7	3	7	9	11	18	20	21
Girls												
90	11	17	19	20	21	20	21	22	21	23	26	28
80	9	13	15	17	19	18	20	17	19	20	22	22
70	7	11	13	15	17	17	15	15	12	18	19	19
60	6	9	11	13	14	15	11	13	10	16	15	17
50	6	8	9	12	13	11	10	11	10	15	12	16
40	5	7	8	10	10	8	8	10	8	13	12	15
30	4	5	7	8	9	7	5	7	5	11	10	12
20	3	4	6	7	8	6	3	5	5	10	5	9
10	2	3	4	5	4	2	1	3	2	5	3	5

Reprinted, by permission, from J. Hoffman, 2006, *Norms for fitness, performance, and health* (Champaign, IL: Human Kinetics), 46; Adapted, by permission, from Presidents Council for Physical Fitness, Presidents Challenge Normative Data Spreadsheet [Online]. Available: www.presidentschallenge.org.

TABLE 8.4 Standard Passing Scores for Police Department Personnel in Push-Ups to Failure

20-29 YEARS		30-39 YEARS		40-49 YEARS		50-59 YEARS	
M	F	M	F	M	F	M	F
29	15	24	11	18	9	13	9

Adapted from Hoffman 2006.

PULL-UPS TO FAILURE

PROCEDURE (HOFFMAN 2006)

1. The subject begins by hanging from the bar with arms straight and an overhand grip (see figure 8.4a).
2. The subject pulls the body upward until the chin is above the bar (see figure 8.4b).
3. The subject returns to the starting position.
4. Any swinging movements during the exercise should be avoided.
5. The number of repetitions before volitional failure is recorded.

RELIABILITY

High test–retest correlation coefficients (>.83) have been reported for the pull-up test in both male and female schoolchildren (Engelman and Morrow 1991). However, there are no published data assessing the reliability of the test for adults. Furthermore, the width that the hands should be placed apart is not always specified in the published literature. This variable could affect the reliability of the test and should be controlled for by the examiner.

VALIDITY

The number of pull-ups completed before failure (nine) was found to be a strong indicator of performance during a specific firefighting task in a group of firefighters (Williford et al. 1999). Elsewhere an increase in pull-ups was reported in prepubescent girls and boys (mean age: 8.4 years) who followed an eight-week resistance training program (Siegel, Camaione, and Manfredi 1989).

A modified version of the test performed on a climbing board has been shown to differentiate among sport climbers of various levels (Grant et al. 1996; 2001). Similarly, a modified version is available for use with children, in which the subject starts lying on the back and pulls up against a bar placed on a stand (figure 8.5). This modified pull-up has been shown to be both a valid and a reliable method of testing muscular endurance in children (Saint Romain and Mahar 2001). Table 8.5 shows normative values for the number of pull-ups achieved before failure in youth; table 8.6 shows the performance evaluation for college-aged men in this test.

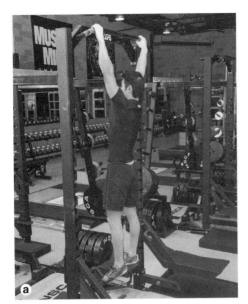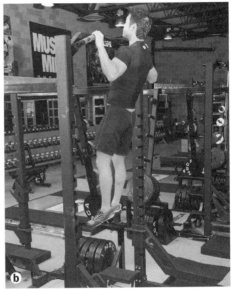

FIGURE 8.4 The starting position and ending position during a successful pull-up.

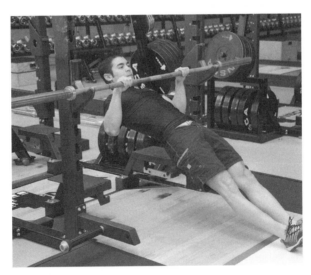

FIGURE 8.5 Modified version of the pull-up test for children. The subject has reached the completion of one repetition here.

TABLE 8.5 Normative Values for Pull-Ups to Failure in Youth

% rank	AGE (YEARS)											
	6	7	8	9	10	11	12	13	14	15	16	17+
Boys												
90	3	5	6	6	7	7	8	9	11	12	12	15
80	1	4	4	5	5	5	6	7	9	10	10	12
70	1	2	3	4	4	4	5	5	7	9	9	10
60	0	2	2	3	3	3	3	4	6	7	8	10
50	0	1	1	2	2	2	2	3	5	6	7	8
40	0	1	1	1	1	1	1	2	4	5	6	7
30	0	0	0	0	0	0	1	1	3	4	5	5
20	0	0	0	0	0	0	0	0	1	2	4	4
10	0	0	0	0	0	0	0	0	0	1	2	2
Girls												
90	3	3	3	3	3	3	3	2	3	2	2	2
80	1	1	2	2	2	2	2	1	1	1	1	1
70	1	1	1	1	1	1	1	0	1	1	1	1
60	0	0	0	0	1	0	0	0	0	0	0	0
50	0	0	0	0	0	0	0	0	0	0	0	0
40	0	0	0	0	0	0	0	0	0	0	0	0
30	0	0	0	0	0	0	0	0	0	0	0	0
20	0	0	0	0	0	0	0	0	0	0	0	0
10	0	0	0	0	0	0	0	0	0	0	0	0

Reprinted, by permission, from J. Hoffman, 2006, *Norms for fitness, performance, and health* (Champaign, IL: Human Kinetics), 44; Adapted with permission from the *Journal of Physical Education, Recreation & Dance,* 1985, 44-90. JOPERD is a publication of the American Alliance for Health, Physical Education, Recreation and Dance, 1900 Association Dr., Reston, VA 20191.

TABLE 8.6 Performance Evaluation of College-Aged Men Performing Pull-Ups to Failure

Classification	Number of pull-ups
Excellent	15+
Good	12–14
Average	8–11
Fair	5–7
Poor	0–4

Reprinted, by permission, from J. Hoffman, 2006, *Norms for fitness, performance, and health* (Champaign, IL: Human Kinetics), 44; Adapted from AAHPERD, 1976, *AAHPERD youth fitness test manual* (Reston, VA: Author).

PARTIAL CURL-UP

TECHNIQUE

The partial curl-up requires the subject to lift the trunk as in the traditional sit-up. This removes the influence of the hip flexor muscles (Baumgartner et al. 2007). Typically, the test requires the subject to perform as many repetitions as possible within a specified time, such as 60 seconds or 120 seconds, and a specific cadence is often set.

PROCEDURE (HOFFMAN 2006)

1. With tape, place two parallel lines on the floor 10 centimeters (4 in.) apart. (Some researchers place the lines 12 centimeters [4.7 in.] apart [Grant et al. 2001]).

2. The subject starts on the back with the knees bent and the arms fully extended at the sides with fingers contacting the first line (see figure 8.6a).

3. The subject starts the exercise by curling the upper back so that both middle fingers touch the second tape mark 10 centimeters (4 in.) away (see figure 8.6b) while keeping the feet on the floor.

4. The subject performs as many repetitions as possible in 60 seconds at a cadence of 20 curl-ups per minute (40 beats per minute). (Some researchers have used a cadence of 50 beats per minute [Grant et al. 2001]).

RELIABILITY

There are no published reliability data for this test.

VALIDITY

The number of curl-ups completed in a 60-second period was shown to differentiate among athletes from diverse sports (Rivera, Rivera-Brown, and Frontera 1998). However, improvements in this test were not reported

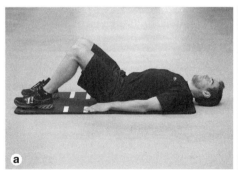
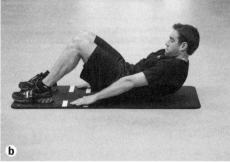

FIGURE 8.6 Starting and finishing positions for the partial curl-up. Notice that the feet are not held by a partner during the exercise.

following an eight-week resistance training intervention completed by prepubescent children (Siegel, Camaione, and Manfredi 1989). Similarly, researchers have reported that the number of repetitions completed before volitional failure was not able to differentiate performance abilities in sport climbers (Grant et al. 1996; 2001) or playing position in rugby league players (Meir et al. 2001). Normative data for this test performed by the adult general population are shown in table 8.7; data for youth are shown in table 8.8; table 8.9 shows standard passing scores for police department personnel in sit-ups achieved in 60 seconds.

Leg Press or Squats to Failure (Load as a Percentage of 1RM)

Studies using isoinertial measures of muscular endurance for the lower body musculature, in which repetitions are performed to volitional failure, tend to be performed on older subjects. The authors have used repetitions with a load relative to the subjects' 1RM, reporting values from 60 to 90% (Adams et al. 2000; Foldvari et al. 2000; Henwood, Riek, and Taafe 2008; Rana et al. 2008). In a group of older women (mean age: 51.0 years), Adams and colleagues (2000) reported that 7 to 18 repetitions were achieved in the leg press movement performed with a load equivalent to 70% of 1RM. Foldvari and colleagues (2000) reported a range of repetitions between 0 and 26 in older women (mean age: 74.8 years) performing the leg press with a load equivalent to 90% of 1RM. One might question the validity of this load for some of the subjects performing a muscular endurance test, particularly given the number of repetitions achieved by some. Interestingly,

TABLE 8.7 Normative Values for Partial Curl-Ups to Failure in the Adult General Population

% rank	20–29 YEARS M	20–29 YEARS F	30–39 YEARS M	30–39 YEARS F	40–49 YEARS M	40–49 YEARS F	50–59 YEARS M	50–59 YEARS F	60–69 YEARS M	60–69 YEARS F
90	75	70	75	55	75	50	74	48	53	50
80	56	45	69	43	75	42	60	30	33	30
70	41	37	46	34	67	33	45	23	26	24
60	31	32	36	28	51	28	35	16	19	19
50	27	27	31	21	39	25	27	9	16	9
40	23	21	26	15	31	20	23	2	9	3
30	20	17	19	12	26	14	19	0	6	0
20	13	12	13	0	21	5	13	0	0	0
10	4	5	0	0	13	0	0	0	0	0

Reprinted, by permission, from ACSM, 2000, *ACSM's guidelines for exercise testing and prescription*, 8th ed. (Lippincott, Williams, and Wilkins), 86.

TABLE 8.8 Normative Values for Partial Curl-Ups to Failure in Youth

% rank	AGE (YEARS)											
	6	7	8	9	10	11	12	13	14	15	16	17+
Boys												
90	23	27	31	41	38	49	100	60	77	100	79	82
80	20	23	27	33	35	40	58	55	58	70	61	63
70	15	20	25	27	29	35	48	48	52	60	48	50
60	12	16	20	23	27	29	36	42	48	50	40	47
50	10	13	17	20	24	26	32	39	40	45	37	42
40	9	12	15	18	20	22	31	35	33	40	34	39
30	8	10	13	15	19	21	27	31	30	32	30	31
20	7	9	11	14	14	18	24	30	28	29	28	28
10	5	7	9	11	10	13	18	21	24	22	23	24
Girls												
90	23	27	31	41	36	44	56	63	51	45	50	60
80	20	23	27	33	29	40	49	52	44	37	41	50
70	15	20	25	27	27	37	40	46	40	35	32	48
60	12	16	20	23	25	32	34	41	33	30	27	42
50	10	13	17	20	24	27	30	40	30	26	26	40
40	9	12	15	18	21	24	26	36	28	25	23	33
30	8	10	13	15	19	21	24	32	25	22	20	30
20	7	9	11	14	17	18	21	27	21	19	19	28
10	5	7	9	11	12	18	16	20	16	13	15	24

Reprinted, by permission, from J. Hoffman, 2006, *Norms for fitness, performance, and health* (Champaign, IL: Human Kinetics), 43; Adapted, by permission, from Presidents Council for Physical Fitness, Presidents Challenge Normative Data Spreadsheet. Available: www.presidentschallenge.org.

TABLE 8.9 Standard Passing Scores for Police Department Personnel in Sit-Ups Achieved in 60 Seconds

20–29 YEARS		30–39 YEARS		40–49 YEARS		50–59 YEARS	
M	F	M	F	M	F	M	F
38	32	35	25	29	20	24	14

Adapted, by permission, from J. Hoffman, 2006, *Norms for fitness, performance, and health* (Champaign, IL: Human Kinetics), 48.

the number of repetitions achieved was not significantly related to subjects' functional status. Henwood and colleagues (2008) reported that the number of repetitions achieved using a load equivalent to 70% of 1RM performed in a leg press machine did not change following a 22-week resistance training program that elicited improvements in functional performance tasks in a mixed group of older (65 to 84 years) men and women. Unfortunately, the number of repetitions achieved was not reported.

In contrast, Rana and colleagues (2008) reported an increase in the number of repetitions performed during the back squat with a load equivalent to 60% of 1RM following a six-week resistance training program in college-aged women. Approximately 15 repetitions were performed in the test prior to the resistance training program, and more than 20 were performed posttraining.

It would appear from this limited sample of studies that a load equivalent to 70% of 1RM or below is required to allow sufficient repetitions for a test of muscular endurance given the range of repetitions required for a resistance training exercise emphasizing muscular endurance. However, no reliability data are reported for any of the tests discussed here.

As mentioned previously, the limitations of using a test of muscular endurance with external loads relative to maximal muscular strength are that such a test requires the subject to perform a 1RM test, and loads relative to maximal strength are not often encountered in activities of daily living or sport. Unfortunately, no data on using muscular endurance tests of the lower body with absolute loads are available.

FLEXED-ARM HANG

The flexed-arm hang field test for muscular endurance differs from those discussed so far in that the outcome is the time a specific posture is held as opposed to the number of repetitions performed. Variations in the technique can be used in this test. For example, the bar can be grasped with an overhand or underhand grip. Similarly, variations in the posture have been reported in the literature, such as requiring that the chin be maintained above the bar or below the bar with various elbow angles (Clemons et al. 2004). The variant discussed here—using an overhand grip and maintaining the chin above the bar—is the most common in the literature (see figure 8.7).

PROCEDURE (HOFFMAN 2006)

1. A bar that is higher than the subject's standing height is required.

2. The subject grasps the bar with an overhand grip wrapping the thumbs around the bar. (Note that there is no mention of the width of the grip to be used.

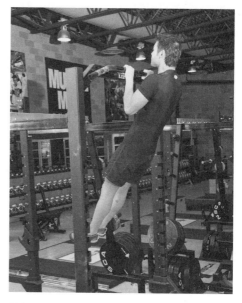

FIGURE 8.7 Starting position used in the flexed-arm hang test.

However, the examiner should record this width and maintain consistency across testing sessions.)

3. With assistance from spotters, the subject is raised to a height at which the chin is above, but not touching, the bar (see figure 8.7).

4. The subject is required to hang without support for as long as possible. The time is recorded from when the spotters remove their support until the chin touches or falls below the bar.

RELIABILITY

A test–retest correlation of .97 was reported for the time achieved in the flexed-arm hang test performed by women (Clemons et al. 2004).

VALIDITY

The flexed-arm hang test has been used to show sex differences among adolescent distance runners (Eisenmann and Malina 2003). Similarly, Siegel, Camaione, and Manfredi (1989) reported that the time of the flexed-arm hang increased following the completion of an eight-week resistance training program in prepubescent girls and boys (mean age: 8.4 years). A modified version of the test has been performed on a climbing board; the time achieved was able to differentiate among elite and recreational sport climbers (Grant et al. 1996).

Other researchers have noted that the performance in the flexed-arm hang is unrelated to other tests of upper body muscular endurance in women and was more strongly related to a test of maximal muscular strength (Clemons et al. 2004). The average time achieved by the subjects in this study was 6.1 seconds, whereas an average of 13.8 repetitions was achieved in the test of muscular endurance (lat-pulldowns to failure with an external load equivalent to 70% of 1RM). This may reflect the importance of determining a minimum time required for a test to be considered a measure of muscular endurance, just as a minimum number of repetitions is required when the endurance test requires the external load to be moved repeatedly.

Normative values for the flexed-arm hang test in youth are shown in table 8.10.

Laboratory Tests for Muscular Endurance

There are many laboratory tests of muscular endurance, all of which require the use of dynamometers. All of these tests are specific to the research question of interest, and few standardized procedures have been published. The laboratory test for muscular endurance discussed here is an isokinetic test requiring a dynamometer. Issues relating to isokinetic dynamometry are addressed in chapter 7.

TABLE 8.10 Normative Values for Flexed-Arm Hang in Youth

% rank	AGE (YEARS)											
	6	7	8	9	10	11	12	13	14	15	16	17+
Boys												
90	16	23	28	28	38	37	36	37	61	62	61	56
80	12	17	18	20	25	26	25	29	40	49	46	45
70	9	13	15	16	20	19	19	22	31	40	39	39
60	8	10	12	12	15	15	15	18	25	35	33	35
50	6	8	10	10	12	11	12	14	20	30	28	30
40	5	6	8	8	8	9	9	10	15	25	22	26
30	3	4	5	5	6	6	6	8	11	20	18	20
20	2	3	3	3	3	4	4	5	8	14	12	15
10	1	1	1	2	1	1	1	2	3	8	7	8
Girls												
90	15	21	21	23	29	25	27	28	31	34	30	29
80	11	14	15	16	19	16	16	19	21	23	21	20
70	9	11	11	12	14	13	13	14	16	15	16	15
60	6	8	10	10	11	9	10	10	11	10	10	11
50	5	6	8	8	8	7	7	8	9	7	7	7
40	4	5	6	6	6	5	5	5	6	5	5	5
30	3	4	4	4	4	4	3	4	4	4	3	4
20	1	2	3	2	2	2	1	1	2	2	2	2
10	0	0	0	0	0	0	0	0	0	1	0	1

Values are time in seconds.

Adapted, by permission, from J. Hoffman, 2006, *Norms for fitness, performance, and health* (Champaign, IL: Human Kinetics), 47; Adapted, by permission, from Presidents Council for Physical Fitness, Presidents Challenge Normative Data Spreadsheet. Available: www.presidentschallenge.org.

ISOKINETIC LABORATORY TEST FOR MUSCULAR ENDURANCE

The specific test discussed here assesses the muscular endurance of the knee flexors and extensors at a velocity of $180° \cdot s^{-1}$. Muscular endurance is determined from the change in peak torque during a series of repeated contractions.

EQUIPMENT AND TECHNIQUE (MAFFIULETTI ET AL. 2007)

The same equipment and technique used in isokinetic tests of maximal muscular strength.

PROCEDURE (MAFFIULETTI ET AL. 2007)

1. The subject completes the procedure outlined for isokinetic tests of maximal muscular strength (refer to chapter 7).

TABLE 8.11 Practical Summary of Tests of Muscular Endurance

Test	Contraction type	Specific resources	Published validity	Published reliability	Published normative/ descriptive data	Ease of administration	Skill require- ments
Bench press to failure	SSC Multijoint	Free weights, bench, and rack	Yes	Yes	Only for YMCA test	If abso- lute load is selected, then easy to admin- ister. Number of test sub- jects limited by equipment.	Familiarity with bench press
Push-ups to failure	SSC Multijoint	None	Yes	Yes	Yes	Easy to admin- ister	Familiarity with push- up
Pull-ups to failure	SSC Multijoint	Pull-up bar or rack when using modified version for chil- dren	Yes	Only for children	Yes	Easy to admin- ister with appropriate equipment	Familiarity with pull-up
Partial curl-ups to failure	SSC Multijoint	Floor markings	Yes	No	Yes	Easy to admin- ister	Familiarity with curl-up
Leg press or squats to failure	SSC Multijoint	Leg press machine, free weights, and squat rack	Yes	No	No	If abso- lute load is selected, then easy to admin- ister. Number of test sub- jects limited by equipment.	Limited with leg press Familiarity with squat exercise
Flexed- arm hang	Isometric Multijoint	Pull-up bar	Yes	Yes	Yes	Easy to admin- ister with appropriate equipment	Limited skill require- ments
Knee flexor and extensor endur- ance	Isokinetic Single-joint	Isokinetic dynamom- eter	No	Yes	No	Time consum- ing	Limited skill require- ments

SSC = stretch-shortening cycle

2. The subject performs 20 reciprocal extension and flexion contractions at an angular velocity of $180° \cdot s^{-1}$.

3. Fatigue is defined in two ways: (a) Peak torque values achieved in contractions 2 through 5 and contractions 17 through 20 are averaged, and the percent difference between these averages (percentage loss) represents fatigue; and (b) the decline in peak torque between contraction 2 and contraction 20 via the negative slope is calculated using linear regression analysis.

RELIABILITY

Maffiuletti and colleagues (2007) reported a test–retest correlation of .81 for fatigue expressed as a percentage loss, while a value of .78 was reported for the negative slope calculation of fatigue in a group of recreationally active men and women.

VALIDITY

There are no published validity data for this test.

Comparing Muscular Endurance Measurement Methods

Table 8.11 summarizes the field and laboratory tests that have been discussed in this chapter and provides a rating of the tests in terms of the type of muscular contraction involved, the resources required, published validity and reliability, published normative data, ease of administration, and potential skill requirements of the subject.

As with most other physical capacities, many tests are available for measuring muscular endurance. The field tests discussed here are easy to administer, and many of them involve no equipment at all. Moreover, the analysis and interpretation of the data should pose no problems to the fitness professional. Certainly, the field tests of muscular endurance appear to be well suited to large groups. However, the fitness professional needs to consider the principle of specificity and choose a test that matches the performance for which the subject is training.

Warm-ups to be used prior to tests of muscular endurance are not adequately addressed in the literature. Based on the order in which tests should be administered as part of a testing battery, Harman (2008) proposed that tests of muscular endurance follow agility, maximal power and strength, and sprint tests. This order should ensure that the subject is sufficiently warmed up prior

Professional Applications

(continued)

(continued)

to the muscular endurance test, although the examiner should avoid fatiguing the subject. (Chapter 7 outlines an appropriate warm-up.)

Tests of muscular endurance of the upper body musculature have been performed in the same session as, but following, tests of maximal muscular strength with well-trained athletes (Baker and Newton 2006). This protocol may be specific to the upper body musculature, which has been shown to recover more quickly than that of the lower body in response to resistance training workouts (Hoffman et al. 1990), and therefore may not apply to muscular endurance tests for the lower body. The examiner needs to consider the fatigue caused by other tests used in a battery, particularly when eccentric and stretch–shortening cycle activities are involved. Consistency in the administration of tests within a battery should always be considered.

With tests of muscular endurance in which submaximal loads are moved repeatedly until volitional fatigue, examiners should stipulate a minimum number of repetitions to complete. Kraemer and colleagues (2002) recommended a minimum of 10 repetitions of an exercise to develop muscular endurance, and so this threshold would seem appropriate for tests of muscular endurance (Baker and Newton 2006). This is an important point given that muscular strength is proposed to lie along a continuum from zero (no force generated) to maximal force production (maximal muscular strength); if an external load, whether absolute or relative, can be moved only once, the test does not provide a valid measure of muscular endurance.

This repetition threshold may bring the validity of some of the tests discussed in this chapter into question (e.g., push-ups to failure, pull-ups to failure) when performed by certain populations. Furthermore, the question arises of how long the subject should hold a specific posture in tests such as the flexed-arm hang for the test to be a valid measure of muscular endurance. For example, if a subject is able to hold the posture for only two seconds, one could argue that this is closer to the maximal force end of the strength continuum than it is to the no force end. Therefore, the test is measuring maximal muscular strength. The need to determine a minimal time threshold for holding a posture for a test to be considered a valid measure of muscular endurance seems fraught with difficulty and may therefore preclude the use of such tests.

The issue of cadence arises when subjects need to perform repetitions to volitional failure. Failure to specify a cadence could reduce the reliability of the test, whereas selecting one may compromise the external validity of the test (rarely do people perform repetitive movements at a constant cadence in activities of daily living or sport). Both of these situations can limit the ability of the test to track changes in a person's performance across time. LaChance and Hortobagyi (1994) reported that a cadence had a significant effect on the number of repetitions performed during strength exercises.

A solution to the cadence problem would be to allow subjects to set their own cadences and so ensuring the external validity of the test while also recording the time taken to achieve volitional failure. These data could provide some information pertaining to the average power output achieved by the subject during the test (the repetitions achieved represent the work performed, which, when divided by the time taken, can provide the rate at which the work was performed). This suggestion would be more appropriate when absolute external loads are used, simplifying the calculations. This would also conform to the suggestion of using absolute external loads given that rarely do people experience loads relative to their levels of maximal muscular strength or their body mass in activities of daily living or sport (Stone et al. 2006).

Despite the proposed validity of using absolute loads in tests of muscular endurance, these protocols may not accurately reflect the specific adaptations following a training intervention. Specifically, a relationship exists between maximal muscular strength and muscular endurance when the endurance test requires that subjects move an absolute external load repeatedly (Stone, Stone, and Sands 2007; Zatsiorsky 1995). This may lead to improvements in muscular endurance simply in response to increases in maximal muscular strength, which appears contrary to the principle of specificity.

As a result of all of these factors, the question could be raised: What useful information is the fitness professional gaining from these tests that would not be gleaned from other tests such as those measuring maximal muscular strength? Given the greater time taken to administer many of the field tests of maximal muscular strength, the reverse argument could be used: Why not just administer a test of muscular endurance using repetitions to failure and calculate maximal muscular strength? Certainly the field tests of muscular endurance are easy to administer and lend themselves to large groups being tested concurrently. However, it was noted in chapter 7 that the available prediction equations are not entirely accurate, and so experts suggested that testing maximal strength is better than predicting it from repetitions with a submaximal load.

The utility of tests of muscular endurance appears to be limited in athletic populations, unless the fitness professional is overseeing the testing of a very large number of athletes. In contrast, field tests of muscular endurance would appear to be well suited for use with the general population.

Finally, although some tests of muscular endurance have been shown to differentiate among athletes of differing performance levels, few of these field tests have been used to track the changes in muscular endurance as a result of specific training interventions, certainly in adults. Validation of strength tests requires the assessment of the relationships between the changes in the test scores and those of performance measures following an intervention (Abernethy, Wilson, and Logan 1995; Murphy and Wilson 1997). As with most other tests of strength, these analyses have not been performed with tests of muscular endurance.

SUMMARY

- Muscular endurance is defined as the ability to voluntarily produce force or torque repeatedly against submaximal external resistances or to sustain a required level of submaximal force in a specific posture for as long as possible.

- Two types of tests are often used to measure muscular endurance, both of which require the subject to resist fatigue:
  1. Repetitions performed to volitional failure against a submaximal external resistance
  2. Maintaining a specified posture for as long as possible

- Tests of muscular endurance are typically administered to large groups of subjects such as schoolchildren, military and law enforcement personnel, and firefighters.

- The field tests used to measure muscular endurance are easy to administer and interpret.

- With field tests that involve repetitions to volitional failure, it would appear that an absolute load rather than a relative load should be used, particularly during the bench press exercise.

- No research has been published investigating the use of absolute external loads with lower body tests of muscular endurance.

- Often, field tests of upper body muscular endurance (e.g., push-up and pull-up tests) allow modifications for use with females and children.

- The fitness professional should determine the utility of a test based on the principle of specificity.

- Once the test has been selected, it should be administered consistently in terms of warm-up procedures, instructions to the subject, time of administration, and so on.

9

Power

Mark D. Peterson, PhD, CSCS*D

The principle of specificity suggests that human performance evaluation be approached as a systematic, discriminatory process in which components of physical fitness are independently tested, scored, and interpreted. This principle is driven by the assumption that fitness attributes are not only distinct but also specifically responsive to training variables. Because training is designed to address the unique conditions of a given sport or activity, testing and evaluation should complement exercise prescription, and form the objective foundation upon which the entire performance enhancement process is monitored. The notion of specificity is particularly complex when managing the factors associated with power production. In fact, muscular power assessment and subsequent development has become one of the most debated and widely deliberated topics across all segments of exercise science.

Power shares a robust association with movement on a continuum from high performance athletics to geriatrics (Bean et al. 2002; Earles, Judge, and Gunnarsson 1997), the measurement of which accounts for neuromuscular subtleties that are often overlooked in other measures of raw force production. Many experts regard power output capacity as the best index of coordinated human movement, chronic function or dysfunction (Evans 2000; Suzuki, Bean, and Fielding 2001; Puthoff and Nielsen 2007), or acute deficiency (e.g., neuromuscular fatigue) (Nordlund, Thorstensson, and Cresswell 2004; Racinais et al. 2007). Many also consider the manipulation of variables to accommodate power adaptation as a principal training objective. To that end, a thorough understanding of the factors that influence power production and explosive movement capacity provides a definitive basis for monitoring, developing, and refining performance enhancement programming.

Operationalizing Power

Among many practitioners and the general public, the term *power* has emerged as a nonspecific designation of movement encompassing factors of speed, strength, or both. In athletic contexts, various permutations of the word *power* are used to characterize movement qualities or capacities ranging from very-high-load, slow movement patterns (e.g., *powerlifting*) to very-low-load, high-velocity activities (e.g., *a powerful tennis serve*). Despite the lack of a mainstream consensus definition for *power*, it is recognized as a clustering of neuromuscular factors related to maximal force production and rate of force development.

The expression of power through coordinated movement is also contingent on external morphological and biomechanical factors including type of muscle action, mass lifted (which may include body mass or limb mass plus an external load), anthropometric characteristics (e.g., limb lengths), muscle architecture (e.g., fiber composition, muscle pennation angle, fiber cross-sectional area, and number of active sarcomeres in series), tendon and connective tissue stiffness, joint range(s) of motion, and movement distance (Cormie et al. 2011a). Despite these many factors that contribute to power, athletes and practitioners have derived arbitrary means of "power training," with the intent to facilitate an adaptive response that translates to augmented explosive movement capacity.

Considering that the term *power* typically evokes the perception of high-speed movement, many people are inclined to take the tenets of specificity to literally mean "train fast, be fast." However, to create the most strategic methods of training and adaptation, it is vital to compartmentalize power into the primary testable and trainable elements.

With the growing popularity of power training among strength and conditioning coaches, personal trainers, and athletes, a standardized evaluation of power output or explosive movement performance is critical. Existing methods range from basic field tests, to elaborate biomechanical assessments in human performance laboratories, to *in vitro* activation and measurement of force development in biopsied muscle fibers. Moreover, the *industry* response to this increased interest in power testing and training has been a surplus of products available to the public. Certainly, greater visibility reflects a positive change in the field of exercise science and the performance enhancement industry; however, methods of evaluating power must be systematic and standardized to ensure the collection of valid, reliable data. Such a system of testing would allow professionals to share norm-referenced standards and to make formal, cross-sectional inspections of physiological and performance attributes (e.g., regression modeling to identify the association between maximal force production and jumping ability across athletic populations, while controlling for age, sex, body dimensions, and training status).

Mechanisms of Power Production and Expression

The mechanisms of power output production have received a great deal of research attention. However, translation of empirical findings to performance enhancement outcomes is a distinct challenge to investigators, and has led to confusion regarding practical application. The expression of power through coordinated movement involves numerous physiological attributes, intrinsic biomechanical factors, and external loading parameters. Thus, although "maximal power" may be defined as the critical threshold interaction between strength and speed (Cronin and Sleivert 2005), this is only true in the specific context for which it is being examined. Depending on the test used, muscular power is documented to be contingent on the following intrinsic physiological factors:

- Availability of adenosine triphosphate (ATP) stores within the specific muscles being tested
- Ratio of fast fibers (i.e., Type II fibers) to slow fibers (i.e., Type I fibers)
- Whole muscle volume or cross-sectional area (CSA)
- Muscle architecture (i.e., pennation angle)
- Intramuscular coordination (i.e., recruitment of fibers within a given muscle)
- Intermuscular coordination (i.e., recruitment of synergistic agonist muscles to perform a movement)
- Coordinated timing and coactivation of antagonist musculature
- Rate coding (i.e., axonal conduction velocity and stimulation frequency)
- Stretch–shortening cycle (i.e., the active stretch of a muscle followed by an immediate shortening)

In many cases it is also necessary to account for differences in body size when examining power changes over time or among individuals. This is because performance in most activities is suggested to be highly contingent on a fitness-to-body-mass ratio (see chapter 1 for ways to normalize or adjust fitness characteristics to body mass).

Although to some extent the principle of specificity is based on theoretical constructs, many professionals use it when generating test batteries and as the basis for training prescriptions. However, when applied to muscular power output, the principle of specificity is complicated by numerous interrelated factors. Therefore, it may be advisable not only to consider the manifestation of power output as it is exhibited through explosive movement, but also to isolate the specific underlying physiological characteristics that could prohibit or potentiate power adaptation. Thus, in contrast to other discrete fitness attributes (e.g., maximal oxygen consumption), power output should be evaluated using a systems approach that incorporates multiple components related to absolute force production, rate of force production, metabolic specificity, movement velocity, work capacity, and body-mass-adjusted power.

Much research has been devoted to investigating the force–velocity relationship. One of the most well-known characteristics of muscle tissue, the force–velocity relationship exemplifies the interactions between muscle contraction velocity and the magnitude of force production. Originally considered by A.V. Hill in 1938 using frog skeletal muscle, and later revised in 1964 (Hill 1964), this relationship was initially examined in, and applied to, isolated muscle. Hill determined that a muscle contracts at a velocity inversely proportional to the load. Many subsequent investigations have confirmed this physiological phenomenon within isolated muscle, as well as within muscle groups during dynamic movement. For the purpose of this chapter, the force–velocity and power–velocity relationships will be illustrated using such Hill-type models (Faulkner, Claflin, and McCully 1986) (see figure 9.1).

Hill-type models do not effectively characterize molecular contributions and muscle architectural characteristics. Cross-bridge models (Wu and Herzog 1999) and anatomically based structural models (Yucesoy et al. 2002) have also been proposed that take into account force responses at the cellular level, as well as fiber arrangement and passive and elastic connective tissue properties, respectively.

Regardless of the interpretive model, the maximal velocity of a given movement depends on the resistance applied to that movement. Specifically, maximal voluntary muscular contraction against a high load produces slower velocities than maximal contractions against a light load. This trade-off between velocity and force for coordinated movement is easily demonstrated during heavy resistance training in which extremely high loads are lifted through a range of motion at slow velocities. At some point along this continuum, the load may be great enough that velocity reaches zero, and an isometric contraction is produced.

Moreover, any applied force that produces movement is defined not only by the load encountered, but also by the velocity at which the dynamic action takes place. For every submaximal exertion (i.e., against relative intensities or loads less than maximal voluntary contraction) there is a distinct maximal velocity that is producible. If the load is decreased to a negligible extent, the potential velocity is maximized. At some point along the force–velocity curve for every muscle action and subsequent movement, there is a force-maximizing load at which velocity is extremely low but dynamic force is at its greatest level. There is also a point along this curve at which the instantaneous product of force and velocity may be maximized. This product is known as muscular peak power, and although associated, it is distinct from absolute strength and maximal movement speed. As noted in figure 9.1, the apex of the power–velocity curve illustrates the expression of

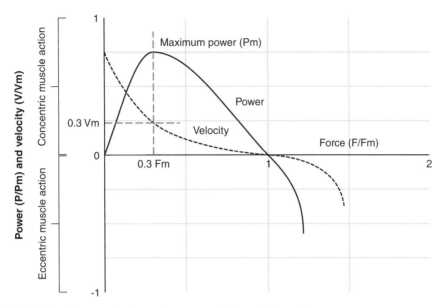

FIGURE 9.1   Force–velocity and power–velocity relationships.

Reprinted, by permission, from National Strength and Conditioning Association, 2008, Speed, agility, and speed-endurance development, by S.S. Plisk. In *Essentials of strength training and conditioning*, 3rd ed., edited by T.R. Baechle and R W. Earle (Champaign, IL: Human Kinetics), 460; Adapted, by permission, from J.A. Faulkner, D.R. Claflin, and K.K. McCully, 1986, Power output of fast and slow fibers from human skeletal muscles. In *Human muscle power*, edited by N.L. Jones, N. McCartney, and A.J. McCornas (Champaign, IL: Human Kinetics), 88.

peak power. Despite overlap among strength, speed, and consequent power output, these parameters are discrete, trainable muscular fitness attributes.

According to Newton's Second Law of Motion, *force* is equal to the product of mass and acceleration (Force = mass × acceleration) of an object, or body. When force is applied to move an object, as in weightlifting, it must not only offset the gravitational force elicited by the mass of the object, but also facilitate movement in the direction opposite to that of gravitational force. In reference to resistance training, a frequently used expression is *muscular strength,* which is defined as the maximal ability to generate force through a specific movement pattern, velocity, or rate of force production (Stone et al. 2000).

Muscle strength and power are often confused as synonymous; however, these attributes are in fact distinct, because high force production may occur in the absence of movement (e.g., isometric muscle action), whereas power cannot. Conversely, dynamic muscle action is a necessary component of power production, and as such, power is the manifestation of work accomplished (i.e., Work = force × distance) per unit of time. In the case of isometric maximal voluntary contraction (MVC), force is very high, but power is zero because no movement occurs and thus no work is accomplished. Ultimately, an increase in power production capacity enables a given muscle to produce the same amount of work in less time, or a greater magnitude of work in the same time. Muscular power is then exhibited by virtually all muscle actions that produce a velocity, and may be more easily defined as the rate of muscular force production (Power = force × velocity) throughout a range of motion (Cronin and Sleivert 2005).

Although this definition generally indicates linear movement, it is important to note that displacement may also be angular, and respective work may be accomplished through angular movement, such as across a joint or with an ergometer (e.g., cycling, rowing). During angular displacement, rotational speed (i.e., angular velocity) and torque are fundamental properties not present with linear displacement. Angular velocity is measured in radians per second (rad/s), and torque is measured in newton-meters, thus yielding this equation for angular work: Work = torque × angular displacement. Although this represents a different computation for determining work, the fundamental principles that apply to quantifying power are still used: Power = work / time. As will be discussed, several tests that use rotational work to derive power estimates have received a great deal of research attention.

Because the topic of muscular power capacity has gained popularity in the world of performance enhancement, it should therefore be examined and delineated with distinct and equitable emphases to that of absolute force production and maximal speed of movement. However, as is the case for both strength and speed, there are a number of task-specific methods to test power that vary considerably with regard to muscle action and the time course over which power is generated (i.e., duration that data collection occurs). These tests should not be used interchangeably because the results may not reflect the same outcome or underlying pathways for generating power output.

When generalizing or applying data for exercise prescription, fitness professionals should keep in mind that power exhibited under one set of conditions may not necessarily translate across other conditions (Atha 1981). Because power reflects the interaction between muscle force production and velocity, anything that alters either of these also directly modifies power production capacity.

This chapter distinguishes between submaximal power output and the ways to measure maximal power. Power ranges from 0 watts (W) in an isometric contraction, to over 7,000 watts when an Olympic-caliber weightlifter performs a clean (Garhammer 1993). The continuum of dynamic muscle actions and respective power outputs varies considerably across this range, and thus it is imperative to differentiate the peak expression capacities that coincide with human movements, as well as the appropriate testing methods.

Types and Factors of Power

The breakdown of overt power output into the fundamental elements is necessary not only for appropriately targeted testing, but also for the design and refinement of sport performance programming (Cormie, McGuigan, and Newton 2011b). Indeed, as is the case for all fitness or performance attributes, pinpointing elements of deficiency is difficult if testing is not broad based and sport specific. Therefore, testing for power requires an understanding of the types of power, as well as the factors that comprise power output and explosive coordinated movement. However, proper evaluation also requires a thorough comprehension of the power-related performance requirements associated with a given sport or activity. Thus, fitness professionals must discriminate among the types of power by compartmentalizing them into categories based on metabolic requirements and the time course through which power is produced (e.g., types of anaerobic power and explosive, or instantaneous, power).

Fitness professionals also need to acknowledge those factors that contribute to power output or explosive coordinated movement, but may not be traditionally considered an outcome of power expression, per se. Two such factors that directly translate to *powerful* performance outcomes and may be distinguished from overt power output are rate of force development and reactive strength capacity. Unraveling these factors is necessary for identifying the needs of the athlete, as well as for ensuring the systematic prescription and refinement of training to maximize performance.

Anaerobic Power

The term *anaerobic power* is often used interchangeably with *maximal power*, but may better reflect the rate of adenosine triphosphate (ATP) use over a single (or multiple) maximal effort against a submaximal load. Anaerobic activity occurs at the onset of exercise and is demonstrated as the accumulation of muscular work not attributable to aerobic metabolism. This "oxygen deficit," which is pronounced in the first minutes of moderate- to high-intensity exercise, has been thoroughly characterized since the early 1910s (Krogh and Lindhard 1913).

Anaerobic activity also occurs at relative intensities that exceed $\dot{V}O_2max$, thus requiring discrete fuel sources that depend directly on the degree of exercise intensity. Specifically, the anaerobic glycolytic (i.e., the lactic acid system) and phosphocreatine systems (i.e., PC system or alactic system) contribute ATP at a much faster rate than is possible by aerobic pathways. The metabolic trade-off to this high rate of ATP turnover is that the energy sources for anaerobic metabolism (glucose and glycogen) are limited and diminish significantly faster than during lower-intensity exercise. The depletion of

TABLE 9.1 Relative Intensity, Energy System, and Respective Power Production Capacity for Various Time Courses of Activity

Time course for anaerobic activity	Relative intensity*	Energy system	Power production capacity
0–6 seconds	Highest	ATP-phosphocreatine	Highest
6–30 seconds	Very high	ATP-phosphocreatine and anaerobic glycolysis	Very high
30 seconds to 2 minutes	Moderate to high	Anaerobic glycolysis	Moderate to high
2–3 minutes	Moderate	Anaerobic glycolysis and aerobic metabolism	Moderate
>3 minutes	Low	Aerobic metabolism	Low

*Relative intensity is expressed per maximal ability, regardless of time course.

energy substrate is particularly rapid for higher-intensity activities fueled by the phosphocreatine system.

Depending on relative intensity (i.e., as expressed relative to maximal force production), the onset of fatigue or muscular failure may occur after a single repetition, or after as long as six seconds, when fueled by the phosphocreatine system. Generally, any high-intensity *anaerobic* exercise that exceeds this time course occurs through the metabolic processes of the anaerobic glycolytic system, for up to approximately two minutes (see table 9.1). Beyond two minutes of exertion, additional work is progressively and incrementally fueled by the aerobic system. Glycogen (i.e., stored carbohydrate), glucose (i.e., blood sugar), ATP, and phosphocreatine (i.e., stored locally in the muscle tissue) are the primary energy sources for anaerobic metabolism. Although they are available only in limited quantities, they are replenished rapidly following bouts of recovery (i.e., three to five minutes for ATP resynthesis, within eight minutes for creatine phosphate, and up to 24 hours for glycogen) (Friedman, Neufer, and Dohm 1991; Harris et al. 1976).

Evaluating maximal anaerobic capacity has been considered an important component of physiological testing. Anaerobic power output may be evaluated on a continuum from instantaneous performance to power production across longer time courses. Thus, the term *peak anaerobic power* may designate the greatest output or production of work per a specific quantity of time.

Of the tests used to determine anaerobic power, several have received the majority of attention from the sport science community. In particular, the 30-second Wingate Anaerobic Test (see page 229) has been the gold standard test for power production capacity; its widespread appeal is largely due to the ease of administration and its documented validity and reliability (Bar-

Or 1987). As will be further discussed, this test allows for the computation of peak power, anaerobic capacity, and anaerobic fatigue. Certainly, these are all important components of anaerobic performance and have direct application to most sporting events. However, this test is inherently limited because it may not be a sufficient predictor of instantaneous performance attributes, which are regulated through neurological pathways. Further, it is not biomechanically specific to any sport other than cycling, so there are inherent limitations in its application to athletic scenarios in which body mass is not supported, a fixed range of angular motion is not repeatedly performed, or both.

Maximal Instantaneous Power

Maximal instantaneous power (Gollnick and Bayly 1986) may be generally defined as the highest potential power attainable in a single movement or repetition. Also known as maximal power, this attribute has been designated as the greatest potential product of force production and velocity.

Given that maximal power is related to the capacity of the neuromuscular system to develop a significant amount of force in a short period of time (i.e., contingent largely on rate of force development), this may be considered the fundamental component of performance in activities requiring maximal velocities with a constant load, especially at the point of impact or release (e.g., kicking, punching, jumping). Further, this has been viewed as an exceedingly important testing parameter and training objective in most sport conditioning programs.

Most research attention has been devoted to the load–power relationship in lower body compound movements such as the squat, clean, jump squat, and vertical jump. Findings demonstrate that maximal power is expressed at various percentages of peak force production, is largely contingent on the type of movement, and may range anywhere from 0% of maximal force production for the jump squat (i.e., no external additional load) (Cormie et al. 2007), to 80% of 1RM for the power clean (Cormie et al. 2007). Conversely, for isoinertial contractions (i.e., constant resistance), maximal power occurs at approximately 30% of maximal voluntary isometric contraction (Josephson 1993). Of particular relevance to lower extremity activity, body mass should be taken into account when measuring power output (i.e., added to, or considered a fraction of, the load lifted).

Rate of Force Development

Rate of force development (RFD)—also called rate of force production (RFP) or rate of torque development (RTD)—may be considered the rate of rise in contractile force (or torque) at the onset of contraction (Aagaard et al. 2002). RFD is illustrated using the slope of the force- or joint moment–time curve (i.e., change in torque / change in time), as depicted in figure 9.2. The

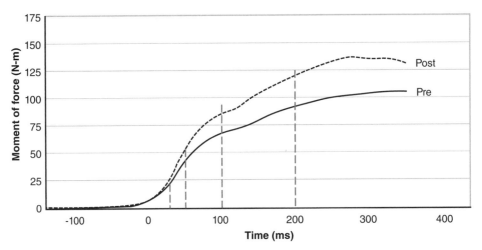

FIGURE 9.2 Rate of force development and moment–time curve.

Adapted from C. Suetta et al. 2004. "Training-induced changes in muscle CSA, muscle strength, EMG, and rate of force development in elderly subjects after long-term unilateral disuse". *Journal of Applied Physiology* 97: 1954-1961. Used with permission.

peak rate of force production (PRFP) is then the steepest point on the slope of the force–time curve, and represents the ability of a muscle (or group of muscles) to rapidly generate force or tension $(N \cdot s^{-1})$. These attributes are particularly significant for coordinated movements that require very fast and forceful muscular contractions, such as sprinting and jumping. Such activities require contractions in as little as 50 milliseconds, which is much shorter than is typically required for maximal force production (i.e., > 400 ms) (Aagaard et al. 2002; Thorstensson et al. 1976). RFD is exceedingly important for tasks associated with postural stabilization and balance, as well as high-force, high-velocity eccentric tasks such as preventing slip-and-fall accidents (Suetta et al. 2007).

An increase in RFD would represent an augmented ability to generate force and ultimately lead to significantly higher absolute force production over the same time course (Aagaard et al. 2002). More important, during conditions that do not permit maximal force or power production (i.e., extremely rapid eccentric or concentric muscle action), the capacity to develop a high degree of muscle force in a short time (i.e., high RFD) may indicate superior performance (Suetta et al. 2004) as compared to absolute strength or power. As demonstrated in figure 9.2, RFD may be significantly improved in as little as 12 weeks of standard resistance training exercise, among aging subjects.

Reactive Strength

The expression of muscular power is also contingent on factors unrelated to the contractile physiology of muscle. Specifically, noncontractile elements of the musculotendinous unit contribute significantly to the storage of elastic energy during eccentric contractions and the subsequent performance of concentric muscle actions and explosive movements (Wilson, Murphy, and Pryor 1994). Further, a direct link has been documented between musculotendinous stiffness (MTS) and the potential energy that may be used as a contributing synergistic factor during such concentric, explosive actions (Chelly and Denis 2001).

Over the last decade a great deal of attention has been devoted to the topic of reactive strength, both from a research perspective and among professionals designing exercise programs. Part of this interest is due to the purported adaptability of this anatomical property through strategic training approaches. Specifically, research has demonstrated that MTS may be specifically adapted based on loading history (Poussen, Van Hoeke, and Goubel 1990) and is particularly responsive to eccentric loading and repetitive plyometric actions. Ultimately, a stiffer musculotendinous system allows for more efficient elastic energy contributions at high countermovement speeds, thereby enhancing force production during the subsequent concentric phase of the movement (Chelly and Denis 2001).

The term *reactive strength* combines the concepts of energy storage and subsequent muscle action performance. Integral to reactive strength, the stretch–shortening cycle (SSC) enhances the capacity of the muscle–tendon unit to produce maximal force in the shortest amount of time (Chmielewski et al. 2006). The rapid loading of muscle during the eccentric, or yielding, phase of muscle action stimulates not only the storage of elastic energy, but also a myostatic stretch reflex, through stimulation of mechanoreceptors (i.e., muscle spindles). Afferent information is sent from the muscle spindles through the monosynaptic reflex loop to provide excitatory feedback to the preloaded (agonist) muscle. Both the rate of loading and the magnitude of the respective load directly influence this reflex and the stimulation of the agonist muscle (Bobbert et al. 1996).

Whereas SSC activity is considered more efficient (i.e., metabolic efficiency) than non-SSC activity (Alexander 2000), it is important to also regard the influence of SSC on peak power output capacities, as it is expressed through plyometric activity (e.g., jumping). The ability to discriminate concentric-only power output (i.e., without SSC) from that which occurs during SSC actions is particularly important among athletes who rely heavily on both attributes.

Sport Performance and Power

Proper assessment of power is vital for translation into sport performance programming and exercise prescription. Following are several additional points related to the application of power data for training and performance.

- *Use of data to prescribe power training.* Various researchers have suggested training be prescribed at a load that accommodates maximal power output (Kaneko et al. 1983). Using this strategy would thus require the acquisition of peak power data from a load–power curve for specific exercises. Conversely, other experts have pointed out that because maximal power is merely a snapshot of the instantaneous product of force and speed, training for improvement in power should instead be structured to address the load–power continuum, and hence a broader range of factors that influence the expression of power (i.e., maximal strength, strength-speed, speed, RFD, and reactive strength). As a simple example of how the expression of power may conceal the interaction between force production and movement speed, consider a situation in which power output is identical for two loads, although the movement velocity is higher for the lighter load and lower for the heavier load (Baker, Nance, and Moore 2001).

- *Influence of body mass.* Although significant debate currently surrounds the appropriate use of power data for exercise prescription (Cronin and Sleivert 2005; Cormie and Flanagan 2008), most experts agree that body mass is a critical variable that should be accounted for, both when testing and training for lower extremity muscular power. Because performance in most sports requires a certain degree of proficiency in manipulating body mass (e.g., jumping, bounding, accelerating, change of direction), it is certainly logical to control for the influence of body mass when evaluating explosive movement. It is also vital to account for changes in body mass over time, which facilitates accurate observations of power-to-body-mass-ratio fluctuations. Power-to-body-mass ratio is considered a critical predictor of performance enhancement across both anaerobic- and aerobic-based sports (Gibala et al. 2006; Lunn, Finn, and Axtell 2009), and should therefore be closely monitored (see the section Practical Applications for a case study of the vertical jump).

- *Hierarchy of performance.* Modeling of athletic performance involves a systematic, qualitative examination of movement to determine which factors most contribute to diminished or enhanced performance (Bartlett 2007; Ham, Knez, and Young 2007). Also known as hierarchical models, this process allows for the decomposition of movement into the contributory biomechanical and physiological factors that explain variability in the performance outcome. At present much debate surrounds the strategies to optimize power output and performance enhancement; and thus, more research is needed to unravel the biomechanical and physiological issues that explain the interrelationships among muscular strength, rate of force development, maximal power output, and the subsequent translation of these to explosive movement. For now, fitness professionals should consider the expression of power within such a hierarchical construct and incorporate a spectrum of sport-specific power tests. Assessing these factors separately ensures a systematic prescription and refinement of training to maximize performance.

Tests for Power

The remainder of this chapter presents several tests for evaluating power and explosiveness that may be easily integrated into a sport conditioning or personal training program. These tests have documented validity and reliability and may be applied according to the specific needs of an athlete. As previously mentioned, a measure of power is specific to the context in which it is executed (e.g., the time course for power production, muscle action specificity), and thus should not be used interchangeably with other tests.

Lower Body Tests

The vast majority of research pertaining to power testing and training has been devoted to the lower extremities. This is intuitive considering the extent that muscles of the lower extremities are needed for producing the ground reactive forces associated with acceleration, deceleration, jumping, landing, and rapid changes of direction.

WINGATE ANAEROBIC TEST

Developed at the Wingate Institute in the 1970s (Ayalon, Inbar, and Bar-Or 1974), the Wingate Anaerobic Test (WAnT) measures peak anaerobic power, anaerobic capacity, and anaerobic fatigue. This test occurs with a 30-second time course using a cycle ergometer. The calculation of peak power is typically acquired within the first five seconds of work, and is expressed in total watts (W), or relative to body mass (W/kg). Further, using the entire 30 seconds of cycling, anaerobic capacity (AC) may be calculated as the total external work performed, and is expressed in kilojoules (kJ). Lastly, anaerobic fatigue is often included in the WAnT and allows for the calculation of the percentage of power output reduction throughout the test (i.e., fatigue index).

EQUIPMENT

- Mechanically braked cycle ergometer. For the WAnT, a Monark cycle ergometer is typically used. Other ergometers (e.g., Fleisch cycle ergometer) require different loading parameters.
- Optical sensor to detect and count reflective markers on the flywheel
- Computer and interface with appropriate software (e.g., Sports Medicine Industries, Inc.)

PROCEDURE

1. Warm-up: After initial familiarization and individual adjustment on the cycle ergometer, the subject performs three to five minutes of light cycling at a load that is 20% of the load used for the actual

test. At the end of each minute of the warm-up, the subject performs approximately five seconds of sprinting.

2. Following the specific warm-up, the subject participates in light dynamic stretching of the quadriceps, hamstrings, and calf muscles. This time may also be used to further explain testing instructions.

3. The test is initiated with the subject pedaling at maximal cadence against no load. A verbal command of "Go" provides the auditory cue to begin pedaling. Once the subject is at maximal cadence (usually in the first one to three seconds), apply the external load for the 30-second all-out test. Load = 0.075 kilogram per kilogram of body mass (Monark cycle ergometer).

4. Following the application of the appropriate resistance, the 30-second test is started, and data collection commences. The subject must remain seated throughout the entire 30 seconds.

5. Flywheel revolutions per minute (rpm) are counted (preferably by photocell and computer interface), and peak power is calculated based on maximal rpm (usually over the first five seconds of work) and angular distance. For the Monark cycle ergometer, each revolution is equal to 1.615 meters.

6. The test is terminated after 30 seconds of all-out work. Following the test, a two- to five-minute cool-down period is recommended before the subject dismounts the cycle ergometer.

OUTCOME MEASURES

1. Peak power (PP) = (flywheel rpm for highest five-second period × 1.615 meters) × (resistance in kilograms × 9.8)

2. Mean power (MP) is calculated as the average of all five-second intervals throughout the entire 30-second test, and is usually regarded as a surrogate descriptor of anaerobic endurance.

3. Anaerobic capacity (AC) is expressed as kilogram-Joules (1 kg-m = 9.804 J) and is calculated by adding each five-second peak power output over the entire 30 seconds.

4. Anaerobic fatigue describes a decline in power output and is calculated as follows: AF = [(highest five-second PP − lowest five-second PP) / (highest five-second PP)] × 100.

5. The fatigue index is also often calculated to characterize the percentage of peak power drop-off: FI = [1 − (lowest power output / peak power) × 100].

ADDITIONAL CONSIDERATIONS AND MODIFICATIONS

A more thorough description of this test may be found in the seminal text by Inbar and colleagues (Inbar, Bar-Or, and Skinner 1996). This test may be modified extensively, depending on the desired outcome. For example, if a person is interested in merely ascertaining peak power output, there is no need to perform the entire 30-second test. A 5- to 10-second test has been used for this purpose. Further, a modified WAnT has been proposed for elderly men and women (Bar-Or 1992), in which maximal pedaling occurs for only 15 seconds. However, for this test, resistance added to the flywheel is equal to 9.5% of whole-body lean mass, which must be ascertained through a valid measurement of body composition (e.g., whole-body plethysmography or hydrodensitometry).

Tables 9.2 and 9.3 provide percentile ranks for males and females for the Wingate Anaerobic Test.

TABLE 9.2 Wingate Anaerobic Test: Percentile Ranks for Physically Active Males and Females (18-28 years old)

Percentile rank	WATTS		WATTS · KG^{-1}	
	Male	Female	Male	Female
95	676.6	483	8.6	7.5
90	661.8	469.9	8.2	7.3
85	630.5	437	8.1	7.1
80	617.9	419.4	8	7
75	604.3	413.5	8	6.9
70	600	409.7	7.9	6.8
65	591.7	402.2	7.7	6.7
60	576.8	391.4	7.6	6.6
55	574.5	386	7.5	6.5
50	564.6	381.1	7.4	6.4
45	552.8	376.9	7.3	6.2
40	547.6	366.9	7.1	6.2
35	234.6	360.5	7.1	6.1
30	529.7	353.2	7	6
25	520.6	346.8	6.8	5.9
20	496.1	336.5	6.6	5.7
15	494.6	320.3	6.4	5.6
10	470.9	306.1	6	5.3
5	453.2	286.5	5.6	5.1

Adapted with permission from *Research Quarterly for Exercise and Sport* Vol. 60, No. 2, 144–151. Copyright 1989 by the American Alliance for Health, Physical Education, Recreation and Dance, 1900 Association Drive, Reston, VA 20191.

MARGARIA-KALAMEN TEST

Margaria, Aghemo, and Rovelli (1966) and Kalamen (1968) devised stair sprinting tests to predict power output. What is commonly used today is representative of the most reliable of the versions and is known as the Margaria-Kalamen Power Test (Fox, Bowers, and Foss 1993; McArdle, Katch, and Katch 2007). This test allows for a simple computation of power output based on vertical distance traveled, total time to complete, and body mass, following a rapid accent of a staircase. This test has been used with various populations and provides a valid measure of peak power that has been demonstrated to be positively associated with performance in other explosive movements.

EQUIPMENT

- Staircase with nine or more steps. The step should be approximately 7 inches (18 cm) high, and the lead-up area should be at least 20 feet (6 m) long (see figure 9.3).
- Scale for body weight measurement
- Measuring stick or tape
- Electronic timer with a start and stop switch. A stopwatch may be used, but this may not yield accurate time or power output calculations.

PROCEDURE

1. The height of each step is measured with a measuring stick or tape, and recorded. The vertical distance from the third step to the ninth step is then determined by multiplying the step height by six steps (i.e., Step height × 6) (see figure 9.4 on p. 235). Height is recorded in meters using this conversion factor: 1 inch = 0.0254 meters.

TABLE 9.3 Wingate Anaerobic Test Classification of Peak Power (W and W/kg^{-1}) and Anaerobic Capacity (W and W/kg^{-1}) for Female and Male NCAA Division I Collegiate Athletes

Classification	Peak power (W)	Peak power (W/kg^{-1})	Anaerobic capacity (W)	Anaerobic capacity (W/kg^{-1})
Females				
Elite	>730	>11.07	>541	>8.22
Excellent	686–730	10.58–11.07	510–541	7.86–8.22
Above average	642–685	10.08–10.57	478–509	7.51–7.85
Average	554–641	9.10–10.07	414–477	6.81–7.5
Below average	510–553	8.60–9.09	382–413	6.45–6.80
Fair	467–509	8.11–8.59	351–381	6.1–6.44
Poor	<467	<8.11	<351	<6.1
Males				
Elite	>1163	>13.74	>823	>9.79
Excellent	1092–1163	13.03–13.74	778–823	9.35–9.79
Above average	1021–1091	12.35–13.02	732–777	8.91–9.34
Average	880–1020	11.65-12.34	640–731	8.02–8.90
Below average	809–879	10.96–11.64	595–639	7.58–8.01
Fair	739–808	9.57–10.95	549–594	7.14–7.57
Poor	<739	<9.57	<549	<7.14

Adapted, by permission, from M.F. Zupan et al., 2009, "Wingate Anaerobic Test peak power and anaerobic capacity classifications for men and women intercollegiate athletes," *Journal of Strength and Conditioning Research* 23 (9): 2598–2604.

2. The timing switch mechanisms are placed on the third step and the ninth step. These will allow for an accurate start time (third step) and stop time (ninth step), respectively.

3. The subject's weight is then taken and converted into newtons. Conversion factors: 1 pound = 4.45 newtons; or 1 kilogram = 9.807 newtons.

4. Warm-up: After initial familiarization with the test procedure, the subject performs approximately five minutes of moderate-intensity aerobic exercise (incline walking or jogging are preferable), followed by several dynamic range of motion exercises for the hip flexors and extensors, hamstrings, quadriceps, and calves. The subject is then allowed two trial runs at approximately 50 and 80% to fully acclimate to the test procedures. This will allow for the most valid measure of maximal power production.

5. The test is initiated with the subject sprinting forward across the lead-up area (see figure 9.4) toward the staircase. A verbal command of "Go" provides the auditory cue to begin sprinting from the starting line.

6. The subject ascends the flight of stairs as quickly as possible, taking three steps at a time (i.e., from the floor to the third step, sixth step, and ninth step).

7. Time is recorded from the third step to the ninth step, to the nearest 0.01 seconds, using the timing system or stopwatch.

8. The test should be repeated once or twice to determine the best possible performance. Recovery between trials should be two to three minutes.

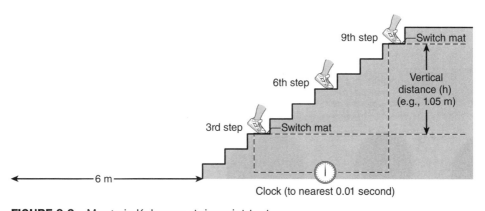

FIGURE 9.3 Margaria-Kalamen stair sprint test.

TABLE 9.4   Margaria-Kalamen Stair Sprint Normative Values (in Watts)

Classification	15–20 years	20–30 years	30–40 years	40–50 years	Over 50 years
Females					
Excellent	>1785	>1648	>1226	>961	>736
Good	1491–1785	1383–1648	1040–1226	814–961	608–736
Average	1187–1481	1098–1373	834–1030	647–804	481–598
Fair	902–1177	834–1089	637–824	490–637	373–471
Poor	<902	<834	<637	<490	<373
Males					
Excellent	>2197	>2059	>1648	>1226	>961
Good	1844–2197	1726–2059	1383–1648	1040–1226	814–961
Average	1471–1824	1373–1716	1098–1373	834–1030	647–804
Fair	1108–1461	1040–1363	834–1088	637–824	490–637
Poor	<1108	<1040	<834	<637	<490

Adapted, by permission, from Fox, Bowers, and Foss, 1993, The physiological basis for exercise and sport, 5th ed. (Dubuque, IA: Wm C. Brown), 676, ©The McGraw-Hill Companies.

OUTCOME MEASURES

Power in watts (W) is calculated using the subject's weight (in newtons), total vertical distance (in meters), and time (in seconds) by the following formula:

$$\text{Power (watts)} = (\text{weight} \times \text{height}) / \text{time}$$

Table 9.4 provides normative values for the Margaria-Kalamen test.

ADDITIONAL CONSIDERATIONS AND MODIFICATIONS

A thorough description of the age-based norms for this test exist (McArdle, Katch, and Katch 2007). In addition, several modifications to the Margaria-Kalamen test have been devised to accommodate certain populations. Because some people cannot safely ascend a staircase by every third step, Clemons and Harrison (2008) devised a modification that requires subjects to ascend a single flight of 11 steps. This modification does not require a sprint lead-up, and so a normal staircase can be used. For the ascent, participants take a single step initially (i.e., onto the first step), followed by two steps each stride thereafter. A vertical distance of 2.04 meters is used for the measurement of power, and time in seconds is recorded to ascend to the top of the staircase (see figure 9.4). Time is recorded from the top of step 1 to the top of step 11, and power is calculated as Power (W) = [(body mass (kg) × 2.04) × 9.81) / time].

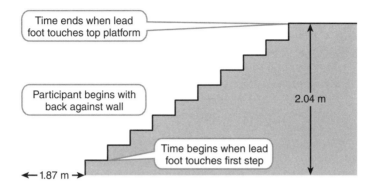

Time ends when lead foot touches top platform

Participant begins with back against wall

2.04 m

Time begins when lead foot touches first step

←1.87 m→

FIGURE 9.4 Modified Margaria-Kalamen stair sprint test.

Reprinted, by permission, from J. Clemons and M. Harrsion 2008, "Validity and reliability of a new stair sprinting test of explosive power," *Journal of Strength and Conditioning Research* 22(5): 1578–1583.

VERTICAL JUMP TEST

The vertical jump (VJ) is one of the most frequently used tests of power and explosiveness in strength and conditioning. The appeal of the VJ test is due, in part, to the ease of test administration, but also to the fact that the results are directly applicable to most sports that require jumping and others in which lower body power output is paramount (e.g., weightlifting). As previously mentioned, numerous underlying factors contribute to VJ performance, and as such, numerous methods of testing jumping ability exist. Some of the most common versions of VJ testing are the basic countermovement VJ, the squat jump, and the approach VJ. The procedures for a standard countermovement vertical jump are provided next, and additional information concerning modifications is presented at the end.

EQUIPMENT

- Commercially available Vertec apparatus (Sports Imports, Columbus, OH) (see figure 9.5)

Or

- A smooth, tall wall (i.e., with ceiling height greater than the subject's jumping ability)
- Chalk to mark hand
- Measuring stick or tape

PROCEDURE USING VERTEC APPARATUS

1. The subject's weight is taken and converted into kilograms (for purposes of peak power estimate). Conversion factor: 1 pound = 0.454 kilograms.

2. The subject's reach height is measured and recorded. To do this, adjust the height of the Vertec plastic vanes to be within the subject's reach. The shaft that holds the vanes is marked with measurements, and the measurement selected should coincide with the bottom vane. Each vane represents 0.5 inches, and each red vane represents an increment of 6 inches. The subject reaches, without lifting the heels (i.e., flat footed) and touches the highest vane possible with the dominant hand. To prevent confounding results, the subject must stand directly beneath the apparatus and reach as high as possible.

3. Warm-up: After initial familiarization with the test procedure and the Vertec apparatus, the subject performs approximately five minutes of moderate-intensity aerobic exercise (incline walking or jogging are preferable), followed by several dynamic range of motion exercises for the hip flexors and extensors, hamstrings, quadriceps, calves, and shoulders. The subject is then allowed several trials without the Vertec apparatus to become familiar with the countermovement jump procedure.

4. The subject's jump height is then measured and recorded. To do this, lift the height of the Vertec stack so that the top vane is higher than the subject's estimated jump height. Again, the measurement on the Vertec shaft must be carefully used to ensure an accurate calculation of jump height.

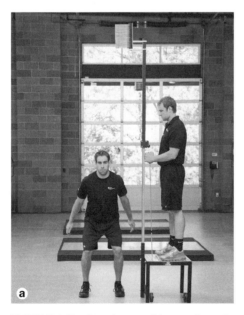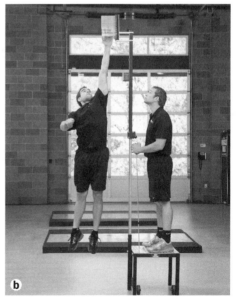

FIGURE 9.5 Starting position and maximal height of the vertical jump using a Vertec apparatus.

5. For a standard countermovement VJ test, the subject is not permitted to take any lead-up steps (i.e., approach). This test requires the subject to perform a rapid countermovement by quickly descending into a squat (i.e., flexion of hips and knees, and forward and downward movement of the trunk) while swinging the arms down and backward (see figure 9.5). This rapid countermovement is immediately followed by a maximal jump in which the dominant hand reaches to touch the highest possible Vertec vane.

6. Following each jump, the vanes are moved out of the way for consecutive trials (i.e., the highest vane touched and all vanes underneath are turned to the opposite direction).

7. The best of three trials is recorded to the nearest 0.5 inch.

8. Vertical jump height is recorded as the difference between the highest jump and the previously recorded reach height.

PROCEDURE USING WALL AND CHALK

General note: The measurement of body weight and procedures for warm-up and countermovement are the same as those used when testing VJ with the Vertec apparatus.

1. The subject's reach height is measured and recorded. To do this, the subject rubs chalk on the middle finger of the dominant hand. Standing with the dominant shoulder adjacent to the wall, the subject reaches as high as possible and makes a chalk mark on the wall.

2. Using a countermovement, the subject then jumps as high as possible and makes a second chalk mark on the wall to designate the height of the maximal jump.

3. The best of three trials is recorded to the nearest 0.5 inch.

4. Vertical jump height is recorded as the difference between the highest chalk mark and the previously recorded reach height.

OUTCOME MEASURES

1. Vertical jump performance = maximal jump height – reach height. Normative data on VJ performance are provided for nonathletic, healthy college students (Patterson and Peterson 2004) as well as for various athletic populations (Hoffman 2006).

2. Estimate of power: Several equations allow for the estimation of power from vertical jump performance. This is an important step to consider, because body mass is associated with jump height and instantaneous power production. For example, if two people have the same absolute vertical jump, but different body masses, they perform different quantities of work to achieve that jump height. Further, this may also apply to repeated bouts of testing for the same person over

an extended period of time. If a person gains or loses weight between bouts of testing, jump height and subsequent power production may be altered. Jump height is therefore a crude proxy for explosive power performance. One frequently used equation is the Sayers equation (1999), which estimates peak power as follows:

$$\text{Peak power (W)} = [60.7 \times (\text{jump height [cm]}) + 45.3 \times (\text{body mass [kg]}) - 2{,}055]$$

This equation has been shown to be highly valid and reliable, and gender differences do not interfere with the accuracy of PP estimates (Sayers et al. 1999). Further, this method has been verified as a valuable means of quan-

TABLE 9.5 Descriptive Data for Vertical Jump Among Female and Male Active College Students

Gender	HEALTHY NONATHLETE COLLEGE STUDENTS		RECREATIONAL COLLEGE ATHLETES		COMPETITIVE COLLEGE ATHLETES	
	Inches	Centimeters	Inches	Centimeters	Inches	Centimeters
Females	14.1	35.81	15–15.5	38–39	16–18.5	41–47
Males	22.2	56.39	24	61.00	25-25.5	64-65

Reprinted, by permission, from J. Hoffman, 2006, *Norms for fitness, performance, and health* (Champaign, IL: Human Kinetics), 60.

TABLE 9.6 Percentile Ranks for Vertical Jump in High School and Collegiate Football Players

Percentile rank	9TH GRADE		10TH GRADE		11TH GRADE		12TH GRADE		NCAA DIVISION III		NCAA DIVISION I	
	Inches	Centimeters	Inches	Centimeters	Inches	Centimeters	Inches	Centimeters	Inches	Centimeters	Inches	Centimeters
90	27.6	70.1	27.4	69.6	28.5	72.4	30	76.2	30	76.2	33.5	85.1
80	25.5	64.8	26	66	26.9	68.3	28	71.1	28.5	72.4	31.5	80
70	24	61	24.6	62.5	25.5	64.8	26.5	67.3	27.5	69.9	30	76.2
60	23.5	59.7	23.9	60.7	25	63.5	26	66	26.5	67.3	29	73.7
50	22.3	56.6	23	58.4	24	61	25	63.5	25.5	64.8	28	71.1
40	21.9	55.6	22	55.9	23.5	59.7	23.5	59.7	24.5	62.2	27	68.6
30	21.2	53.8	21	53.3	22	55.9	22.5	57.2	23.5	59.7	25.5	64.8
20	19.3	49	19	48.3	20.5	52.1	21.5	54.6	22	55.9	24	61
10	17.7	45	18	45.7	18.8	47.8	19.5	49.5	20	50.8	21.5	54.6

Adapted, by permission, from J. Hoffman, 2006, *Norms for fitness, performance, and health* (Champaign, IL: Human Kinetics), 60.

TABLE 9.7   Percentile Ranks for Vertical Jump Among NCAA Division I Female Volleyball, Softball, and Swimming Athletes

Percentile rank	VOLLEYBALL		SOFTBALL		SWIMMING	
	Inches	Centimeters	Inches	Centimeters	Inches	Centimeters
90	20	50.8	18.5	47	19.9	50.5
80	18.9	48	17	43.2	18	45.7
70	18	45.7	16	40.6	17.4	44.2
60	17.5	44.5	15	38.1	16.1	40.9
50	17	43.2	14.5	36.8	15	38.1
40	16.7	42.4	14	35.6	14.5	36.8
30	16.5	41.9	13	33	13	33
20	16	40.6	12	30.5	12.5	31.8
10	15.5	39.4	11	27.9	11.6	29.5

Adapted, by permission, from J. Hoffman, 2006, *Norms for fitness, performance, and health* (Champaign, IL: Human Kinetics), 62.

tifying lower body PP and weightlifting ability among elite athletes (Carlock et al. 2004). Harman and colleagues (1991) developed another commonly used equation that allows for an estimate of both peak and mean power, with the following computations:

$$\text{Peak power (W)} = [61.9 \times (\text{jump height [cm]}) + 36 \times (\text{body mass [kg]}) + 1,822]$$

$$\text{Mean power (W)} = [21.2 \times (\text{jump height [cm]}) + 23 \times (\text{body mass [kg]}) - 1,393]$$

There are no normative data across multiple populations using these equations. Therefore, they should be used to estimate power output within subjects (clients or athletes) to enhance internal validity, rather than to make comparative inferences to a norm-reference standard. Tables 9.5, 9.6, and 9.7 provide percentile ranks for the vertical jump test.

ADDITIONAL CONSIDERATIONS AND MODIFICATIONS

A static squat jump (SJ) test may be used as a modification of the counter-movement VJ test. This test requires the same basic procedures as the VJ test, except that the countermovement is removed. The subject descends into a full squat position (i.e., thighs approximately parallel to the floor, or knees at a 90° angle), where a one- to two-second isometric contraction occurs. Following a "Go" command, the subject jumps as high as possible, without a countermovement. Depending on the procedure, some experts do not recommend using an arm action when performing the SJ (e.g., hands are on hips or fingers are interlaced behind the head). Specifically, if a contact mat or force platform is used then an arm action may not be advisable, because doing so artificially augments jump performance and confounds the measurement accuracy of lower body power production.

The SJ is an effective test for evaluating concentric-only explosive movement, and many strength and conditioning coaches use it as a supplement to the traditional VJ. The Sayers equation may also be used for this test, because it has been demonstrated to be valid and reliable (Sayers et al. 1999). Some coaches prefer to have subjects start by sitting down in a chair when testing SJ, to prevent a countermovement from occurring. This can be dangerous, however, because the chair may interfere with a safe landing.

An approach VJ allows the subject to take several lead-up steps prior to a maximal countermovement jump. Many strength and conditioning coaches use an approach VJ, because it is representative of sport-specific explosive movement. Variations of this test exist (e.g., single-leg take-off versus double-leg take-off; one-step approach versus multiple-step approach); however, to collect reliable data, fitness professionals should adopt a single procedure and replicate it over multiple repeated bouts (i.e., between subjects, as well as for multiple trials for a single subject).

REACTIVE STRENGTH INDEX (RSI)

Reactive strength performance may account for the stretch–shortening cycle (SSC) that occurs during explosive movement in many performance tasks. Specifically, in movements that involve high force and high-speed muscle and joint actions (e.g., the vertical jump), the force–velocity curve is affected by the preceding loading phase (i.e., countermovement) such that at any given speed of movement, a greater force production is possible (i.e., the force–velocity curve shifts to the right). Because of the neuromuscular adaptation and alteration in musculotendinous stiffness that occurs in conjunction with plyometric and eccentric exercise (Poussen, Van Hoeke, and Goubel 1990), this parameter is considered to be a trainable entity, thus requiring a valid, reliable system to assess it.

Although various approaches have been used, most are performed to compare the countermovement jump and the static squat jump heights (Walshe, Wilson, and Murphy 1996). A slightly different approach, the reactive strength index (RSI), has recently been used to quantify plyometric or SSC performance (Flanagan and Harrison 2007); it is derived from performance in the depth jump. RSI calculation uses jump performance and time spent on the ground (i.e., the *amortization phase* is the time spent to decelerate from the landing in which muscle lengthening occurs, to the time of take-off in a subsequent maximal jump), and has demonstrated to be a valid and reliable means of expressing explosiveness (Flanagan, Ebben, and Jensen 2008).

EQUIPMENT

- Various plyometric boxes or risers of different heights. This test has documented validity and reliability at a box height of 30 centimeters (11.8 in.) (Flanagan, Ebben, and Jensen 2008).
- Commercially available contact mat

PROCEDURE

1. Warm-up: After initial familiarization with the test procedure and the contact mat, the subject performs approximately five minutes of moderate-intensity aerobic exercise (jogging or running is preferable), followed by several dynamic and rapid range of motion exercises for the hip flexors and extensors, hamstrings, quadriceps, and calves. The subject is then allowed several depth jump trials at a submaximal effort. Because this test is stressful to the muscles and joints of the lower body, fully acclimating subjects to this test is very important.

2. To initiate this test, the subject steps off the box and lands with both feet on the contact mat simultaneously. Immediately following this landing, the subject jumps as high as possible. Particular emphasis should be made to reduce eccentric action and contact time from the depth jump prior to the concentric action.

3. The subject should perform two or three trials at each box height, with a minimum of 90 seconds of recovery between trials.

OUTCOME MEASURES

1. The subject's jump height and contact time are measured and recorded from the contact mat. Using the flight time, jump height is calculated using the following equation: Jump height = $(9.81 \times \text{flight time}^2) / 8$.

2. Ground contact time may be calculated as the time between initial foot contact and take-off (Flanagan, Ebben, and Jensen 2008).

3. Reactive strength index (RSI) is calculated using the following equation: RSI = jump height / contact time.

ADDITIONAL CONSIDERATIONS AND MODIFICATIONS

Other methods allow fitness professionals to examine the effects of the SSC and its relation to explosive movement or athletic performance. An alternative to the RSI test involves comparing the eccentric utilization ratio (EUR) by simply examining the ratio of countermovement jump height to squat jump height (McGuigan et al. 2006). Using these two factors, prestretch augmentation can be calculated as follows:

$$(\text{Countermovement jump height} - \text{squat jump height}) / \text{squat jump height}) \times 100$$

Each of these measures may provide reliable data to account for changes in SSC and musculotendinous stiffness that occurs with training.

STANDING LONG JUMP

The standing long jump (SLJ) is another frequently used test of lower body explosive performance. This test may be used in conjunction with the VJ test, because it provides information about vertical and horizontal displacement. This test is particularly important to administer when SLJ exercises (e.g., bounding) are included in athletes' exercise prescriptions. Data on maximal SLJ distance help fitness professionals prescribe specific percentages of this performance for subsequent training dosages (e.g., three repetitions at 90% SLJ max).

EQUIPMENT

- Flat jumping surface, at least 20 feet (6 meters) long. Gym floors (i.e., basketball or volleyball courts), rubber tracks, and artificial turf field are recommended.
- Tape measure
- Roll of masking tape
- Several commercially available standing long jump mats (e.g., Gill Athletics, Champaign, IL) may be used for this test.

PROCEDURE

1. Designate a starting line. This may be done using a 3-foot (1 m) piece of masking tape.
2. Warm-up: After initial familiarization with the SLJ test procedure, the subject performs approximately five minutes of moderate-intensity aerobic exercise (jogging or running is preferable), followed by several dynamic and rapid range of motion exercises for the hip flexors and extensors, hamstrings, quadriceps, calves, and shoulders. The subject is then allowed several SLJ trials at less-than-maximal effort. Like the RSI test, this test is stressful to the muscles and joints of the lower body, which makes fully acclimating subjects to this test exceedingly important.
3. The subject's jump distance is measured and recorded. With the toes behind the starting line, the subject uses a rapid countermovement and then jumps forward as far as possible. A marker is placed behind the subject's rearmost heel, using a small piece of masking tape.
4. The best of three trials is recorded to the nearest 0.5 inch.
5. Standing long jump performance is recorded as the difference from the starting line (i.e., the 0-inch mark) and the longest jump.

OUTCOME MEASURES

Standing long jump = maximal jump distance from the 0-inch mark / starting line. Table 9.8 shows percentile and ranking data for elite and 15- and 16-year-old male and female athletes (Chu 1996).

TABLE 9.8 Percentile and Ranking Data for Standing Long Jump Among Elite and 15- and 16-Year-Old Male and Female Athletes

Percentile rank	ELITE MALE ATHLETES		ELITE FEMALE ATHLETES	
	Inches	Centimeters	Inches	Centimeters
90	148	375.9	124	315
80	133	337.8	115	292.1
70	122	309.9	110	279.4
60	116	294.6	104	264.2
50	110	279.4	98	248.9
40	104	264.2	92	233.7
30	98	248.9	86	218.4
20	92	233.7	80	203.2
10	86	218.4	74	188
	15- AND 16-YEAR OLD MALE ATHLETES		15- AND 16-YEAR OLD FEMALE ATHLETES	
Classification	Inches	Centimeters	Inches	Centimeters
Excellent	79	200.7	65	165.1
Above average	73	185.4	61	154.9
Average	69	175.3	57	144.8
Below average	65	165.1	53	134.6
Poor	<65	<165	<53	<135

Adapted, by permission, from J. Hoffman, 2006, *Norms for fitness, performance, and health* (Champaign, IL: Human Kinetics), 58; Adapted, by permission, from D.A. Chu, 1996, *Explosive power and strength* (Champaign, IL: Human Kinetics), 171.

ADDITIONAL CONSIDERATIONS

Because this test has an increased risk for injury, it should be reserved for well-trained people with no existing injuries or musculoskeletal discomfort. As mentioned, it is exceedingly important that subjects warm up properly prior to this test. Further, several preliminary trials are typically needed to serve as a specific warm-up.

Upper Body Tests

The majority of tests and training protocols emphasize lower extremity muscular power. However, upper extremity power production and performance are also exceedingly important for most sports and activities. Two primary tests to examine maximal upper extremity anaerobic capacity and power are the Upper Body Wingate Anaerobic Test and the Medicine Ball Put. Each of these tests has been validated numerous times and has proven reliable across multiple populations.

UPPER BODY WINGATE ANAEROBIC TEST

Similar to the traditional WAnT for the lower body, the Upper Body Wingate Anaerobic Test is generally performed in a laboratory setting and has the advantage of providing several outcomes related to upper body anaerobic capacity. This test occurs with a 30-second time course using a modified cycle ergometer with an arm crank. The calculation of peak power is typically acquired within the first three to five seconds of work, and is expressed in total watts (W), or relative to body mass (W/kg). Further, using the entire 30 seconds of arm cranking, anaerobic capacity (AC) may be calculated as the total external work performed, and is expressed in kilojoules (kJ). Lastly, anaerobic fatigue is often reported, which allows for the calculation of the percentage of power output reduction throughout the test (i.e., fatigue index).

EQUIPMENT

- Mechanically braked cycle ergometer with additional adjustment for an arm crank (i.e., a cycle ergometer with handles where the pedals normally are)

- Table for mounting the ergometer for testing. This should be higher than 70 centimeters (27.6 in.) and have room for legs underneath.

- Additional weight (80 to 100 kg, or 176 to 220 lb) to load the ergometer to prevent movement during the test

- Optical sensor to detect and count reflective markers on the flywheel

- Computer and interface with appropriate software (e.g., Sports Medicine Industries, Inc.)

PROCEDURE

1. The subject should be seated comfortably in a chair placed behind the cycle ergometer so that the feet are flat on the floor. This allows the subject to pedal with no restrictions.

2. Warm-up: After initial familiarization with and individual adjustment of the upper body ergometer, the subject performs three to five minutes of light arm cranking, with no load or a load that is less than 20% of the load used for the actual test. At the end of each minute of the warm-up, the subject should perform approximately five seconds of maximal arm cranking.

3. Following the specific warm-up, the subject should participate in light dynamic stretching of the entire shoulder joint, pectoral musculature, and muscles of the biceps, triceps, and forearms. This time may also be used to further explain testing instructions.

4. The test is initiated with the subject cranking at maximal cadence against no load. A verbal command of "Go" provides the auditory cue

to begin arm cranking. Once the subject is at maximal cadence (usually in the first one to three seconds), apply the external load for the 30-second all-out test. Load = 0.050 kilogram per kilogram of body mass (Monark cycle ergometer) (Nindl et al. 1995).

5. Following the application of the appropriate resistance, the 30-second test is started, and data collection commences. The subject must remain seated throughout the entire 30 seconds.

6. Flywheel revolutions per minute (rpm) are counted (preferably by photocell and computer interface), and peak power is calculated based on maximal rpm (usually over the first five seconds of work) and angular distance. Each revolution is equal to 1.615 meters.

7. The test is terminated after 30 seconds of all-out work. Following the test, a two- to five-minute cool-down period is recommended.

OUTCOME MEASURES

See the section Wingate Anaerobic Test. Table 9.9 provides typical values for peak mean power in males and females for the Upper Body Wingate Anaerobic Test.

MEDICINE BALL PUT

The field test most frequently used to measure power of the upper body is the seated medicine ball put (Clemons, Campbell, and Jeansonne 2010). The widespread popularity of this test is due not only to the ease of administration, but also to the direct specificity of this movement to a functional task such as the chest pass in basketball, or even the rapid punching of combat athletes. Moreover, because this exercise is commonly used in training, test data may easily be extrapolated to training prescription.

EQUIPMENT

- 45° incline bench
- High-durability medicine ball: 6 kilograms (13.2 lb) for females, 9 kilograms (19.8 lb) for males (Clemons, Campbell, and Jeansonne 2010)
- Gymnastics chalk (i.e., carbonate of magnesium)
- Measuring tape
- Room or gymnasium with at least 8 meters (26 feet) of clearance

PROCEDURE

1. The measuring tape is placed on the floor with the end positioned under the front frame of the bench, to anchor it.

2. The tip of the tape should be positioned so it is aligned with the outside of the medicine ball while it rests on the subject's chest (i.e., in

TABLE 9.9 Upper Body Wingate Anaerobic Test: Typical Values for Peak Power and Mean Power in Males and Females

Classification	AGE (YEARS)							
	<10	10–12	12–14	14–16	16–18	18–25	25–35	>35
Male peak power								
Excellent	205	192	473	473	575	658	565	589
Very good	164	171	389	411	484	556	501	510
Good	143	159	343	379	438	507	469	471
Average	122	148	298	348	393	458	437	433
Below average	101	137	253	316	347	409	405	394
Poor	80	126	207	284	301	360	373	356
Very poor	60	115	162	252	256	311	341	317
Male mean power								
Excellent	161	159	333	380	409	477	415	454
Very good	136	142	276	321	349	403	375	395
Good	118	133	248	293	318	366	355	366
Average	100	124	220	264	288	329	335	337
Below average	83	116	192	236	258	292	315	308
Poor	65	107	165	207	227	255	294	279
Very poor	47	98	137	179	197	218	274	249
Female peak power								
Excellent	201	176	214	–	–	–	–	–
Very good	152	159	199	–	–	–	–	–
Good	135	141	184	–	–	–	–	–
Average	119	124	170	–	–	–	–	–
Below average	102	106	155	–	–	–	–	–
Poor	86	89	140	–	–	–	–	–
Very poor	53	55	110	–	–	–	–	–
Female mean power								
Excellent	153	158	194	–	–	–	–	–
Very good	130	137	165	–	–	–	–	–
Good	118	126	151	–	–	–	–	–
Average	107	116	137	–	–	–	–	–
Below average	6	105	122	–	–	–	–	–
Poor	84	94	108	–	–	–	–	–
Very poor	73	83	93	–	–	–	–	–

Adapted, by permission, from J. Hoffman, 2006, *Norms for fitness, performance and health* (Champaign, IL: Human Kinetics), 56; Adapted from O. Inbar, O. Bar-Or, and J.S. Skinner, 1996, *The Wingate anaerobic test* (Champaign, IL: Human Kinetics), 82, 84, 91, 92.

the ready position, prior to putting the ball) (Clemons, Campbell, and Jeansonne 2010; see figure 9.6).

3. The tape should be extended outward from the bench for at least 8 meters (26 feet), and secured to the floor.

4. Warm-up: After initial familiarization with the bench orientation and putting procedure, the subject performs five minutes of moderate-intensity aerobic exercise, followed by several dynamic range of motion exercises for the shoulder and elbow joint (e.g., modified or regular push-ups or hand walk-outs). The subject is then allowed several submaximal trials with the appropriate medicine ball.

5. For the test, the subject should be seated comfortably on the incline bench with feet flat on the floor and the medicine ball against the chest.

6. The subject grasps the medicine ball with both hands, one on each side.

7. Without any additional bodily movement (e.g., trunk or neck flexion, arm countermovement), the subject attempts to propel (i.e., "put") the medicine ball at an optimal trajectory of 45°, for maximal horizontal distance.

8. Every attempt should be made to propel the ball in a straight line, to yield valid data.

9. Three to five attempts are permitted, with a minimum of two minutes of rest between attempts.

OUTCOME MEASURES

Each test attempt should be measured by the closest chalk mark (i.e., in the direction of the bench) and recorded to the nearest centimeter or inch.

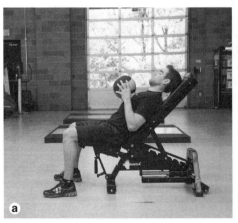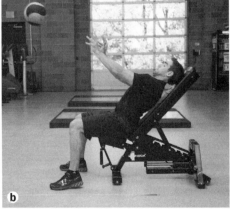

FIGURE 9.6 Starting position and trajectory for the medicine ball put.

Adapted from Clemons, J.M., B. Campbell, and C. Jeansonne. 2010. Validity and reliability of a new test of upper body power. *Journal of Strength and Conditioning Research* 24 (6): 1559-1565.

MODIFICATIONS

This test has been used extensively with various loading parameters and across populations. Further, many studies have reported the use of upright benches (i.e., seated upright at 90°) instead of 45° incline benches. To maintain test quality, examiners should use the same protocol each time a given subject is tested.

Warm-Up and Postactivation Potentiation (PAP): A Special Consideration for Testing Power

When designing an exercise prescription for improved muscular perfor-mance, the prescription of independent exercises and variables must account for both acute physiologic responses (i.e., immediate response), as well as the chronic adaptive response to training. Likewise, when designing a test battery to evaluate baseline performance and enhancement, the acute responses of warm-ups, testing procedures, and testing sequences should be considered, as these factors may strongly influence test outcomes.

According to the Fitness-Fatigue Model (Bannister 1991; Chiu and Barnes 2003), the stressors that manifest in a testing or training session produce distinct physiological responses that affect immediate performance, as well as chronic adaptive-responses. Essentially, the model is based on two tenets: an enhanced fitness after-effect and a suppressed fatigue after-effect. Rela-tive to this chapter, the first tenet is specific to the immediate, heightened physiological response as elicited by acute stimuli (i.e., through strategic warm-up procedures). If applied appropriately, this acute stimulus may have a direct influence on the power production capacity of the neuromuscular system, particularly in tests of instantaneous maximal power.

Most research on this topic has examined the effect of electrically stimu-lated muscle fiber and the consequent "potentiated" effect on muscle twitch and force production, in animal models. Interestingly, a considerable amount of recent evidence in humans demonstrates an immediate enhancement of force production following voluntary muscle action at high relative loads (Baudry and Duchateau 2007). The mechanisms for this time-dependent increase in performance are largely unexplained, but have been attributed to an increased rate of cross-bridge attachment as a result of an enhanced sensitivity of the contractile proteins to calcium (Ca^{2+}) (Baudry and Ducha-teau 2007). This acute response elicits improvement in performance through increases in twitch force and rate of force development. From a practical standpoint, postactivation potentiation (PAP) following highly intense stimuli has also been found to increase the rate of force development, jump height, and sprint performance (Chiu and Barnes 2003; Chatzopoulos et al. 2007).

Clearly, the application of PAP through strategic warm-up approaches may offer a neurological advantage in acute competitive or testing scenarios. Progressive dynamic warm-up protocols should incorporate successive movements ranging from low intensity to high intensity, to adequately prepare the body to produce maximal power.

The effects of PAP are not uniform across all athletes. A given stimuli that is appropriate for one athlete may actually induce fatigue in another. Therefore, it is important to offer a variety of progressive warm-ups to accommodate people at different levels of training and degrees of muscular fitness.

Professional Applications

Power is expressed across virtually all dynamic muscle actions and shares a robust association with movement on a continuum from basic activities of daily life to high-level performance. The measurement of power output accounts for neuromuscular subtleties that are not captured when examining raw strength capacity or speed of movement. Thus, power may be a superior indicator of coordinated movement, chronic functional capacity, or acute deficiency. A thorough comprehension of the factors that contribute to power production and translation to explosive movement will provide a foundation for monitoring, developing, and refining performance enhancement programming.

The assessment of power should be not only a principal element of any athlete or client profile (i.e., during a needs analysis), but also as an index of fitness or performance adaptation over time. Because the overt expression of power involves numerous physiological factors, conducting a battery of tests to capture the range of maximal capacities across various time-course intervals (e.g., RFD, maximal instantaneous power, peak power over 5 to 10 seconds of exertion, maximal and mean anaerobic power over 15 to 30 seconds) provides an accurate picture of a person's true strengths and weaknesses. Conversely, by limiting power assessment to a single test, a fitness professional would greatly reduce the likelihood of pinpointing underlying deficiencies. Such an omission may occur because the expression of power is influenced by more than a single factor, and can thus become convoluted either through changes in a single factor, or any combination of multiple factors. By using a comprehensive approach that accounts for the fundamental requirements of a given activity or sport (i.e., energy-system, biomechanical, and muscle-action specificity), fitness professionals can use strategic testing and targeted training to address clients' deficiencies, maximize adaptations, and significantly improve their performance.

However, as is the case with other muscular fitness components, methods of testing power are task specific, and vary considerably in biomechanical attributes and the time alloted for data collection. These tests should not be used interchangeably, because the results do not always reflect the same outcomes

(continued)

(continued)

and thus may not be relevant to a given training agenda or sport-specific performance. Further, power exhibited under one set of conditions may not necessarily translate across other conditions. Therefore, fitness professionals should isolate and assess the specific "trainable" attributes that could prohibit or potentiate power output adaptation. As outlined in this chapter, power should be evaluated using a systems approach that incorporates multiple components related to absolute force production, rate of force production, metabolic specificity, movement velocity, work capacity, and body-mass-adjusted power.

Because power is reflective of the interaction between muscle force and velocity, anything that alters either of these two parameters also directly modifies power production capacity. However, because performance in most sports requires a certain degree of proficiency in manipulating body mass (e.g., jumping, bounding, accelerating, cutting), fitness professionals should also consider the influence of body mass when evaluating explosive movement. Accounting for changes in body mass over time may also allow for the accurate observation of body-mass-adjusted power fluctuation.

Body-mass-adjusted power (a.k.a. power-to-weight ratio) has been suggested as a fundamental predictor of performance in most sports. This is intuitive considering that the load being manipulated in most activities is the mass of the body; thus, performance can be improved by increasing power, decreasing body mass, or doing a combination of both. Although weight loss, per se, is not generally a goal in most performance enhancement programs, in certain cases body fat reduction may be warranted. A person with excess body fat who reduces absolute fat mass may experience augmented performance and realize a positive adaptation for long-term cardiometabolic health.

The following case study demonstrates the contribution of body mass and peak power to vertical jump performance. Although hypothetical, this is a realistic example of how manipulating one or more variables can translate to augmented performance in explosive movement. Such an example may also serve as a paradigm for other explosive and nonexplosive efforts that require manipulating body mass.

Athlete Profile

Sex: Male

Age: 18 years

Sport: Division I American football

Position: Linebacker

Body mass: 235 lbs (106.6 kg)

Height: 6 feet 1 inch (185.4 cm)

Body mass index: 31 kg · m^{-2}

Body composition: Body fat percentage: 18%; absolute body fat mass: 42.3 lb (19.2 kg)

Strength: 1RM squat: 365 lb (165.5 kg)

Vertical jump: 25 inches (63.5 cm)

Using the Sayers equation, it is possible to estimate the peak power (PP) in watts for this athlete.

$$\text{Peak power (W)} = [60.7 \times (\text{jump height [cm]}) + 45.3 \times (\text{body mass [kg]}) - 2{,}055]$$

$$PP = (60.7 \times 63.5 \text{ cm}) + (45.3 \times 106.6 \text{ kg}) - 2{,}055$$

$$PP = 3{,}854.5 + 4{,}828.9 - 2{,}055$$

$$PP = 6{,}628.4 \text{ watts}$$

By algebraically rearranging the regression formula for PP, it is possible to set jump height as the dependent variable. Using this strategy, PP and body mass become independent variables, and the constants remain the same.

$$\text{Jump height [cm]} = [(2{,}055 + PP) - (45.3 \times \text{body mass [kg]})] / 60.7$$

Based on this new equation, it is possible to predict jump height when a change in body mass occurs. Therefore, if the athlete in this case study were to maintain muscle power output capacity and lose 5% body fat (e.g. ~5% loss of body fat = 11.75 lb [5.3 kg]), he would weigh 223.3 lb (101.3 kg). By entering this new value into the model, it is possible to predict change in jump height with the following equation:

$$\Delta \text{ jump height} = [(((2{,}055 + 6{,}628.4) - (45.3 \times \text{post body mass [kg]})) / 60.7)) - (((2{,}055 + 6{,}628.4) - (45.3 \times \text{pre body mass [kg]})) / 60.7)]$$

$$\Delta \text{ jump height} = [(((2{,}055 + 6{,}628.4) - (45.3 \times 101.3 \text{ kg})) / 60.7)) - (((2{,}055 + 6{,}628.4) - (45.3 \times 106.6 \text{ kg})) / 60.7)]$$

$$\Delta \text{ jump height} = (67.5 \text{ cm} - 63.5 \text{ cm})$$

$$\Delta \text{ jump height} = 4 \text{ cm } (1.58 \text{ in})$$

It is also plausible to speculate on how changes in PP may influence jump height, independent of changes in body mass. Although the original regression equation was formulated using force plate analyses of vertical ground reaction force during the squat jump and countermovement vertical jump (Sayers 1999), ample evidence confirms the utility of both high-intensity strength training and high-speed power training to improve PP during jumping (Cormie, McCaulley, and McBride 2007; Cormie, McGuigan, and Newton 2011b). Therefore, by using this logic, several viable options exist to alter power and jump height:

Viable Performance Enhancement Options

Strength increase only. Method: High-intensity strength training

Speed increase only. Method: High-speed plyometric and power training

Body mass decrease only. Method: Closely monitored and gradual decreases in absolute body fat

(continued)

(continued)

Strength increase + speed increase. Method: Combined multimodality, traditional periodized training, or both

Strength increase + body mass decrease

Speed increase + body mass decrease

Strength increase + speed increase + body mass decrease

This simplistic example demonstrates the fact that many choices are available for achieving the desired outcome of increased VJ performance. Because most performance enhancement programs are not designed to elicit changes in absolute fat mass (on the contrary, relative decreases in fat mass are expected when hypertrophy occurs), fitness professionals should instead regard the trainable muscular fitness parameters as the priority. Clearly, other variables such as RFD and reactive strength capacity may also influence VJ performance. Moreover, the influence of these factors on VJ is likely not uniform across populations (i.e., sex, age, training status). However, this example is intended merely to serve as a discussion point for emphasizing the multidimensional nature of power and explosive movement performance. Ultimately, using a comprehensive approach to evaluate these attributes will provide ample opportunity to optimize performance.

SUMMARY

- Muscular power is robustly associated with movement on a continuum that spans performance at all levels.
- The measurement of power output accounts for neuromuscular and energy transfer properties that are often overlooked with other raw measures of strength or speed.
- Power output is an excellent indicator of coordinated movement capacity, deficiency, or both, and its expression is contingent on numerous interrelated physiological attributes and biomechanical aspects.
- Evaluation of power output in the professional setting requires a broad-based, systematic examination of the requirements of the population being tested.
- Although numerous tests exist to measure muscular power production, each is specific to the context in which it is implemented.
- A thorough needs analysis should precede any performance testing and should account for the requisite underlying physiological, biomechanical, and external factors that go into the specific available tests, as well as an evaluation of how well these tests coincide with the needs of a given athlete.
- Body mass should be taken into consideration to gauge power-to-weight ratio.

10

Speed and Agility

N. Travis Triplett, PhD, CSCS*D, FNSCA

Speed and agility are important components of nearly every athletic performance (Hoffman 2006). Both involve moving the body as rapidly as possible, but agility has the added dimension of changing direction. Sport coaches typically spend time working with athletes on developing speed and agility by focusing on movement technique and reaction time in drills (Plisk 2008). Tests for speed are simple and straightforward, but agility tests vary greatly from those that involve little movement and mostly footwork to those that involve sprinting with multiple changes of direction, with and without a reaction to a varying stimulus. However, speed and agility tests are easily customizable to the sport or desired task.

Measuring speed and agility can help the fitness professional spotlight weaknesses in sport or task performance, which can help direct training goals (Harman and Garhammer 2008). For example, because speed, agility, or both are direct components of many sport movements, testing for either or both can provide information about the effectiveness of drills or other activities in practice, as well as serve as a measure of an athlete's abilities compared to those of other athletes in the same sport or position. The fitness professional can then use the information to alter the prescribed training program, or individualize aspects of a training program for a particular athlete.

Speed

Speed is classically defined as the shortest time required for an object to move along a fixed distance, which is the same as velocity, but without specifying the direction (Harman and Garhammer 2008). In practical terms, it refers to the ability to move the body as quickly as possible over a set distance. However, in reality, the issue is slightly more complex because speed is not constant over the entire distance and can therefore be divided into phases for most people (Plisk 2008). The first phase is acceleration, or the rate of change in speed up to the point at which maximum speed is reached. The second phase is maintenance, in which the top speed is maintained for the remainder of the distance of interest. This varies with the distance to be tested. For example, the acceleration phase for a 40-meter sprint is approximately 10 meters, whereas the acceleration phase for a 100-meter sprint is approximately 30 to 40 meters (Plisk 2008).

If the distance is too long (>200 m), a deceleration phase may also occur, which should be avoided if possible (Harman and Garhammer 2008). Because acceleration and deceleration can occur during maximal running, tests of speed provide information about average speed over the distance of interest. Given the fact that people cannot maintain maximal speed for a long period of time, tests of speed must be shorter than 200 meters, and most are 100 meters or shorter (Harman and Garhammer 2008). This ensures that significant deceleration does not occur, and that the test is not a measurement of aerobic or anaerobic capacity (Harman and Garhammer 2008), which are better measured by other methods (see chapters 5, 7, and 8, respectively).

Agility

Agility is most often defined as the ability to change direction rapidly (Altug, Altug, and Altug 1987). This can take many forms, from simple footwork actions to moving the entire body in the opposite direction while running at a high speed. Thus, agility has a speed component, but it is not the most important component of this trait. The basic definition of agility is too simplistic, because it is now thought to be much more complex involving not only speed, but also balance, coordination, and the ability to react to a change in the environment (Plisk 2008). Some tests of agility may even involve some muscular or cardiorespiratory endurance, but those fall into the category of anaerobic capacity tests (see chapter 8).

The primary difference between tests of speed and tests of agility is that during the agility test, the body movement is stopped and restarted in a different direction. To accomplish this, the subject has to decelerate and then accelerate in the new direction, something that is avoided in speed tests. The goal in agility tests is to accomplish the deceleration and acceleration as quickly and efficiently as possible. In contrast, the goal in speed tests is not to decelerate at all but rather to reach and maintain top speed as quickly as possible. These parameters are interrelated, however, because speed is a component of agility performance.

A person may be able to change direction very quickly, but if the intervening phases of the agility test are performed slowly, the overall test will be compromised. Thus, the examiner must have an understanding of and be able to communicate proper acceleration and deceleration techniques to the subject so the test results are not limited by poor running technique.

In general, proper acceleration to top speed involves increases in both stride length and stride frequency with an accompanying decrease in the degree of body lean (Plisk 2008). The primary difference between accelerating in a speed test and accelerating in an agility test is that often the subject has much less distance in which to accelerate in an agility test, and the body position from a prior deceleration and direction change may limit the subject's ability to reach full stride length and stride frequency. Regarding deceleration, in general, the degree of body lean should increase, and the entire foot should make contact with the running surface (Plisk 2008).

The degree of directional change is influenced by the test setup; some tests require a hard directional change (e.g., a power cut on a line to reverse direction), and others allow for a less severe directional change (e.g., rounding a cone). In any case, the more severe the directional change, the lower the speed and the greater the body lean at that point, so proper deceleration is essential to maximize time efficiency (Plisk 2008).

At the end of any test, the subject should be instructed not to slow down, but rather to run through the finish line or gate, to minimize deceleration. Other technique points are to have the subject visually focus on the target (e.g., cone, line) when performing the test, unless instructed otherwise, such as when shuffling to the side while facing forward.

A component of agility tests that can make them more sport specific is reactive ability to a stimulus that dictates the new direction of movement, instead of letting the subject know the directions of the test beforehand. This technique is not used in every agility test; it is most commonly used as an advanced method to increase the specificity to actual sport environments.

Agility tests that do not involve any change in stimuli are considered closed-skill tests (Plisk 2008). These tests are performed in a stable environment in which the subject knows the test course and which direction to go. Conversely, open-skill tests are unpredictable; the direction is determined by another person, such as a coach or other trainer. Reactive ability is emphasized in open-skill tests, as are balance and coordination, because the movement direction cannot be anticipated. Closed-skill tests are used more often because the conditions can be standardized and norms exist. Additionally, closed-skill tests have greater test–retest reliability because the test format can be the same for each subject every time. Because of their variability, open-skill tests are more often used for training drills or for a quick assessment of athlete performance on a given day without regard to improvements in the test over a period of time.

Sport Performance and Speed and Agility

Most sports, even endurance sports, have speed or agility as a component. Except in sports such as track or swimming where there is minimal or no change in direction, speed and agility are both important aspects of sport performance. The most successful American football lineman, for example, is the one who can react most quickly to the snap of the ball and get off the line toward the opposing player the quickest. Similarly, the best soccer or ice hockey players can change direction and take off with the ball or puck the fastest. Assessing speed and agility in a controlled environment with a test that is similar to the actual demands of the sport of interest is therefore highly useful in helping to design training in order to improve sport performance.

Test Selection

One of the most important steps in using performance tests occurs before the subject even reports to the testing area. Test selection is vital because it affects the validity of the results. The first consideration is that the test represent the physiological demands of the sport. Thus, the fitness professional must have an understanding of the basic energy systems and other physiological traits that would affect sport performance, such as body size. Because many sports require a variety of abilities (e.g., speed, agility, power, anaerobic capacity), a battery of tests is often used to address each of the abilities separately.

Biomechanical factors, such as movement pattern specificity, are important to consider when selecting a test; one agility test may be better for ice hockey, and another, for tennis, for example. Training level is also an important consideration. Tests that involve a higher level of skill or fitness may not be appropriate for novice subjects because their poor technique or conditioning could limit their test performance. Similarly, the sex or age of participants has an impact on test selection; some tests would be difficult for females to complete (i.e., a chin-up test), and others may be inappropriate for prepubescent children.

Testing parameters may be modified to mimic sport characteristics. For example, subjects undertaking an agility test for American football can be required to carry the ball during the test. Tests can also be designed to be more specific to a certain sport movement, but the basic principle of validity must be followed to ensure that it measures what it is supposed to.

Tests of speed and agility should be short, usually less than 20 seconds; longer tests may target the wrong energy systems, and fatigue may affect the results. If an agility test course is too complex, for example, subjects won't be able to build up speed between turns. In any instance, if a test is modified in any way, the published norms are no longer applicable. New

TABLE 10.1 Summary of Speed and Agility Test Characteristics

Test	Ease	Resources	Reliability	Specific trait
40-yard	Easy	Timing system Track or court	.89-.97	Speed
10-yard	Easy	Timing system Track or court	.89	Acceleration
60-yard sprint with flying 30 yard	Moderate	Timing system with multiple gates Track	NA	Acceleration Top speed Speed Maintenance
Pro-agility (5-10-5)	Easy	Stopwatch Cones Field or court	.91	Agility (forward)
T-test	Moderate	Stopwatch Cones Field or court	.93-.98	Agility (forward, backward, lateral)
Three-cone	Difficult	Stopwatch Cones Field or court	NA	Agility (forward)
Edgren side step	Moderate	Stopwatch Court Line markers	NA	Footwork agility
Hexagon	Moderate	Stopwatch Court Line markers	.86-.95	Footwork agility

norms have to be developed by testing numbers of subjects over time. Table 10.1 provides a summary of speed and agility test characteristics.

Methods of Measurement

Both speed and closed-skill agility tests require very little equipment. These tests can typically be accomplished with a stopwatch, a tape measure to set the course, and markers of the course, such as cones. Using automated timing devices can increase the accuracy of the tests, but having the same person time each subject may be all that is necessary to ensure reliable results. Open-skill agility tests are more difficult to standardize because the testing environment is unpredictable. Standardization of procedures, such as how many direction changes there will be per test, and fixing the distance to be moved when a directional change is indicated, will increase the test reliability.

The subject should be adequately warmed up before beginning any testing procedure. Although there are no set guidelines for a warm-up, it is generally recommended that subjects first perform three to five minutes of a low-intensity, large-muscle-group activity such as jogging or riding a stationary bicycle to increase circulation to the whole body. Then, more specific warm-up activities can be performed such as executing the movement or test at half or three-quarter speed.

If the participant has range of motion limitations in the lower body, some light dynamic stretching may be recommended so that the appropriate range of motion can be attained for the activity (Bandy, Irion, and Briggler 1998; Hedrick 2000; Mann and Jones 1999). Because other types of stretching, especially static stretching, have been shown to compromise performance in speed, strength, and power activities, the focus should remain on the warm-up and stretching should be minimal prior to performance (Behm, Button, and Butt 2001; Church et al. 2001; Fletcher and Jones 2004; Nelson and Kokkonen 2001; Power et al. 2004; Young and Behm 2003).

Factors Influencing Test Performance

For test results to be reliable, many things must be taken into consideration in addition to properly planning for test administration (i.e., training examiners). Factors such as environmental conditions may affect test performance and should be noted, particularly when tests are administered outside where weather (temperature, humidity, precipitation) is variable. Other, more controllable factors include subjects' hydration and nutritional status. Instructions can be given to subjects regarding water consumption and pretest meals, which can be replicated for repeat test sessions. Dehydration is known to adversely affect performance, and subjects should consume a pretest meal that is well tolerated. Finally, subjects should be well rested following training sessions (at least 48 hours), and should be given adequate rest periods (5 to 20 minutes) between tests when a battery of tests is being performed.

Tests of Speed

In order to determine a person's maximum speed, tests of speed should be short (<200 meters) and not involve changes of direction. Additionally, the acceleration phase of movement should be accounted for by setting a test length that allows the subject to attain maximum speed and maintain it for several seconds. Thus, the shortest speed tests are in the 30- to 40-yard range. This method of testing reduces the influence of factors such as fatigue or deceleration and will result in the most accurate determination of speed.

40-YARD SPRINT TEST

The most common test of speed is the 40-yard sprint. It is used in the NFL Combine, as well as in many collegiate sport programs in the United States. It is also used in laboratory methods classes in exercise science and physical education academic programs. This test is most appropriate for sports that may have an extended run, such as soccer, field hockey, and lacrosse, in addition to American football. It is also short, fast (<7 seconds), and simple to time. This test is also easily modified to shorter and longer distances to be even more specific for sports such as baseball and basketball. Norms for some of these distances are provided in table 10.2. As with all tests of speed, the main objective is to cover the distance as quickly as possible, and usually no more than three attempts are performed to minimize the decline in performance caused by fatigue.

EQUIPMENT

- Track or field where the distance can be measured
- Tape measure
- Stopwatch or timing gates
- Cones or tape to indicate start and finish lines
- Personnel at the finish line or at both the start and finish lines

PROCEDURE

After instructing the subject on the correct performance of the test, follow these steps:

1. The subject lines up behind the start line, facing forward. Sport-specific stances can also be used, such as a three-point stance as in American football (see figure 10.1a) or a four-point stance as in track (see figure 10.1b).

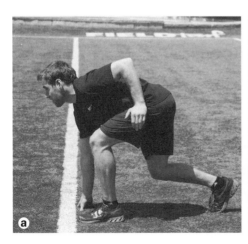 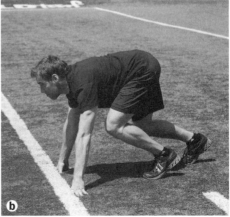

FIGURE 10.1 Three-point and four-point stances for the 40-yard sprint test.

2. The subject should be given a countdown, either verbally or, if using timing gates, by using the beeps programmed into the timing gate unit. Alternatively, an electronic switch activated by the subject's movement can be used.

3. The subject should be allowed two or three trials, with three- to five-minute rests between to ensure nearly full recovery.

4. If using a stopwatch, start the watch at the subject's first movement. Times are typically recorded to the nearest 0.01 second. Hand timing can result in times that are 0.24 second faster (Harman and Garhammer 2008) than the time recorded using a timing gate. Thus, consistency in equipment from test to test and with repeated tests of the same subject is essential.

5. Modifications to the distance can include the 30-yard sprint (basketball) or the 60-yard sprint (baseball), which are more specific to those sports. Any distance can be used, but norms for performance may not be available.

RELIABILITY

The 40-yard sprint is a highly reliable test with test–retest reliabilities typically above .95, but ranging from .89 to .97.

NORMS

See table 10.2.

10-YARD SPRINT TEST

The short 10-yard sprint test is used to determine a person's ability to accelerate, because the acceleration phase in the 40-yard sprint is approximately 10 yards. Although this test is less commonly used, it can provide information about an athlete's ability to accelerate quickly, because much time can be lost during this phase. This test is good for any sport that requires a lot of short sprints, such as American football, bobsled, speedskating, gymnastics, basketball, rugby, baseball, and tennis, because it mimics very closely a start off the line or sprint for the ball. Again, the main objective is to cover the distance as quickly as possible. Four or five trials with two- or three-minute rests between them may be performed because fatigue is less of a factor than in the 40-yard sprint.

EQUIPMENT

- Track or field where the distance can be measured
- Tape measure
- Stopwatch or timing gates
- Cones or tape to indicate start and finish lines
- Personnel at the finish line or at both the start and finish lines

TABLE 10.2 Speed Test Norms for Various Sports (in seconds)

Population	Sex	10 yards	30 yards	40 yards	60 yards
Baseball—NCAA DI	M				7.05 ± 0.28
Baseball—Major League	M		3.75 ± 0.11		6.96 ± 0.16
Basketball—NCAA DI	M		3.79 ± 0.19	4.81 ± 0.26	
Field hockey*	F			6.37 ± 0.27	
American football—NCAA DI	M			4.74 ± 0.3	
Defensive line (DL)				4.85 ± 0.2	
Linebackers (LB)				4.64 ± 0.2	
Defensive backs (DB)				4.52 ± 0.2	
Quarterbacks (QB)				4.70 ± 0.1	
Running backs (RB)				4.53 ± 0.2	
Wide receivers (WR)				4.48 ± 0.1	
Offensive line (OL)				5.12 ± 0.2	
Tight ends (TE)				4.78 ± 0.2	
Football—NFL draftees	M			4.81 ± 0.31	
Lacrosse—NCAA DIII[4]	F			5.40 ± 0.16	
Rugby*	M			5.32 ± 0.26	
Rugby*[2]	F	2.00 ± 0.11		6.45 ± 0.36	
Soccer—NCAA DI[1]	M	1.63 ± 0.08		4.87 ± 0.16	
Soccer—NCAA DIII	M			4.73 ± 0.18	
Soccer—NCAA DIII	F			5.34 ± 0.17	
Tennis—NCAA DI[5]	M	1.79 ± 0.03			
Volleyball—NCAA DI	F			5.62 ± 0.24	
Volleyball—Junior National*[3]	F	1.90 ± 0.01			
Volleyball—Junior National*[3]	M	1.80 ± 0.02			

* indicates that distance is in meters instead of yards.

Abbreviations: NCAA: National Collegiate Athletic Association; DI: Division I (NCAA); DII: Division II (NCAA); DIII: Division III (NCAA).

[1]Cressey et al. 2007, [2]Gabbett 2007, [3]Gabbett and Georgieff 2007, [4]Hoffman et al. 2009, [5]Kovacs et al. 2007.

Adapted, by permission, from J. Hoffman, 2006, *Norms for fitness, performance, and health* (Champaign, IL: Human Kinetics), 111, 112.

PROCEDURE

After instructing the subject on the correct performance of the test, follow these steps:

1. The subject lines up behind the start line, facing forward. Sport-specific stances can also be used, such as a three-point stance as in American football or a four-point stance as in track.

2. The subject should be given a countdown, either verbally or, if using timing gates, by using the beeps programmed into the timing gate unit or the electronic switch.

3. The subject should be allowed two or three trials, with three- to five-minute rests between them to ensure nearly full recovery.

4. If using a stopwatch, start the watch at the subject's first movement. Times are typically recorded to the nearest 0.01 second. Hand timing can result in times that are faster than the times recorded using a timing gate. Thus, consistency in equipment from test to test and with the same subject performing repeated tests is essential.

RELIABILITY

The test–retest reliability for the 10-yard sprint test is .89.

NORMS

See table 10.2.

60-YARD SPRINT WITH FLYING 30 YARD

The "flying" refers to the fact that the 30-yard measurement is taken between yards 10 and 40 of the distance, after the person has accelerated and is in motion (i.e., not from a standing or 3- or 4-point stance). This longer sprint test is used to determine a person's ability to accelerate and to maintain top speed, as well as the person's top speed without taking into account the acceleration phase. It can therefore provide a multitude of data about how the person reaches and maintains speed. This test is most appropriate for athletes in sports that require extended runs, such as baseball, soccer, field hockey, and lacrosse. The main objective is to cover the distance as quickly as possible, and usually three trials or fewer are performed to minimize the decline in performance caused by fatigue, because this is a bigger factor than in the 40-yard sprint.

EQUIPMENT

- Track or field where the distance can be measured
- Tape measure
- Stopwatch or timing gates

- Cones or tape to indicate start and finish lines, as well as the intermediate lines

PROCEDURE

After instructing the subject on the correct performance of the test, follow these steps:

1. The subject lines up behind the start line, facing forward. Sport-specific stances can also be used, such as a three-point stance as in American football or a four-point stance as in track.

2. The subject should be given a countdown, either verbally or, if using timing gates, by using the beeps programmed into the timing gate unit or the electronic switch.

3. The subject should be allowed two or three trials, with three- to five-minute rests between them to ensure nearly full recovery.

4. Personnel should be at the finish line or at both the start and finish lines, as well as at the intermediate lines. For example: the start line, the timer or gate at 10 yards, the timer or gate at 40 yards, and the timer or gate at 60 yards (finish). They should record times for:
   - 0-10 yards = acceleration
   - 0-40 yards = 40-yard time (top speed)
   - 10-40 yards = flying 30-yard time
   - 0-60 yards = 60-yard time (speed maintenance)

5. If using a stopwatch, start the watch at the subject's first movement. Times are typically recorded to the nearest 0.01 second. Hand timing can result in times that are faster than those recorded using a timing gate. Thus, consistency in equipment from test to test and with the same subject performing repeated tests is essential.

NORMS

See table 10.2.

Tests of Agility

Determining a person's agility can be complex because agility involves acceleration, speed, deceleration, balance, and coordination. Agility tests should be very short (<40 yards) and must involve multiple changes of direction. Agility test results can be greatly affected by a person's ability to accelerate and decelerate, so coaching proper acceleration and deceleration technique is necessary to obtain the most accurate test results.

5-10-5 OR PRO-AGILITY TEST

A common test of agility is the 5-10-5, or pro-agility test, also known as the 20-yard shuttle run. It is used in the NFL Combine, as well as in many collegiate sport programs in the United States. It is also used in laboratory methods classes in exercise science and physical education academic programs. This test is best suited for athletes in sports requiring short sprints and a reversal of direction, including basketball, baseball, softball, soccer, and volleyball, in addition to American football. Like the tests of speed, the main objective is to cover the distance (and thereby change direction) as quickly as possible. Three trials or fewer are usually performed to minimize the decline in performance caused by fatigue.

EQUIPMENT

- Track or field where the distance can be measured
- Tape measure
- Stopwatch or timing gates
- Cones or tape to indicate course layout (see figure 10.2)

PROCEDURE

After instructing the subject on the correct performance of the test, follow these steps:

1. The subject lines up straddling the start line, which is the middle line. An upright stance is typically used, and the subject should face forward.

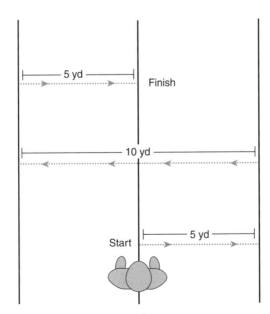

FIGURE 10.2   5-10-5 or pro-agility test.

Reprinted, by permission, from M.P. Reiman and R.C Manske, 2009, *Functional testing in human performance* (Champaign, IL: Human Kinetics), 193.

2. The subject is given a countdown, either verbally or, if using timing gates, by using the beeps programmed into the timing gate unit.

3. The subject starts the test by turning to the left and sprinting for 5 yards; then turning to the right and sprinting for 10 yards before turning back to the left and sprinting for 5 yards. This returns the subject to the start line. The lines marking the distance must be contacted by the foot.

4. The subject should be allowed two or three trials, with three- to five-minute rests between them to ensure nearly full recovery.

5. Personnel should be at the start/finish line. The test starts and finishes on the same line.

6. If using a stopwatch, start the watch at the subject's first movement. Times are typically recorded to the nearest 0.01 second. Hand timing can result in times that are faster than those recorded using a timing gate. Thus, consistency in equipment from test to test and with the same subject performing repeated tests is essential.

7. Modifications to the test can include performing the test while holding a football, or starting the test in a three- or four-point stance. However, the listed norms will not be applicable, and new norms will have to be generated.

RELIABILITY

The test–retest reliability for the pro-agility test is .91.

NORMS

See table 10.3.

T-TEST

A common test of agility is the T-test. It is used in many collegiate sport programs, and in laboratory methods classes in exercise science and physical education academic programs in the United States. This test is best suited for athletes in sports that require that they sprint forward, move laterally, and backpedal, including American football, soccer, basketball, baseball, softball, and volleyball. Like the tests of speed, the main objective is to cover the distance and change direction as quickly as possible. Three trials or fewer are usually performed to minimize the decline in performance caused by fatigue.

EQUIPMENT

- Track or field where the distance can be measured
- Tape measure
- Stopwatch or timing gates
- Cones or tape to indicate course layout (see figure 10.3)

TABLE 10.3 Agility Test Norms for Various Sports (in seconds)

Population	Sex	Pro-agility	T-test	Three-cone	Edgren[#]	Hexagon
Baseball—NAIA	M		10.11 ± 0.64			
Basketball—NCAA DI	M		8.95 ± 0.53			
Competitive college athletes[3]	F					5.5
Competitive college athletes[3]	M					5.0
American football— NCAA DI	M	4.53 ± 0.22				
Offensive and defensive line		4.35 ± 0.11				
Wide receiver and defensive back		4.35 ± 0.12				
Running back, tight end, and linebacker		4.6 ± 0.2				
American football—NFL draftees	M			7.23 ± 0.41		
Ice hockey[2]	M				29.0 ± 2.4	12.6 ± 1.1
Lacrosse—NCAA DIII[4]	F	4.92 ± 0.22	10.5 ± 0.6			
Soccer—elite youth U16	M		11.7 ± 0.1			
Soccer—NCAA DIII	F	4.88 ± 0.18				
Soccer—NCAA DIII	M	4.43 ± 0.17				
Volleyball—NCAA DI	F		11.16 ± 0.38			
Volleyball—NCAA DIII	F	4.75 ± 0.19				
Volleyball—Junior National[1]	F		10.33 ± 0.13			
Volleyball—Junior National[1]	M		9.90 ± 0.17			

# indicates that the test result is the number of lines crossed, not a time value.

Abbreviations: NAIA: National Association of Intercollegiate Athletics; NCAA: National Collegiate Athletic Association; DI: Division I (NCAA); DII: Division II (NCAA); DIII: Division III (NCAA); U16: under 16 age group.

[1]Gabbett and Georgieff 2007, [2]Farlinger, Kruisselbrink, and Fowles 2007, [3]Harman and Garhammer 2008, [4]Hoffman et al. 2009.

Adapted, by permission, from J. Hoffman, 2006, *Norms for fitness, performance, and health* (Champaign, IL: Human Kinetics), 114–115.

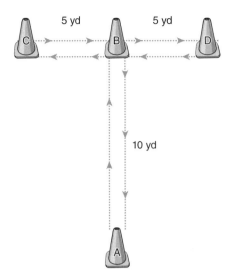

FIGURE 10.3 T-test.

Reprinted, by permission, from M.P. Reiman, 2009, *Functional testing in human performance* (Champaign, IL: Human Kinetics), 192.

PROCEDURE

After instructing the subject on the correct performance of the test, follow these steps:

1. The subject lines up at the start line, at the base of the T (cone A). An upright stance is typically used, and the subject should face forward.

2. The subject should be given a countdown, either verbally or, if using timing gates, by using the beeps programmed into the timing gate unit or the electronic switch.

3. The subject starts the test by sprinting straight ahead for 10 yards and touching the base of cone B with the right hand. The subject then shuffles left for 5 yards and touches the base of cone C with the left hand. Next, the subject shuffles 10 yards to the right, all the way to the farthest cone (D), and touches the base of the cone with the right hand. Finally, the subject shuffles left back to the middle cone (B), touches it with the left hand, and then backpedals to the starting point (cone A). The subject faces forward at all times during the test and is not allowed to cross the feet during the shuffling. Also, the middle cone (B) is not touched when shuffling between the two farthest cones (C and D).

4. The test can also be performed in reverse, going to the right first instead of to the left, and the hand that touches the cone would switch as well. Other modifications to the test can include suspending a tennis ball at cones C and D and having the subject use forehand and backhand strokes to strike the ball (whichever is appropriate depending

on whether the subject plays right- or left-handed) at each cone.

5. The subject should be allowed two or three trials, with three- to five-minute rests between them to ensure nearly full recovery.

6. Personnel should be at the start/finish line. The test starts and finishes on the same line.

7. If using a stopwatch, start the watch at the subject's first movement. Times are typically recorded to the nearest 0.01 second. Hand timing can result in times that are faster than those recorded using a timing gate. Thus, consistency in equipment from test to test and with the same subject performing repeated tests is essential.

RELIABILITY

The T-test has a test–retest reliability range of .93 to .98.

NORMS

See table 10.3.

THREE-CONE TEST

Another test of agility is the three-cone test. It is used in the NFL Combine, as well as in some collegiate football programs in the United States, but norms are available only for American football because the test was developed for that sport. Similar to the other tests of agility, the main objective is to cover the distance as quickly as possible, and change direction without losing much time. Three trials or fewer are usually performed to minimize the decline in performance caused by fatigue.

EQUIPMENT

- Track or field where the distance can be measured
- Tape measure
- Stopwatch or timing gates
- Cones or tape to indicate course layout (see figure 10.4)

PROCEDURE

After instructing the subject on the correct performance of the test, follow these steps:

1. The subject lines up at the start line (cone A). An upright stance is typically used, and the subject should face forward.

2. The subject should be given a countdown, either verbally or, if using timing gates, by using the beeps programmed into the timing gate unit or the electronic switch.

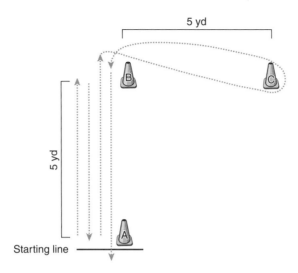

FIGURE 10.4   Three-cone test.

Reprinted, by permission, from M.P. Reiman, 2009, *Functional testing in human performance* (Champaign, IL: Human Kinetics), 196.

3. The subject start the test by sprinting forward 5 yards to cone B (1) and touching the cone; then turning around and sprinting back to cone A (2) and touching that cone. Without stopping, the subject should turn around and sprint back to cone B (3), but this time run around cone B and head to cone C (4), circling around it and coming back around cone B (5) on the outside before returning to cone A (6), the starting point. The only time the cones are touched are in the first part of the test, as described.

4. Modifications to the test can include performing the test while holding a football, or starting the test in a three- or four-point stance. However, the listed norms will not be applicable, and new norms will have to be generated.

5. The subject should be allowed two or three trials, with three- to five-minute rests between to ensure nearly full recovery.

6. Personnel should be at the start/finish line. The test starts and finishes on the same line.

7. If using a stopwatch, start the watch at the subject's first movement. Times are typically recorded to the nearest 0.01 second. Hand timing can result in times that are faster than those recorded using a timing gate. Thus, consistency in equipment from test to test and with the same subject performing repeated tests is essential.

NORMS

See table 10.3.

EDGREN SIDE STEP TEST

The Edgren side step test is an agility test that measures footwork. It is not commonly used, but norms are available for ice hockey players. The main objective is to cover the distance and change direction as quickly as possible. Three trials or fewer are usually performed to minimize the decline in performance caused by fatigue.

EQUIPMENT

- Track or field or court where the distance can be measured
- Tape measure
- Stopwatch
- Cones or tape to indicate course layout (see figure 10.5)

PROCEDURE

After instructing the subject on the correct performance of the test, follow these steps:

1. The subject lines up straddling the start line, which is the middle line. An upright stance is used, and the subject should face forward.
2. The subject should be given a countdown and should start the test by sidestepping to the right until the farthest line is crossed by the right foot. The subject then sidesteps left until the left foot crosses the farthest left line. Count the number of lines crossed while the subject repeats this procedure for 10 seconds.
3. The subject is not allowed to cross the feet; doing so results in a 1-point deduction in the score.
4. The subject should be allowed two or three trials, with three- to five-minute rests between them to ensure nearly full recovery.
5. Personnel should be at the start line.
6. Start the stopwatch at the subject's first movement. Times are typically recorded to the nearest 0.01 second.

NORMS

See table 10.3.

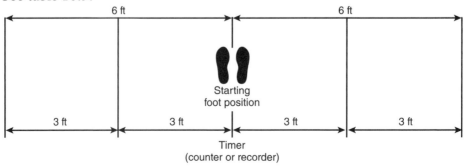

FIGURE 10.5   Edgren side step test.

Reprinted, by permission, from M.P. Reiman, 2009, *Functional testing in human performance* (Champaign, IL: Human Kinetics), 196.

HEXAGON TEST

Another agility test that measures footwork is the hexagon test. It can be used in sports in which foot placement in all directions and cutting movements are common, such as basketball, soccer, rugby, and American football; norms are available for ice hockey players. The main objective is to cover the course and change direction as quickly as possible without losing one's balance. Three trials or fewer are usually performed to minimize the decline in performance caused by fatigue.

EQUIPMENT

This test is best performed indoors.

- Court where the distance can be measured
- Tape measure
- Stopwatch
- Cones or tape to indicate course layout (see figure 10.6)
- Personnel to time and watch for accuracy of course completion

PROCEDURE

After instructing the subject on the correct performance of the test, follow these steps:

1. The subject stands in the middle of the hexagon in an upright stance and faces forward.
2. The subject should be given a countdown and starts the test by double-leg hopping from the center of the hexagon across one side of the hexagon and back to the center. This is performed in a clockwise direction until each side of the hexagon is crossed and the entire hexagon is traversed a total of three times.
3. The subject must face the same direction for the entire test and should not land on a line or lose balance and take an extra step or fail to cross a line. If this occurs, the trial is stopped and restarted.
4. Start the watch at the subject's first movement and stop it when the subject returns to the center of the hexagon for the last time.

RELIABILITY

The range of test–retest reliability for the hexagon test is .86 to .95.

NORMS

See table 10.3.

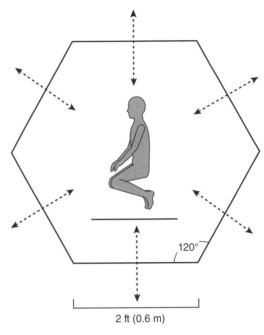

FIGURE 10.6   Hexagon test.

Reprinted, by permission, from M.P. Reiman, 2009, *Functional testing in human performance* (Champaign, IL: Human Kinetics), 194.

Professional Applications

The primary purpose of performing any test should be to gain information about where a person is compared to performance standards in the field or sport. The information can be used for a multitude of purposes, which include the establishment of a baseline value for a new athlete, the measurement of progress as a result of targeted training to improve a particular performance characteristic, and the determination of changes over the course of a competitive season or a phase of training. The test results should then be used to design the next phase of training.

Test selection is vital to this process because not all tests for a particular trait, such as speed or agility, are the most appropriate for specific performance characteristics of a sport or activity. For example, although the 40-yard sprint is the most common test of speed, for a sport such as rugby, in which the runs are very short before being tackled, a 10-yard sprint test may be more appropriate. In contrast, a longer sprint test such as the 60-yard may be more appropriate for baseball players, especially outfielders, or even to simulate running two bases.

Tests of agility can be even more sport or activity specific. The pro-agility test would be very appropriate for tennis, for example, because it closely mimics baseline play. The T-test would also be a good test for tennis because it consists of forward, lateral, and backward movements, such as would occur when coming forward to play the net, moving in the front of the court, and returning to the baseline to resume a rally. However, the three-cone test is most appropriate for American football because it most resembles a play in football in which the player runs forward but then turns around and runs in the opposite direction or to the left or right after the ball carrier.

Most sports consist of several performance variables, and speed and agility are rarely mutually exclusive, except in track, which includes races that are purely based on speed (and endurance). Multiple tests may therefore be selected to provide the best overall physical profile of an athlete or individual. If multiple tests are necessary, the testing order becomes extremely important to ensure the best performance while minimizing the effects of fatigue.

Because speed and agility tests are very close in energy system demands, there are not specific recommendations for testing order. The main concern would be to provide adequate rest between tests and to make sure the subject is warmed up. This may mean a 10- to 15-minute delay between tests, depending on how many attempts are required. Because speed and agility tests are very short, providing adequate rest between repeat attempts (usually two to five minutes) is easily accomplished.

The testing environment is also critical to ensure the best performance results. Safety is of primary concern, and the results that fit published norms are those from tests performed on the least variable surfaces, such as tracks and courts. However, the most sport-specific results are obtained in the conditions in which the athlete performs in training and competition. Although performing speed tests on a track is desirable in terms of the ease of marking the distance and providing the most consistent surface, it would also be acceptable to perform a 40-yard sprint on a soccer field for soccer athletes, as long as enough subjects could be tested to generate new norms. However, if the test is to be primarily used for goal setting, it should be performed on the least variable surface, leaving the replication of competition conditions to the sport practices.

Finally, once test results are obtained, they must be properly interpreted. It is of little use to compare athlete values to published norms if the testing was performed under vastly different conditions than those used to establish the norms. Other factors such as training experience can influence test performance because familiarity with a test can increase performance. The time of the training year in which the test is done can strongly influence test results as well. For example, the results of an agility test done with a group of basketball athletes after the off-season or after a maintenance phase of training would not be as good as those from a test performed after the preseason conditioning.

Understanding the sport or activity from a physiological and mechanical perspective is necessary for proper test selection, and performing the tests in a safe and controlled environment will result in the clearest results. Ultimately, the information can be used to design better training and exercise programs.

SUMMARY

- Tests of speed and agility are used in a multitude of environments, from the exercise science research laboratory to the physical education or exercise science classroom, strength and conditioning facility, and fitness club.

- Speed and agility tests are simple to administer, do not require expensive equipment, and can provide valuable information about clients' strengths and weaknesses or progress with a training program or phase of a program.

- Test selection should be based on the abilities and limitations of the client and the goals of the client's training, sport, or both.

- Also, these tests lend themselves easily to modification, which allows for a great degree of flexibility in test administration and application of the information obtained from the test.

Mobility

Sean P. Flanagan, PhD, ATC, CSCS

Mobility, or ease of movement, is a fundamental requisite of human movement. A certain minimal amount of mobility is necessary for accomplishing any task, be it an activity of daily living or a sport. Mobility is determined by the composite motion available at all of the joints involved in the movement, known as a kinematic chain.[1] Too much (hypermobility) or too little (hypomobility) mobility can have negative consequences for performance and increase the potential for injury. Therefore, a comprehensive evaluation of joint motion should be part of any assessment of a personal training client or athlete.

This chapter examines some of the fundamental concepts associated with mobility and the effects of hyper- and hypomobility on performance and injury potential. Finally, methods used to measure it and how to interpret the results are examined.

Before beginning the discussion, we need to distinguish between mobility and flexibility, and address the current controversy of, and misconceptions about, static stretching. Mobility is the amount of motion available at a joint (or series of joints) and the ease with which the joint(s) can move through the range of motion (ROM). Flexibility refers to the extensibility of the periarticular structures (i.e., muscle, tendon, and fascia) and is but one of the factors that can limit ROM and impede mobility. A growing body of literature (Haff et al. 2006) suggests that static stretching may not improve

---

[1]Most people realize that the body acts like a chain of rigid body segments that are attached to each other and operate together. In engineering, such a system is called a kinematic chain because it describes the motions of these segments without regard for the forces that cause those motions. In exercise science, the term *kinetic chain* is often used interchangeably with *kinematic chain,* even though the term *kinetic chain* does not exist in engineering. *Kinetics* refers to the forces that cause motion. While there is utility in examining how forces are transferred throughout the chain, when discussing mobility the more correct term *kinematic chain* should be used.

performance or decrease injury. Several studies have also shown that static stretching may actually decrease peak force, rate of force development, and power output (Stone et al. 2006) for up to an hour after stretching.

Although findings seem to suggest that there is no need to improve flexibility (or mobility), two important points need to be addressed. First, the acute effects of stretching have to be separated from the chronic effects of stretching (Stone et al. 2006). Just because the acute effects of static stretching appear to have no benefit in terms of injury reduction and may have detrimental effects on performance, this does not mean that static stretching cannot have beneficial effects over time. Second, most of the conclusions about the chronic effects of stretching on injury and performance may be based on a faulty premise (i.e., more is better). If a cake recipe calls for two cups of sugar, adding only one cup will certainly degrade the quality of cake, but adding four cups will not make for a better cake.

Each activity requires a certain amount of mobility for optimal performance. If the person performing that activity does not have an adequate amount of mobility, decreased performance and increased potential for injury could surely result. Even the most ardent proponents of flexibility training seem to concede this point (Haff et al. 2006). Therefore, fitness professionals must understand mobility, determine the mobility demands of a sport or task, and assess the mobility of the athlete to ensure adequate performance for that sport or task.

Fundamental Concepts of Mobility

Individual joint motion has two parts: osteokinematics and arthrokinematics (Levangie and Norkin 2001). The rotation of the two bones in a plane about a common axis is referred to as osteokinematics, whereas arthrokinematics refers to the relative motion (sliding, spinning, and rolling) that occurs between the joint surfaces (see figure 11.1). Osteokinematics is the major component of joint motion and is the focus of this chapter.

Range of motion (ROM) is the amount of rotation available at a joint, or a measure of the osteokinematics. A joint has ROM in each plane of movement in which that joint can rotate, known as a degree of freedom (DOF). If a joint has rotation available only in the sagittal plane, it will have only a single DOF; a joint that allows triplanar motion will have three DOFs. For each DOF, motion is available in two directions (e.g., flexion and extension in the sagittal plane). The DOF of the entire kinematic chain is the sum of the DOFs at each joint in the chain.

The number of DOFs and the amount of ROM in each DOF for each joint are determined by several factors, including the following:

- Shape of the articular structures
- Arthrokinematic motion

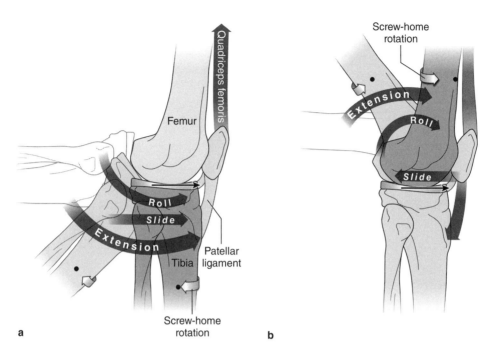

FIGURE 11.1   Arthrokinematic motion (rolling and sliding) associated with the osteo-kinematic motion of knee extension with the tibia moving on the femur *(a)*, and with the femur moving on the tibia *(b)*.

Reprinted from *Kinesiology of Musculoskeletal System: Foundations for Rehabilitation,* 2nd ed,. D.A. Neumann, pg. 530, copyright 2010, with permission from Elsevier.

- Extensibility of the periarticular structures
- Number of joints involved in the movement

The shape of the articular surfaces will largely dictate the number of DOFs (Levangie and Norkin 2001), and the cartilaginous and ligamentous structures will guide the motion in that DOF. For example, the sutures of the skull are joints with virtually no movement, whereas the synovial joints of the limbs allow a relatively large amount of motion. Additionally, hinge and pivot-type synovial joints (e.g., elbow and forearm, respectively) have only one DOF, whereas ball and socket joints of the shoulder and hip have three. Most other types of synovial joints have two DOFs. Understanding the joint shape is important in knowing which motions to test and which would be considered abnormal, so the examiner should have an appreciation for the type of joint that is being tested. The motions available at the joints are presented in tables 11.1 and 11.2 for the extremities and spine, respectively.

As mentioned earlier, arthrokinematic motion is small, accessory motion that occurs at the joint surfaces, such as sliding and spinning (Levangie and Norkin 2001). It influences the amount of osteokinematic motion available. As one bone rotates relative to another (fixed) bone, a certain amount of

TABLE 11.1 Characteristics of and Goniometer Placements for the Joints of the Extremities

Joint	Planes of motion	Movement	Axis of rotation	Stationary arm	Moving arm	End-feel	Normal range (°)
Toe inter-phalangeal	Sagittal	Flexion	Midline of IP joint	Midline of proximal phalanx	Midline of distal pha-lanx	Soft	90
		Extension				Firm	0
Metatarsal-phalangeal	Sagittal	Flexion	Midline of MTP joint	Midline of metatarsal	Midline of proximal phalanx	Firm	20
		Extension				Firm	80
	Transverse	Abduction	Midline of MTP joint	Midline of metatarsal	Midline of proximal phalanx	Firm	20
		Adduction				Firm	0
Subtalar	Frontal	Inversion	Over calca-neal tendon in line with malleolus	Midline of leg	Midline of calcaneus	Firm	35
		Eversion				Hard	20
Ankle	Sagittal	Plantar flex-ion	Lateral mal-leolus	Midline of fibula	Parallel to midline of fifth meta-tarsal	Firm	50
		Dorsiflexion				Firm	20
Knee	Sagittal	Flexion	Lateral epi-condyle	Midline of femur	Midline of fibula	Soft	145
		Extension				Firm	0
	Transverse	Internal rotation	Mid calca-neus	Along the shaft of the second metatarsal at start	Along the shaft of the second metatarsal at end	Firm	20
		External Rotation				Firm	30
Hip	Sagittal	Flexion	Greater tro-chanter	Midline of trunk	Midline of femur	Soft	120
		Extension				Firm	20
	Frontal	Abduction	Ipsilateral ASIS	Contralat-eral ASIS	Midline of femur	Firm	45
		Adduction				Firm	30
	Transverse	Internal rotation	Midpoint of patella	Perpendicu-lar to the floor	Midline of tibia	Firm	40
		External rotation				Firm	40
Shoulder	Sagittal	Flexion	Acromion process	Midline of thorax	Midline of humerus	Firm	165
		Extension				Firm	160
	Frontal	Abduction	Acromion process	Parallel to sternum	Midline of humerus	Firm	165
		Adduction				Firm	0
	Transverse	Internal rotation	Olecranon process	Perpendicu-lar to the floor	Ulnar border of forearm	Firm	70
		External rotation				Firm	90
		Horizontal abduction	Acromion process	Perpendicu-lar to trunk	Long axis of humerus	Firm	45
		Horizontal adduction				Soft	135

Joint	Planes of motion	Movement	Axis of rotation	Stationary arm	Moving arm	End-feel	Normal range (°)
Elbow	Sagittal	Flexion	Lateral epicondyle	Midline of humerus	Midline of radius	Soft	140
		Extension				Hard	0
Forearm	Transverse	Pronation	Head of third metacarpal	Perpendicular to floor	Parallel to pencil held in hand	Firm	80
		Supination				Firm	80
Wrist	Sagittal	Flexion	Triquetrum	Midline of ulna	Midline of fifth metacarpal	Firm	80
		Extension				Firm	70
	Frontal	Radial deviation	Capitate	Midline of forearm	Midline of third metacarpal	Hard	20
		Ulnar deviation				Firm	30
Metacarpal-phalangeal	Sagittal	Flexion	Midline of MCP joint	Midline of metacarpal	Midline of proximal phalanx	Hard	90
		Extension				Firm	20
	Transverse	Abduction	Midline of MCP joint	Midline of metacarpal	Midline of proximal phalanx	Soft	25
		Adduction				Firm	0
Finger interphalangeal	Sagittal	Flexion	Midline of IP joint	Midline of proximal phalanx	Midline of distal phalanx	Firm	100
		Extension				Firm	10

Data from Berryman Reese and Bandy 2002; Kendall et al. 1993; Norkin and White 1995; Shultz et al. 2005; Starkey and Ryan 2002.

sliding is necessary for maintaining congruency between the articular surfaces; a restriction in the amount of sliding will limit the amount of rotation. For example, extending the wrist requires the proximal carpal row to slide toward the palm. A restriction of sliding in the palmar direction will limit the amount of wrist extension.

Arthrokinematic motion is determined by the joint structures themselves: the shape of the articular surfaces and cartilaginous and ligamentous structures. Excessive arthrokinematic motion is termed joint laxity, whereas an abnormally low amount of motion is a joint restriction. Evaluation of arthrokinematic motion is beyond the scope of this chapter; people suspected of having abnormal arthrokinematic motion should be referred to the appropriate health care provider for further assessment and treatment, if necessary.

The extensibility of the periarticular structures (e.g., muscle, tendon, fascia) limits the amount of motion in a DOF. In the absence of joint pathology (an assumption made throughout the rest of this chapter, unless otherwise indicated), ROM is often considered a measure of the extensibility of those periarticular structures. Extensibility of the periarticular structures is joint specific. It is generally accepted that flexibility is not a general characteristic

TABLE 11.2 Characteristics and Measurements of the Spine

Joint	Planes of motion	Move- ment	End- feel	INCLINOMETER METHOD Superior land- mark	Inferior land- mark	Normal range (°)	TAPE MEASURE METHOD Superior landmark	Inferior landmark	Tape measure (cm)
Thoraco- lumbar spine	Sagittal	Flexion	Firm	Spinous process C7	Spinous process S2	60	Spinous process C7	Spinous process S2	6-7
		Extension	Hard			30			
	Frontal	Lateral bending	Firm	15 cm above S2	Spinous process S2	30			
	Trans- verse	Rotation	Firm	Spinous process T12	Spinous process T1	6			
Cervical spine	Sagittal	Flexion	Firm	Vertex of skull[1]	Spinous process T1	50	Chin	Sternal notch	1-4
		Extension	Hard			60	Chin	Sternal notch	20
	Frontal	Lateral Bending	Firm	Vertex of skull[1]	Spinous process T1	45	Mastoid process	Acromion process	15
	Trans- verse	Rotation	Firm	N/A[2]	Base of forehead	80	Chin	Acromion process	10

[1] Halfway between the bridge of the nose and the base of the occiput.

[2] Performed in the supine position.

Data from Berryman Reese and Bandy 2002; Kendall et al. 1993; Norkin and White 1995; Shultz et al. 2005; Starkey and Ryan 2002.

of a person (Berryman Reese and Bandy 2002), but rather, is joint specific. Therefore, no one test can determine how "flexible" a person is.

It is important to understand that the joints of the body rarely act in isolation. Rather, they act as part of a kinematic chain. When the distal end of a limb is free to move (i.e., open kinematic chain), a muscle's extensibility will affect the ROM of each joint it crosses in the direction opposite its anatomical classification of action.

A monoarticular (single) muscle crosses one joint and affects the ROM of that joint (e.g., the gluteus maximus crosses the hip joint and affects hip flexion ROM). Multijoint muscles cross two (biarticular) or more (polyarticular) joints. A biarticular muscle affects both joints that it crosses (the hamstring crosses both the hip and the knee and affects the ROM of hip flexion and knee extension). Polyarticular muscles (such as the long head of the biceps brachii) affect each joint they cross. When a muscle's action creates joint rotations in multiple planes, its extensibility affects the ROM of each rotation in the opposite direction of its anatomical action. For example, the gluteus maximus both extends and externally rotates the hip joint. Therefore, its extensibility affects both hip flexion and hip internal rotation.

When the distal end of a segment is fixed or constrained to move in some way (i.e., closed kinematic chain), the extensibility of a muscle will affect the ROM of every joint in the limb, whether it crosses them or not. For example, if the foot is flat and the trunk is vertical (as in a single-leg wall squat), the amount of knee flexion is determined by the amount of ankle and hip flexion (Zatsiorsky 1998). A limitation in the ROM at either the hip, knee, or ankle can affect the amount of motion at the other two joints because of this coupling of joint rotations. Similarly, bilateral movements (such as the squat) involve two limbs moving in parallel. To maintain bilateral symmetry, joint motion is coupled not only between the joints of the same limb but also between the joints of the opposite limb.

Sport Performance and Mobility

Relating performance or injury potential to any one variable is difficult because, by its very nature, human movement is multifactorial (involving mobility, strength, power, endurance, and neuromuscular control). Additionally, the outcome (performance, injury) involves complex interactions among the performer, task, and environment. While the optimal result in a task requires a specific movement pattern that is performed in a stereotypical manner (Bobbert and van Ingen Schenau 1988), there is a range of acceptable deviations and the performer should have enough mobility to be able to exploit the use of those deviations when necessary. Based on a preponderance of the evidence, it appears reasonable to conclude that every task requires an optimal ROM from the performer so that correct posture can be maintained, energy can be generated or absorbed by the muscles, and the end effector (hand, foot) can be positioned properly in space.

Rather than being limited to a particular angle, acceptable mobility probably spans several degrees in either direction for a given task. Increasing or decreasing mobility within this range will not affect performance or injury potential (Thacker et al. 2004). However, hyper- and hypomobility can have negative implications for performance and may lead to musculoskeletal injury if not corrected. Hypermobility may lead to an unstable joint if that motion cannot be controlled (stability is discussed in chapter 12). Hypomobility can lead to the negative consequences discussed next.

Posture

When ideal posture is maintained, intersegmental reaction and inertial forces flow through the segments that are structurally best able to deal with them. For alignment to be ideal, the tension on all of the muscles crossing the joints must be balanced. Greater tension of muscles on one side of a joint, and corresponding laxity on the other, could pull the body segments out of alignment and require other structures (such as ligaments) to bear a larger proportion of the stresses. For example, people with increased curvature of the low back (hyperlordosis) were found to have increased strain on the ligaments of the lumbar spine, which decreased with postural stability exercises that included stretching (Scannell and McGill 2003).

Additionally, because posture is the position from which all movement begins and ends, faulty posture can predispose a person to injury as a result of increased stress on tissues that are ill equipped to deal with it. For example, subtalar pronation and hip internal rotation are part of the normal energy-absorbing motions that occur during landing. People who start a landing with more subtalar pronation or more hip internal rotation (or both) are more likely to end the landing with more subtalar pronation or more hip internal rotation (to achieve the same amount of motion). But this excessive ROM can lead to increased strain on the anterior cruciate ligament, and subsequently tear it (Sigward, Ota, and Powers 2008).

Energy Generation and Absorption

Energy generation and absorption require that the joints involved produce a force through a certain ROM. If the necessary motion of that joint in that plane is inadequate, motion may occur at either a different joint, or at the same joint in a different plane, to compensate for the deficiency. If a muscle can produce force while acting concentrically over a larger ROM, it can generate greater energy, improving performance. For example, the ROM of shoulder external rotation in baseball pitchers is twice what is considered normal (Werner et al. 2008). However, that amount of motion is necessary because of the high correlation between shoulder external rotation and the velocity of the ball at release (Whiteley 2007). Increased external rotation means that force can be generated over a larger ROM of internal rotation, increasing the amount of energy transferred to the ball.

Similarly, if a muscle can produce force while acting eccentrically over a larger ROM, it can absorb more energy. Muscles have the largest energy-absorbing capability of any structure in the body (e.g., bone, cartilage, ligaments). It is not surprising, then, that decreased shoulder internal rotation ROM in baseball pitchers predisposes them to glenoid labral tears (Burkhart, Morgan, and Kibler 2003). This is because the external rotators (teres minor, infraspinatus) acting eccentrically to slow the arm down will be able to absorb less energy after the ball is released.

These effects are not limited to the joints that a muscle crosses. As explained earlier, flexion of the hip, knee, and ankle are coupled during weight-bearing activities (Zatsiorsky 1998), and a limitation in the ROM of any one joint may cause a decrease in the ROM of the other joints in the chain. Limited ankle plantar flexion can decrease forward progression of the tibia, limiting the amount of energy that can be absorbed by the plantar flexors. In an attempt to absorb the energy further up the chain, increased motion may occur in the frontal plane (Sigward, Ota, and Powers 2008), collapsing the knee into a valgus position (see figure 11.2). Unfortunately, this position increases the energy absorbed by the ligaments of the knee (Markolf et al. 1995). Likewise, proper jumping requires energy to be transferred from the proximal thigh to the distal foot (Bobbert and van Ingen Schenau 1988). Limiting the ROM in the sagittal plane would decrease energy generated by the leg muscles and, as a result, jump height; and energy "leaking" into the frontal plane, in addition to increasing injury risk, would not be useful in increasing jump height.

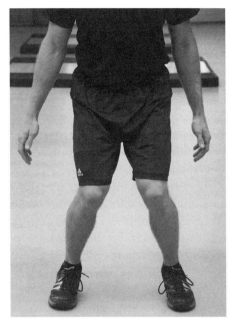

FIGURE 11.2   Valgus collapse position.

Position of the End Effector

Activities of daily living and sport often require the hand or foot to be positioned somewhere in space. Restrictions in hip mobility may lead to injuries of the low back. Decreased hip flexion as a result of tight hamstrings can cause someone to make up that deficit with increased spinal flexion in activities such as a deadlift. However, spinal flexion decreases the ability of the erector spinae to produce a posterior shear force by 60% (McGill, Hughson, and Parks 2000) and limit the ability of the hip musculature to push or pull a load (Lett and McGill 2006). Similarly, decreased ROM at the glenohumeral joint requires compensatory motion at the thoracolumbar spine (Fayad et al. 2008) during reaching tasks, which could potentially move the spine out of the position in which it is best able to transfer forces.

Mobility Testing

Mobility is often assessed by determining the ROM of each DOF involved in a movement. ROM can be tested either actively or passively and either in isolation or integrated with the rest of the kinematic chain, giving four possible permutations. Each permutation has a unique ROM value. Because the utility of a value lies in comparing it to something else, fitness professionals must decide up front how they want to evaluate ROM so they can make appropriate comparisons.

ROM is often classified as either active (AROM) or passive (PROM). AROM is often thought of as the person moving his own joint, whereas during PROM an evaluator (such as a personal trainer, strength coach, or athletic trainer) moves the joint for the person. However, these definitions are not entirely correct. AROM is more accurately defined as when the muscles responsible for moving a joint perform the movement. Conversely, PROM is when a force other than those muscles moves the joint. For example, actively contracting the hamstring to flex the knee would be an example of AROM. If an evaluator flexes the knee, or if a person flexes her own knee using her arms, it is PROM. Although touching the toes from a standing position is often considered AROM, it could be argued that it is PROM because the force of gravity is involved in flexing the hips and spine. In general, a joint usually has greater PROM than AROM because of the ability of the external force to apply overpressure at the end range of motion (Shultz, Houglum, and Perrin 2005), but this is not always the case (Berryman Reese and Bandy 2002).

Both AROM and PROM are used to assess the motion of a joint. AROM provides information about both the motion available at the joint and the muscles' ability to produce it. But because AROM requires the muscles to generate sufficient torque to produce movement, it is not possible to differentiate among limited ROM due to weakness or pain of the muscle, lack of flexibility, and some other pathology in the joint. This is why the American Medical Association recommends testing both AROM and PROM (Berryman Reese and Bandy 2002) for those suspected of a physical impairment.

With a person who is healthy and asymptomatic, it is usually sufficient to test either AROM or PROM, and not both. Corkery and colleagues (2007) argued that AROM eliminates tester bias and standardizes measurements because the person being tested is asked to move the joint to tolerance. It would seem reasonable to test only AROM with healthy, asymptomatic subjects, but this is a matter of the fitness professional's personal preference. Either way, the examiner just needs to be consistent about which one is used, and annotate accordingly.

After determining whether to test AROM or PROM, the fitness professional has to decide whether to test the muscle in isolation or as part of the kinematic chain and how to test them. A comparison of various mobility tests is presented in table 11.4 (page 292). Testing the mobility of the kinematic chain can be done by simply watching the task (e.g., gait, throwing) or by administering multijoint movement screens designed for the specific purpose of examining the mobility of the chain (Cook 2001). Filming the activity with a high-speed digital camera allows for a slow-motion playback that can alert the examiner to an aberrant motion that may be missed by the naked eye. Analyzing the digital images with commercially available software allows the examiner to quantify the movement at each joint with a high degree of accuracy, which makes this test highly reliable and valid (Kadaba et al. 1989).

Movement screens, developed by Cook (2001), include a battery of tests for evaluating the mobility of the kinematic chain: the deep squat, hurdle step, in-line lunge, shoulder mobility, active straight-leg raise, trunk stability push-up, and rotary stability of the trunk tests. As of this writing, neither the validity nor the reliability of these screens has been published in peer-reviewed journals, but the use of these screens might hold some promise for predicting injury (Kiesel, Plisky, and Voight 2007). Further investigation is warranted.

Isolated tests include single-joint tests and muscle length tests. With single-joint tests, all muscles crossing multiple joints are put in a shortened position across all joints they cross except the joint being tested. For example, in testing hip joint flexion, the knee is also flexed so that the multijoint hamstrings are shortened across the knee while being lengthened across the hip. Such a test can be used to assess the flexibility of the monoarticular hip extensors (Kendall, McCreary, and Provance 1993).

Muscle length tests are used to assess the flexibility of the multijoint muscles by lengthening the muscle across all the joints it crosses (Kendall et al. 1993). For example, to test the flexibility of the hamstrings, the hip is flexed and the knee is extended, lengthening the muscle across both joints. Single-joint muscles normally possess enough flexibility to allow a joint to move through its full ROM, whereas multijoint muscles usually do not unless they are shortened at the other joints they cross (Kendall et al. 1993).

A cross between isolated and integrated testing is composite testing, in which motion is measured in two or more joints, albeit in a nonfunctional pattern (Berryman Reese and Bandy 2002). The most popular example of a composite test is the sit-and-reach test, which measures the composite motion of hip and lumbar flexion. Other composite tests include the shoulder lift test, fingertip-to-floor test, and Apley scratch test (Berryman Reese and Bandy 2002). The problem with such tests is that they do not reveal the contributions each joint makes to the movement. In the sit-and-reach test, hypermobile hip extensors can compensate for hypomobile trunk extensors, and vice versa. Therefore, the utility of these tests is limited.

A full assessment of mobility in a healthy, asymptomatic population is a two-step process (see figure 11.3). The first step involves the analysis of joint motion that is part of an integrated kinematic chain activity, which is usually performed actively. Because of the number of tests that would have to be performed to test every joint in the body, these screens can save time by alerting the examiner to the presence of an aberrant movement pattern in need of further attention. If an aberrant pattern is noted, the examiner could have the person mimic the pattern in a gravity-eliminated position, or move the person passively. This eliminates the need for strength, power, or neuromuscular control, allowing the examiner to determine whether the problem is indeed one of mobility.

To ascertain the exact location of the problem (if one exists), the next step involves examining each joint in the kinematic chain in isolation. Isolated testing requires both single-joint and muscle length tests. Isolated testing should also be performed on all "problem" joints, which are sus-

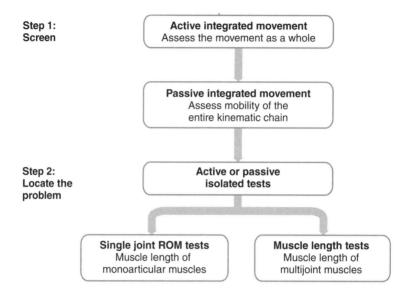

FIGURE 11.3 Assessing mobility. The process flows from examining the movement as a whole to see if a problem exists, to examining the movement in a gravity-eliminated position or passively to determine if it is in fact a problem with mobility. If it is, isolated joint testing is performed to determine which joint (or joints) is the problem within the kinematic chain.

ceptible to either hyper- or hypomobility because of either past history or tasks performed on a regular basis. For example, a hurdler with a history of hamstring strains should have hamstring flexibility assessed regularly. A baseball pitcher, even when injury free, should have his glenohumeral internal rotation ROM assessed regularly as part of an injury prevention program.

Range of Motion Tests

There are too many functional movement patterns to include all of them in a chapter of this size. Fitness professionals need to be familiar with the biomechanics of the activities they are training their clients or athletes to perform to appreciate what is normal or abnormal for that activity, and to screen for abnormal movement patterns accordingly. Although movement screens (Cook 2001) may hold promise, scientific evidence is not sufficient to merit making recommendations concerning their use at this time. Conducting composite tests to assess flexibility is not recommended. Therefore, the remainder of this chapter focuses on isolated ROM tests of muscle flexibility.

When measuring ROM, the examiner should have an appreciation of the DOF quality, quantity, and end-feel. Each of these provides a unique piece of information and should be considered part of the full assessment.

The quality of the ROM is how the motion feels to both the examiner and the subject and is therefore evaluated subjectively. Normal motion should be full and fluid. Irregular, hesitant, jerky, or painful motion would signal a problem with that movement (Houglum 2005).

The quantity of ROM is simply how much motion is available at a joint. It can be measured either subjectively or objectively. However, several authors have determined that objective measures are more accurate and more reliable than subjective ones (Brosseau et al. 2001; Croxford, Jones, and Barker 1998; Youdas, Bogard, and Suman 1993). With a qualitative test, the evaluator examines the rotation and subjectively determines whether the ROM is within normal limits, hypermobile, or hypomobile. With a quantitative test, the evaluator measures the actual joint angle at the end range of motion with a goniometer, inclinometer, or tape measure (described in the next section). Normal ranges of motion for each joint are presented in tables 11.1 and 11.2 for the extremities and spine, respectively.

The end-feel is what limits the range of motion. It is measured subjectively. Normal end-feels can be soft, firm, or hard (Norkin and White 1995). A soft end-feel occurs when two muscle bellies come in contact (e.g., when a person flexes the elbow, the muscles of the forearm and upper arm contact each other and limit further motion). A firm end-feel occurs when resistance from the soft tissue prevents further motion, such as the hamstrings or joint capsule preventing further motion when extending the knee. A hard end-feel occurs when two bones come in contact, such as during elbow extension when the olecranon process comes in contact with the olecranon fossa. Normal end-feels for the joints are also presented in tables 11.1 and 11.2.

Abnormalities in either the quality or end-feel of the ROM are often serious, and are beyond the scope of practice of a fitness professional. If these problems are noted, the person in question should be referred to the appropriate health care provider. Changing the quantity of motion is within the scope of most fitness professionals, so it is important that they know how to properly perform the tests and interpret the results. Table 11.4 on page 292 provides a comparison of mobility evaluations.

SINGLE-JOINT TESTS

ROM of a single joint can be measured qualitatively by visually inspecting the joint in question as it reaches its end range of motion or by quantifying it through the use of specialized instruments, including goniometers, inclinometers, and tape measures (see figure 11.4). In either case, the joint being tested is moved through its full ROM while every other joint is stabilized. The examiner must ensure that each multijoint muscle is stabilized in its slack (or shortened) position. Both end ROMs for each DOF are then recorded.

EQUIPMENT

Goniometers, inclinometers, or tape measures

PROCEDURE

1. The goniometer has two arms with a 360° marked circle in the center. The arm with the circle is the fixed arm and should be placed along a reference line on the heavier (proximal) segment.
2. The axis of rotation of the goniometer is placed coincident with the axis of rotation of the joint. The other arm is the moving arm. and it is placed along a reference line on the lighter (usually proximal) segment.
3. During either AROM or PROM, the joint is moved to the end of its ROM, and the angle is measured on the goniometer.
4. The locations of the proximal arm, distal arm, and axis of rotation are listed in table 11.1 for the extremities.

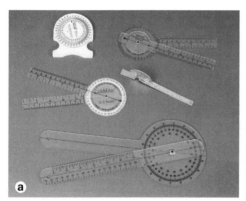

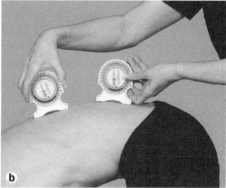

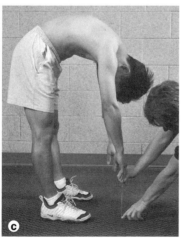

FIGURE 11.4 Common measuring apparatuses: (a) goniometers of various sizes, (b) inclinometer, and (c) tape measure.

Figure 11.4a reprinted, by permission, from P.A. Houglum, 2011, Therapeutic exercise for musculoskeletal injuries, 3rd ed. (Champaign, IL: Human Kinetics), 136, 137. Figure 11.4b reprinted, by permission, from V. Heyward, 2010, Advanced fitness assessment and exercise prescription, 6th ed. (Champaign, IL: Human Kinetics), 272.

Figure 11.4c Reprinted, by permission, from P.A. Houglum, 2011, Therapeutic exercise for musculoskeletal injuries, 3rd ed. (Champaign, IL: Human Kinetics), 137.

ADDITIONAL CONSIDERATIONS

With some joints, such as the spine, using a goniometer is difficult. In these instances, either a tape measure or an inclinometer can be used. Here, the absolute distance (tape measure) or segment angle (inclinometer), rather than the relative joint angle, is measured between the moving segment and some fixed reference point. The tape measure is used to determine the distance between two vertebrae, and although it is appropriate for all motions in the cervical spine, it is usually appropriate to measure only spinal flexion in the thoracolumbar spine. The inclinometer makes use of the difference between a segment's beginning and ending position in relation to gravity, similar to a carpenter's level (Berryman Reese and Bandy 2002). The ROM is determined by subtracting the reading at the inferior landmark from the reading at the superior landmark. The thoracolumbar spine and cervical spine are usually measured as different segments, with representative values presented in table 11.2.

MUSCLE LENGTH TESTS

Muscle length tests are used to measure the flexibility of multijoint muscles.

PROCEDURE

Although the procedures for muscle length tests are the same as those for single-joint tests, the positioning of the joints is different. With single-joint tests, each multijoint muscle is stabilized in its slack (or shortened) position, and lengthened only across the joint being measured. With muscle length tests, the process is repeated with the muscle in its lengthened position at both its proximal and distal joints. In the case of polyarticular muscles, the muscle is in its lengthened position at all of the joints that it crosses. The positioning of the joints for both single-joint and muscle length tests of the lower extremities are presented in table 11.3.

NORMS

For muscle length tests, Kendall, McCreary, and Provance (1993) suggested that the norm is for the muscle length to be approximately 80% of the total range of motion for the two joints. An example is given for the muscle length of the hamstrings. The hip joint has an approximate ROM of 135° (10° of extension to 125° of flexion), and the knee joint has an approximate ROM of 140° (0° of extension to 140° of flexion). The combined ROM of the joints is the sum of 135 and 140, or 275°. With the hip flexed to 80°, the knee's ROM should still be 140° (or 80% of 275°). If the hip was flexed to 90°, then the knee's ROM should be 130° (from 10° to 130° of flexion).

Currently, no normative or reliability data are available for muscle length tests of the upper extremities. These tests may be more appropriate for health care practitioners, and interested readers are referred elsewhere (Berryman Reese and Bandy 2002; Kendall, McCreary, and Provance 1993).

TABLE 11.3 Positioning for Single-Joint and Muscle Length Tests of the Lower Extremities

| Joint motion | SINGLE-JOINT TEST | | MUSCLE LENGTH TEST | | | |
	Position or movement of proximal joint	Position or movement of distal joint	Position or movement of proximal joint	Position or movement of distal joint	Muscle tested	ROM of distal joint (°)
Ankle dorsiflexion	Knee flexed	Dorsiflexion	Knee extended	Dorsiflexion	Gastrocnemius	4
Knee flexion	Hip flexed	Knee flexed	Hip extended	Knee flexed	Rectus femoris	53
Knee extension	Hip extended	Knee extended	Hip flexed	Knee extended	Hamstrings	28
Hip flexion	Hip flexed	Knee flexed	See rectus femoris test above			
Hip extension	Hip extended	Knee extended	See hamstrings test above			

Data from Berryman Reese and Bandy 2002; Kendall et al. 1993; Corkery et al. 2007.

Interpretation of Results

After the measurement of ROM has been conducted, the results need to be interpreted. Interpretation usually involves comparing the values obtained to normative data or the minimum values required to perform an activity. Values can also be compared bilaterally, or over time.

Values obtained during the test can be compared to normative data, such as those presented in tables 11.1 through 11.3. However, these comparisons should be made with care, because there is no universal standard for ROM. For example, although 90° of external rotation of the shoulder is considered normal, baseball pitchers may have (and require) twice that amount (Werner et al. 2008).

Values can also be compared to those normally considered required for a given task. For example, the normal range of dorsiflexion is 20°, but 10° is required for normal walking gait and 15° is required for normal running gait, although a recent investigation (Weir and Chockalingam 2007) has shown that the actual requirements for walking gait are highly variable, between 12 and 22°. An appreciation of the biomechanics and variability of various tasks is required to understand the ROM requirements of those tasks.

Bilateral comparisons (i.e., comparing the right and left sides) of the same person is another way to interpret the results. There is no general consensus about how much difference between the two is acceptable. However, some authors suggest that the two sides should be between 10% (Burkhart, Morgan, and Kibler 2003) and 15% (Knapik et al. 1991) of each other. For most people, this appears to be a reasonable standard.

Finally, the values of a joint can be compared to values of the same joint taken earlier. Comparing the same test on the same person over time is an excellent way to quantify changes resulting from exercise, aging, or injury. Because of the effects of temperature (Robertson, Ward, and Jung 2005) and activity (Wenos and Konin 2004) on flexibility, examiners need to ensure that pretest conditions are similar for comparisons to be valid. When pretest conditions are standardized, these comparisons are among the best ways to determine the effectiveness of an intervention program.

Mobility should be assessed to identify ROM deficits; athletes without deficits will probably realize little benefit from increasing their mobility (Haff et al. 2006). A decreased ROM should be considered a deficit under the following conditions:

- The decreased ROM alters the mechanics of a movement (either sport specific or fundamental).

- The joint ROM is not within normal limits for an athlete's sport. Athletes at or below the acceptable ROM, even if it does not appear to affect their mechanics, should probably improve ROM to within these limits.

- A decreased ROM is the result of an injury, and the ROM is not restored to preinjury levels.

- A decreased ROM creates asymmetry bilaterally. Except in some rare instances, the ROM should be comparable bilaterally (side-to-side differences should be less than 10%).

Deficits are corrected by using stretching exercises that increase the ROM of a joint. Biarticular muscles need to be lengthened across both ends while being stretched. Techniques such as static stretching and PNF (proprioceptive neuromuscular facilitation) can be used. Stretches should be held for approximately 30 seconds, with 10 seconds of rest between them. Four or five repetitions should be performed, and stretching can be done twice or three times per day.

Athletes with no deficits should be tested only periodically (perhaps annually). Athletes with identified deficits should be tested more regularly. Once the deficit has been corrected, occasional tests should be performed to ensure that mobility is maintained at adequate levels.

Comparing Mobility Measurement Methods

Table 11.4 summarizes and compares the tests that have been discussed in this chapter.

TABLE 11.4 Comparisons of Mobility Evaluations

Test type	Validity	Reliability	Equipment	Time	Major advantages	Major disadvantages
3-D biomechanical analysis	High	High	3-D motion analysis system	High	Reliably and accurately collect 3-D data while the athlete is performing the activity	Cost; training of evaluator; processing time; not prescriptive
Movement screen	Unknown	Unknown	Camcorder; dowel rod; 2 × 6; or none	Moderately low	Athlete is performing real-world activities; multiple joints are assessed simultaneously	Validity and reliability not established; lack of norms; potential for no universal screen for all athletes; not prescriptive
Composite tests	Low	Moderate to high	Sit-and-reach box	Moderately low	Easy to perform and low cost	Unable to distinguish which joint is limiting ROM
ROM and muscle length	High	Moderate to high	Goniometer; tape measure; or none	Moderately high	Cheap; minimal equipment and training	Mobility not assessed during activity; takes time to assess each individual joint

Professional Applications

The first step in assessing the mobility of an athlete is to conduct a needs analysis for the athlete's sport, determining the joints involved and the amplitude and directions of the movements necessary for that sport. This information is available for many popular sports in biomechanics texts and journals. For example, baseball pitchers require approximately 170° of external rotation, whereas American football quarterbacks require about 160° of external rotation during a throw (Fleisig et al. 1996). Running requires 20° of hip extension, 70° of hip flexion, 110° of knee flexion, 30° of dorsiflexion, and 20° of plantarflexion (Novacheck 1998), but the positions of the hip and knee immediately prior to contact place the biceps femoris at 100% of its resting length (Thelen et al. 2006). Similar data should be found for other sports of interest.

The next step is to determine whether the athlete is performing the sporting movements correctly. If possible, this should be done by observing the athlete performing the sport. The gold standard would be a three-dimensional biomechanical analysis, which is expensive and time consuming (making it impractical in a lot of situations). Watching with the human eye is the least preferred method because people are unable to detect small changes, can view the performance only once, and are hampered by the movement speed, leading to poor reliability and validity (Knudson and Morrison 1997). An alternative may be to record the movement with a high-speed camcorder and view the recording multiple times at slow speeds. The point is to compare the ranges of motion that the athlete uses to normative data or some exemplary performance to determine whether too little (or too much) motion is occurring at the various joints.

Even the process of observing recorded performances may be too time-consuming for a large number of athletes. Screening of a more fundamental movement pattern (such as a squat or lunge) may provide some information, but the transfer of these movements to higher-level tasks (such as running and cutting) has not been established. Different types of sporting activities may require different fundamental movement patterns. For example, a baseball pitcher may not need the same movement qualities as a wrestler.

The initial evaluation provides an assessment of movement quality. This alerts the fitness professional to a problem, but does not reveal the cause of that problem. A movement screen should not be prescriptive, because of the multiple causative factors that could potentially be involved. A reasonable next step would be to identify the cause of the problem by evaluating each potential cause individually. This would start with the mobility of each joint in the chain.

Consider a case in which an athlete exhibits valgus collapse during drop landings from a box (see figure 11.2). This is considered a faulty movement pattern. This problem could be a result of a lack of mobility, strength, power, endurance, or neuromuscular control of any of the joints in the lower extremity. The athlete performs a squat in a gravity-eliminated position (such as on a Total Gym or sled machine), which reveals signs of valgus collapse. This suggests the need for an evaluation of the mobility of the joints in the chain, specifically looking for any of the following factors: restricted hip external rotation (Sigward, Ota, and Powers 2008; Willson, Ireland, and Davis 2006), limited ankle plantarflexion (Sigward, Ota, and Powers 2008), or restricted supination of the subtalar joint (Loudon, Jenkins, and Loudon 1996). Determining the problem joint can only be accomplished by examining the mobility of each joint individually using the ROM tests described in this chapter and comparing the results to the norms in table 11.1. If the ROM appears to be within normal limits, the problem is either with another joint or with another motor quality (strength, power, endurance, neuromuscular control). This will require further testing.

Potential or previous problem areas should also be examined when conducting ROM testing. Shoulder injury is always a potential problem for pitchers, and a deficit in glenohumeral internal rotation can be a contributing factor. Each athlete should be examined for a deficit in internal rotation using either absolute (ROM < 25°) of relative (bilateral differences > 25°) measures (Burkhart, Morgan, and Kibler 2003). A previous injury will alter the material properties of the hamstrings, subjecting them to greater strains and making them more susceptible to injury in the future (Silder, Reeder, and Thelen 2010). Athletes with known previous hamstring injuries should be evaluated using a muscle length test of the hamstrings, and the results should be compared both to normative data (table 11.1) and to the hamstrings on the unaffected side.

(continued)

(continued)

Mobility testing should be aimed at identifying deficits. A deficit should be considered any decrease in ROM that alters the mechanics of the movement (either a sport-specific skill or fundamental movement pattern), does not fall within the normal limits required for the specific sport or activity, creates a bilateral asymmetry, or all of these. These deficits should then be targeted for intervention using stretching techniques such as static stretching or PNF (proprioceptive neuromuscular facilitation). Each stretch should be held for approximately 30 seconds and repeated four or five times with 10 seconds of rest between them. Stretching exercises can be performed twice or three times a day, but because of the decreases in neuromuscular performance (Stone et al. 2006), they should not be performed before activities with high force or power requirements. Athletes with no identified ROM deficiencies will likely receive little to no benefit from a stretching program, and should focus their efforts on the other motor abilities discussed in this book.

SUMMARY

- Mobility is a fundamental component of effective and efficient human movement.
- A thorough assessment of mobility requires an examination of the quality, quantity, and end-feel of every joint in the kinematic chain of an aberrant movement pattern, as well as those areas prone to injury either for the person or for that activity.
- Values obtained from a mobility test should be compared to established norms, to values of the same joint on the opposite side of the body, to values of the same joint taken earlier, or all of these.
- Although human movement is complex and multifactorial, less-than-optimal mobility in a given task can impair performance and increase the potential for injury.

Balance and Stability

Sean P. Flanagan, PhD, ATC, CSCS

When thinking about balance, many images can come to mind: a surfer, a gymnast, and a figure skater are a few of the more dramatic examples of athletes requiring balance. However, almost every athlete, and certainly any athlete that spends time on one foot, needs balance.

Many people equate balance and stability, but this is erroneous. Stability is the ability to return to a desired position or motion after a disturbance. Anytime athletes come in contact with opponents, objects, or even unexpected variations in terrain, they are exposed to disturbances. Thus, stability is an important concept in athletics.

The examination of any motor quality or attribute requires that we first define it in an unambiguous way and then construct a test that eliminates all other variables except the one being tested. Measuring a fundamental quality such as strength or $\dot{V}O_2max$ is (relatively) straightforward. In contrast, several fundamentally different motor qualities may have been examined when someone is said to have good balance or be stable. By their very nature, these qualities involve multiple joints and multiple systems (skeletal, muscular, and nervous), which makes testing a difficult proposition. The purpose of this chapter is to provide a theoretical background on the concepts of balance and stability, discuss their effects on performance and injury, categorize various types of tests, and describe three field tests in detail.

Training is all about improving abilities that enhance performance (such as mobility, strength, power, endurance, or neuromuscular control). To do so, we must first identify them through a comprehensive test battery. Other chapters deal with fundamental qualities such as mobility and strength. Performance is not simply the sum of all of these qualities; it is also a function of how they interact to create planned or reactive movements. Balance and stability testing is one way of assessing these interactions during reactive events.

Body Mechanics

Many people have misconceptions about balance and stability. Added to this confusion is the fact that some terms that have very different mechanical meanings are used interchangeably in popular jargon. What follows is a review of some principles of mechanics and control theory to establish a common terminology and framework for balance and balance-like measures that will be used throughout this chapter.

Center of Gravity

To simplify the description of any rigid body (e.g., thigh, forearm), all of its mass is assumed to be concentrated at one imaginary point known as the center of mass. The mass of the body is evenly distributed about this point in all directions. In the (vertical) direction of gravity, this point is known as the center of gravity (COG). For any rigid body, the location of the center of mass, and thus the COG, is fixed.

In a multisegmented body such as the human body, the COG is the weighted sum of the COG of each segment. Unlike in a rigid body, the location of the COG in a multisegmented body moves depending on the configuration of the segments. In an adult male standing in the anatomical position, the COG is located anterior to the second sacral vertebra (Whiting and Rugg 2006), but raising the right arm overhead shifts the COG up and to the right. To complicate matters even further, the location of the COG can even be outside of the body during certain configurations. Determining the location of the COG in space at any moment in time is no easy task, yet the central nervous system appears to be able to accomplish this task in most situations without much difficulty.

Ground Reaction Force

Two bodies in contact with each other produce equal and opposite reaction forces. If you are not moving, your weight will produce a force onto the ground, which will produce an equal and opposite force back onto you (the ground reaction force, or GRF). These forces are distributed over the areas of contact.

Center of Pressure and Base of Support

Another simplifying assumption in the analysis of movement is that all of the contact forces are concentrated at a single point, known as the center of pressure (COP). The COP is not a static point but, being a representation of the GRF, must reside within an area outlined by all contact areas. This area is known as the base of support (BOS). For example, if only one foot is in contact with the ground, the BOS is the contact area of the foot. If two feet are in contact with the ground, the BOS includes the contact areas of both feet plus the area between them (Whiting and Rugg 2006). Spreading the feet apart (anterior–posterior, laterally, or both) or adding another point of contact increases the size of the BOS. If body weight and the GRF are of equal magnitudes, and the COP is located directly below the COG, then no net forces or moments are acting on the body. The body is standing still. It is in static equilibrium, or balanced.

Being a biological system, the human body does not remain perfectly motionless for very long, if at all. Rather, the location of the COG in space is constantly deviating from a central location, and the body automatically corrects for it by relocating the COP to bring the COG back to the central point. Although constantly in flux, the location of the COG (and thus, the COP) is at this central point during quiet standing when integrated over time.

Balance

Balance is the ability to maintain the COG over the BOS without taking a step. Taking a step creates a loss of balance (Horak and Nashner 1986). Interestingly, accelerating the COM during gait involves a projection of the COG away from the BOS, which is why walking and running are sometimes referred to as controlled falling.

Movement of the COG (and thus, the COP) within the BOS is termed *sway*. Two measures have been used to quantify sway (see figure 12.1). The first is the angle that intersects a line that runs vertically through the center of the BOS and a line that runs from the COG to the center of the BOS (Nashner 1997b). The second is the excursion of the COP from its central location (Lafond et al. 2004), usually measured with a force plate. Although both are essentially measuring the same thing, excursion of the COP is more precise because of the difficulties in pinpointing the location of the COG in a multisegmented, moving body.

Steadiness

Steadiness refers to the amount of sway that occurs while maintaining a static posture. Several measures have been used to quantify steadiness, including the root mean square error (RMS) of the COP, COP range, mean COP position, mean median power frequency (MPF), sway area, mean COP velocity, and COP path length (Lafond et al. 2004). In general, the more people move, the farther they move; or, the faster they move their COP while maintaining a static posture, the less steady they are (see figure 12.1).

In a slow-moving situation, if the COG moves beyond the BOS, the COP cannot create a counter-moment, and the person must take a step (i.e., loses balance). If the COG remains within the confines of the BOS, muscular activity can move the COP and return the COG to the more central location. However, this requires a certain amount of strength and a sufficient

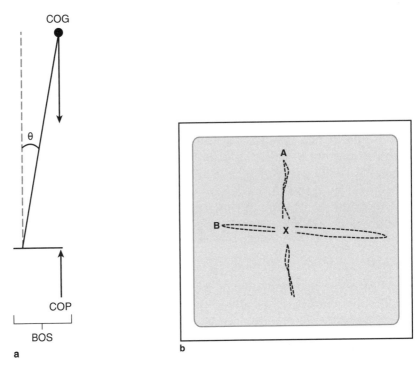

FIGURE 12.1 The center of pressure and balance. The relation between the center of gravity (COG), center of pressure (COP), base of support (BOS), and angle of sway (θ) is depicted on the left side. Note that the COP cannot be outside the BOS. If the COP is not directly under the COG, a moment will exist about the ankle, and the body will sway. The right side shows the BOS (white area), the limit of sway (gray area), the location of the COP (marked with an X), and the anterior–posterior (A) and medial–lateral (B) COP excursions. Note that the limit of sway cannot exceed the BOS, and the COP excursions will not exceed the limit of sway.

reaction time. The farthest a person can move the COG and COP while keeping the feet stationary is the limit of sway, and is also used to quantify balance (see figure 12.1).

In a static position, the limit of sway will always be within the confines of the BOS (Nashner 1997b). This is not necessarily the case with a moving body. If the center of mass is moving fast enough, momentum may require the person to take a step even if the COG is centered over the BOS, or momentum may return the COG to a central position even if it is outside of the BOS (Pai et al. 2000).

Stability

The terms *steadiness,* the ability to maintain a particular static posture (Mackey and Robinovitch 2005), and *balance,* the ability to maintain the COG over the base of support, are often used interchangeably with the term *stability.* But this is not always correct. Stability is the ability to maintain a desired position (static stability) or movement (dynamic stability) despite kinematic (motion), kinetic (force), or control disturbances (Reeves, Narendra, and Cholewicki 2007). Steadiness is how well one can "stand still," whereas stability is how well one can return to a position or movement following a perturbation. This is a subtle but important distinction. Balance can be used in both instances: the ability to maintain the COG over the BOS either in the absence (steadiness) or presence (static stability) of a perturbation. Because these qualities are fundamentally different, specifying which ability is being tested is important.

Implicit in the definition of *balance* is that the feet remain stationary. As mentioned earlier, walking and running involve projecting the center of mass away from the BOS. If the feet are moving, the center of mass is following a certain trajectory, and the ability to maintain that trajectory should be referred to as dynamic stability. It is a bit of a misnomer to use the term *dynamic balance,* because keeping the COG over the BOS may actually impair the ability to perform the task.

Control Theory

Controlling the COG, GRF, and COP is necessary for the completion of any task. Even the simple act of standing still involves the interaction of several complex systems (muscular, skeletal, and nervous) with the environment. Reeves, Narendra, and Cholewicki (2007) suggested that understanding such interactions would be greatly improved through the application of control theory from a systems engineering perspective, a schematic of which is presented in figure 12.2.

To begin with, the system needs some reference, which is the desired output. If the goal of the task is static equilibrium (i.e., standing still), then the desired posture is the reference. If the goal of the task involves movement, then the trajectory of the end effector (the hand, foot, or body's center of mass) is the reference. The controller (i.e., the central nervous system) provides inputs (i.e., muscle activations) to the plant (i.e., the musculoskeletal

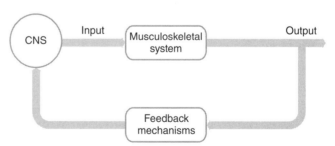

FIGURE 12.2 Control theory schematic. The central nervous system sends inputs to the musculoskeletal system, producing a desired output (position or trajectory). Feedback, via intrinsic properties of the musculoskeletal system and proprioceptors, is used to compare the output to the reference. Further inputs to the musculoskeletal system by the CNS are based on this feedback.

system), which produces a certain output. The output is measured against the reference by the controller via feedback (the intrinsic properties of the musculoskeletal system and proprioception). Proprioception, or sensory feedback, is provided by the integration of vision, vestibular, muscle, and tendon receptors (spindles and Golgi tendon organs); joint mechanorecep- tors; and cutaneous receptors. The nervous system uses this feedback to produce a new set of inputs for the musculoskeletal system.

If the system can maintain a reference position or trajectory, or return to a reference position or trajectory following a perturbation, the system is said to be stable. From this definition of stability, it should be evident that stability is a binary quality: a system is either stable or it is not. There are no varying degrees of stability (Reeves, Narendra, and Cholewicki 2007). If a system is unstable, it will be rather obvious. What's probably of more interest is the system's performance and robustness. Performance refers to how quickly the system can return to the desired position or trajectory fol- lowing a perturbation, while robustness refers to how large a perturbation the system can withstand.

Figure 12.2 shows three potential sources of "failure" in the system; places that can lead to poor performance or a lack of robustness. First, the central nervous system (CNS) could provide faulty input to the musculo- skeletal system. Second, the inputs required for the task could be outside the capability of the musculoskeletal system to achieve the task. In other words, the body may not have the requisite mobility, strength, power, or endurance to be successful. Third, faulty proprioception, altered intrinsic properties, or both, of the musculoskeletal system could provide either incorrect or delayed information to the CNS. Pinpointing which of these areas is responsible for failure is difficult.

Tests of mobility, strength, power, and endurance are described in detail in other chapters of this book and should be included in any assessment. Because deficiencies in these areas impede balance and stability, they should be identified and corrected. Proprioception tests require specialized training and equipment, and are limited to reposition tests and movement detection tests. Reposition tests require the subject to return to a reference position without the aid of vision, whereas movement detection tests determine how quickly the subject can detect passive changes in position.

Proprioceptive deficits are known to occur with injury and can be improved during the rehabilitation process, but there is no evidence to sup- port the ability to improve proprioception in healthy, asymptomatic people (Ashton-Miller et al. 2001). Under most circumstances, fitness professionals would not be involved with, or have the need for, proprioceptive testing. By process of elimination, any decrements in performance not attributable to the plant (musculoskeletal system) or feedback (proprioception) would be assumed to be the fault of the controller (central nervous system; CNS).

Balance training can improve the performance of the musculoskeletal system, proprioception, and the CNS, albeit to different degrees. Improvements to the plant would occur only in the most deconditioned people. For example, balance training would provide eccentric loading to the musculature, but at relatively low levels. It would lead to improvements in strength only if it were above the threshold stimulus for overload. Proprioception is unlikely to be a factor in healthy, asymptomatic people but could be a factor in a person rehabilitating from an injury. Balance improvements in athletes are therefore most likely a result of changes within the CNS.

Tests of balance are sometimes called proprioception tests. As noted in the preceding discussion, this is incorrect: proprioception is just the feedback. Balance tests involve feedback, input, and output; they are more correctly referred to as tests of neuromuscular control because all three areas are being tested and cannot be isolated with these tests.

This discussion contains another layer of complexity. Because the human body is multisegmented, every joint affects the location of the COG. Moreover, movement of any joint affects every other joint in the chain (Zajac and Gordon 1989). Yet certain joints appear to play a more critical role in postural control than others do. In the sagittal plane, small perturbations in the anterior–posterior direction are usually corrected by the ankle, whereas larger perturbations are usually corrected by the hip (Horak and Nashner 1986). Even larger corrections may require the use of the arms (Hof 2007) or a step (Horak and Nashner 1986). In the frontal plane, the location of the COG is controlled by the invertors and evertors of the subtalar joint, abductors and adductors of the hip, and lateral flexors of the trunk (MacKinnon and Winter 1993). This means that the CNS must provide outputs to, as well as integrate feedback from, several joints simultaneously.

Just as balance tests do not measure one isolated system (input, output, feedback), they cannot be used to measure one isolated joint. If an athlete has poor balance, isolated testing of each joint in the chain may be necessary for determining the exact location of the deficit and providing the appropriate corrective exercises.

With this background information in mind, it is possible to describe a number of tests and classify them according to the qualities they measure.

Balance and Stability Tests

Balance and stability are binary qualities: people either have balance (or stability) in a particular situation or they do not. Either they maintain their COG over their BOS, or they do not; there is no balance index. People are either stable or they are not; they either return to the desired position or movement, or they do not. There is no stability index (Reeves, Narendra, and Cholewicki 2007). Rather, when performing balance-like tests, we are measuring either the robustness or performance of the system (person). Robustness reflects the tolerance to change in parameters (Reeves, Narendra, and Cholewicki 2007). Tests measuring the length of an excursion or the steadiness under various conditions are thus measuring robustness. Tests that measure how quickly and accurately the person can return to a reference following a perturbation are measuring the performance. So, what is called a balance test could be measuring one of the following six quantities:

- Steadiness
- Limit of sway
- Performance during a static test
- Robustness during a static test
- Performance during a dynamic test
- Robustness during a dynamic test

Unfortunately, what makes deciphering the literature so challenging is that each measure is often referred to as balance. Because of the variety of ways people use the terms *balance* and *stability*, it is important to understand what the authors are implying. The following sections classify tests based on outcome measures. Where possible, reliability measures are included. Because no gold standard exists, validity data are lacking. The utility of the tests lies in their ability to allow the examiner to discriminate performance or injury potential.

Postural Steadiness Tests

In a postural steadiness test, the subject assumes a particular position and the examiner measures the amount of sway, either subjectively (visually) or objectively (with the aid of sophisticated equipment). Postural steadiness tests can be performed under a variety of base of support (two feet parallel, two feet tandem, one foot), surface (firm, soft), or proprioceptive (eyes open, closed, impaired) conditions, which would measure the robustness of the system. Following are some common postural steadiness tests:

- *Romberg test.* This test has many variations and is commonly used in field sobriety tests. In one version of the test, the subject is asked to close her eyes, tilt her head back, abduct both arms to 90°, and lift one foot off the ground (Starkey and Ryan 2002). Steadiness is subjectively evaluated by the examiner. There are no known published data concerning the validity, reliability, or normative values of this test.

- *Balance error scoring system (BESS).* During this test, the subject has three foot positions (double leg parallel, double leg tandem, single leg) and two surface conditions (firm, soft). Throughout the test, the hands remain on the hips and the eyes are closed. Each position is held for 20 seconds. Points are added each time the subject moves out of position. As in golf, a lower score is better. The test has high reliability (ICCs = .78 to .96) (Riemann, Guskiewicz, and Shields 1999).

- *Unstable platform tests.* Various types of tests have been developed in which the subject stands on an unstable platform, such as a balance board or wobble board; the ability to balance the platform at a central position is quantified by either the amount of time the edges of the platform are in contact with the ground (Behm et al. 2005) or the number of times the edges contact the ground. The reliability of such tests has been reported to be high ($r = .80$ to $.89$; Behm et al. 2005).

- *Computerized tests.* Steadiness can be measured using a force platform integrated with a personal computer. These systems can range from a force platform embedded into the floor, to a system constructed specifically to evaluate steadiness, to a system probably best described as a computerized balance board. The NeuroCom Balance Master System includes a fixed platform interfaced with a computer. Various measures of steadiness can be readily determined using such a system (Blackburn et al. 2000). An example of the computerized balance board is the Biodex Stability System. The amount of movement allowed by the board can be increased, making balancing more difficult. A computer algorithm then determines the standard deviations around the horizontal (level) position (Arnold and Schmitz 1998). The reliability of these measures is low to moderate ($r = .42$ to $.82$) (Schmitz and Arnold 1998).

Reach Tests

Reach tests examine the distance a subject can extend the COG over the BOS for the purpose of quantifying the boundaries of the limit of sway. These tests measure the robustness of the system. Following are common reach tests:

- *Functional reach test.* As the name implies, a functional reach test measures how far the subject can reach forward with an arm while maintaining a BOS in the standing position (Duncan et al. 1990). The subject raises an arm up to a leveled yardstick, which is fixed to a wall at the height of the acromion process. The subject makes a fist, and the location on the yardstick of the third metacarpal is noted. The subject then leans forward as far as possible without taking a step, and the position of the third metacarpal on the yardstick is again noted. The functional reach is the distance between the two positions. Although the reliability of this test is excellent (ICC = .92; Duncan et al. 1990), its utility with a young, healthy population appears limited.

- *Star excursion balance test (SEBT).* The SEBT is analogous to the functional reach test, but the reaching is done with one leg while maintaining single-limb support with the other. Additionally, instead of reaching only in the forward direction, the subject reaches in eight directions: anterior, posterior, medial, lateral, anterolateral, anteromedial, posterolateral, and posteromedial (Hertel, Miller, and Denegar 2000). This test has excellent intra- and intertester reliability (ICCs = .67 to .96 and .81 to .93, respectively), provided both examiners and subjects have had adequate practice (Hertel, Miller, and Denegar 2000; Kinzey and Armstrong 1998). Similar to postural stability tests, tests measuring the response to perturbations of various magnitudes or directions measure robustness, whereas those measuring the time to return to the reference movement measure performance. The extensive equipment and training required to conduct these tests limit their applicability in a field setting.

Postural Stability Tests

With a postural stability test, a subject assumes a position, a perturbation is applied, and the response to that perturbation is measured. The perturbation may be self-motivated (as in landing from a jump), be provided by a mechanical force external to the body (Duncan et al. 1990), or involve altered sensory feedback (Nashner 1997a). Tests measuring the response to perturbations of various magnitudes and from various directions measure robustness, whereas those measuring the time to return to the reference posture measure performance.

- *Landing tests.* In landing tests, subjects either jump up and land or fall from a predetermined height. With the modified Bass test, subjects jump from mark to mark over a predetermined zigzag course (Johnson and Nelson 1986). At each mark, the subject must stick the landing and hold it for five seconds. As in the BESS, points are added for errors during the landing (failing to stop, touching the floor with anything other than the ball of the support foot, and failing to completely cover the mark) or failure to maintain the five-second hold (touching the floor with anything other than the ball of the support foot or moving the supporting foot). When adjusting the distances between marks for subject height and performing the test using only a single leg, the reliability is moderate (ICC = .70 to .74; Riemann, Caggiano, and Lephart 1999) to high (ICC = .87; Eechaute, Vaes, and Duquet 2009). Various protocols have been used to evaluate the postural stability of a person landing on a force platform. These include various heights, distances, and directions. The overall amount of sway (as measured by a COP excursion), the amount of time requiring the GRF to return to body weight, or both, have been measured (Ross and Guskiewicz 2003).

- *Mechanical perturbation tests.* Mechanical perturbation tests usually come in two forms: Either the subject is tethered and a release is conducted (Mackey and Robinovitch 2005), or the platform moves and tilts under the subject's feet (Pai et al. 2000; Broglio et al. 2009). The latter are also referred to as motor control tests (Nashner 1997a). The size of the response in relation to the perturbation and the time to return to the reference position has been measured. The extensive equipment and training required for these tests limit their applicability in a field setting.

- *Sensory perturbation tests.* Sensory perturbations can be as simple as removing visual input by having subjects close their eyes or by altering proprioceptive feedback. One such test commonly found in the literature is referred to as a sensory organization test. It involves tilting either the support surface or the visual surroundings of the subject, or both (Nashner 1997a). The extensive equipment and training required for these tests limit their applicability in a field setting.

Dynamic Stability Test

With a dynamic stability test, a subject performs a particular movement, usually walking. A mechanical perturbation is applied, and the response to that perturbation is measured (Mackey and Robinovitch 2005; Shimada et al. 2003). Similar to postural stability tests, tests measuring the response to perturbations of various magnitudes or directions measure robustness, whereas those measuring the time to return to the reference movement measure performance. The extensive equipment and training required for these tests limit their applicability in a field setting.

Composite Tests

Composite tests involve the examination of multiple abilities simultaneously, of which balance or stability is a major component. Single-leg hop tests for distance, in their various forms, are examples of composite tests. Computerized dynamic posturography is not a composite test per se, but combines a motor control test and a sensory organization test. By examining the information provided by each test, examiners can ascertain the contributions of the biomechanical, sensory, and motor coordination components of balance (Nashner 1997a).

Correlations among balance and stability tests are poor; investigators report either low or nonsignificant correlations among steadiness, static stability, dynamic stability, and composite test scores (Blackburn et al. 2000; Broglio et al. 2009; Hamilton et al. 2008; Mackey and Robinovitch 2005; Shimada et al. 2003). This suggests that each test measures a different quality and that, therefore, multiple balance tests may need to be administered.

Sport Performance and Balance and Stability

Because of the multifactorial nature of balance, establishing a clear link to either performance or injury potential is difficult (table 12.1). Low balance measures could be a result of faulty central processing, deficits of the musculoskeletal system, improper or delayed proprioceptive feedback, or an interaction of the three. Additionally, different tests, measurements, and study designs can make ascertaining the link between balance and performance confusing.

TABLE 12.1 Comparisons of Balance and Stability Evaluations

Test type	Examples	Reliability	Equipment	Major advantages	Major disadvantages
Steadiness	Romberg test	Unknown	None	Easy to perform	Not discriminating for an athletic population
	Balance error scoring system test	High	Airex pad	Easy to perform	Applicability to athletic activities
	Unstable platform tests	Unknown	Platform	Greater perturbations	No standardized tests or norms
	Computerized tests	High	Force plate; computer	Accurate reading of disturbance and response	Costs, equipment, and time
Reach	Functional reach test	High	Yardstick	Easy to perform	Not discriminating for an athletic population
	Star excursion balance test	High	Athletic tape to mark directions	Test performance linked to injury	Test performance not linked to athletic performance
Postural stability	Modified Bass test	Moderate	Athletic tape to mark course	Test performance linked to injury	Test performance not linked to athletic performance
	Mechanical perturbation test	High	Force plate; movable platform	Accurate reading of disturbance and response	Costs, equipment, and time
	Sensory perturbation tests	High	Sensory alteration equipment	Accurate reading of disturbance and response	Costs, equipment, and time

Considering the following questions can help to clarify the effects of steadiness, balance, and stability on performance and injury potential:

- What is the relation between balance performance or robustness, and athletic performance or injury?
- Does balance training lead to improved athletic performance and decreased injuries?

Very few studies have examined the relation between balance performance or robustness, and athletic performance. Using a wobble board test, Behm and colleagues (2005) found a positive correlation between skating speed and steadiness in hockey players under the age of 19 ($r^2 = .42$), but not for those over the age of 19 ($r^2 = .08$). No significant correlation occurred between postural steadiness and pitching accuracy, but a small, positive correlation did occur between sway in unilateral stance with eyes closed and pitching velocity ($r^2 = .27$) (Marsh et al. 2004). Finally, single-leg steadiness was not related to unilateral strength production during a single-leg squat (McCurdy and Langford 2006).

A few more studies examined the effect of balance training on athletic performance. One reported improved measures of steadiness and limits of sway following four weeks of balance training (Yaggie and Campbell 2006). Although these changes transferred to improvements in shuttle run ability, they did not lead to improvements in the vertical jump (Yaggie and Campbell 2006). Similarly, 10 weeks of balance training improved performance on the T-test, as well as 10- and 40-yard sprint times, but it did not improve vertical jump performance (Cressey et al. 2007). Moreover, these improvements were less than what was attained with traditional strength training (Cressey et al. 2007).

With the dearth of information concerning balance performance or robustness, and athletic performance, it is difficult to draw any definitive conclusions. It would seem logical to conclude that balance is task specific, and that activities with greater balance demands require greater balance ability. Yet neither postural steadiness (as measured by the balance error scoring system, or BESS) nor limits of postural sway (as measured by the star excursion balance test, or SEBT) were different between soccer players and gymnasts (Bressel et al. 2007), calling this assumption into question.

Balance requires adequate proprioception, CNS processing, and eccentric strength. The strength levels required to maintain balance are probably low. Proprioceptive ability does not appear to be related to performance (Drouin et al. 2003), and studies have not demonstrated that it can even be improved in healthy adults (Ashton-Miller et al. 2001). The process of elimination would seem to lead to the conclusion that if balance affects performance in healthy adults, it would most probably do so at the level of the CNS. But this hypothesis requires further investigation.

In contrast to performance, more research has been conducted examining the effect of balance performance or robustness on injury, although most of these studies have focused on the lower extremities. Do those whose balance performance is low or less robust have higher injury rates? Do those with injuries have lower balance performance, are they less robust, or both? What is the effect of balance training on injury rates?

Prospective studies in which balance measurements are made in the preseason and related to injuries throughout the season are the gold standard of evidence. In a prospective study of 235 U.S. female high school basketball players, Plisky and colleagues (2006) found that girls with a composite reach distance less than 94.0% of their limb length on the SEBT were 6.5 times more likely to have a lower extremity injury. Similarly, steadiness measures predicted ankle injury in Australian-rules football players (Hrysomallis, McLaughlin, and Goodman 2007), although these same measures did not predict knee injury. Even labral tears in the shoulder have been associated with poor preseason steadiness measures of the nondominant leg of pitchers (Burkhart, Morgan, and Kibler 2000), but these findings are equivocal (Evans, Hertel, and Sebastianelli 2004).

Additionally, several studies have shown that those who have had a knee (Herrington et al. 2009) or ankle (Docherty et al. 2006; Evans, Hertel, and Sebastianelli 2004; Hertel and Olmsted-Kramer 2007; Olmsted et al. 2002; Ross et al. 2009; Ross and Guskiewicz 2004) injury had poorer balance performance and robustness than healthy controls, and measures of performance may be more discriminatory than measures of robustness (Ross et al. 2009). While it is hard to determine if poor balance measures are a cause or consequence of injury, balance performance and robustness are clearly impaired following lower extremity injury. Additionally, these measures are improved with rehabilitation (Lee and Lin 2008; McKeon et al. 2008). These results are not unexpected, considering that, unlike healthy controls, people with an injury have decreased strength, decreased proprioception, and altered central programming.

Numerous studies have examined the effect of balance training on injury rates. In a recent systemic review of randomized controlled trials, Aaltonen and colleagues (2007) reported that the evidence of ability of balance training by itself to prevent injuries was equivocal. This is not surprising given the numerous protocols and balance measures used in the investigations. However, when balance training was just one component of an intervention program, strong evidence suggested that injuries were reduced. Taken together, the results suggest that balance should be one component of a comprehensive testing program.

Measuring Balance and Stability

Fitness professionals should first establish the purpose of the test, pick a category that would fulfill that purpose, and then select a test based on the level of precision required and the resources available. Three tests, the balance error scoring system (BESS), the star excursion balance test (SEBT), and the modified Bass test, were selected for detailed discussion here because they represent different categories (postural steadiness, reach, and postural stability) and require minimal specialized equipment. Additionally, the BESS and SEBT have excellent reliability and a large body of literature supporting them. Interested readers should consult the original literature cited in the reference section for detailed procedures on conducting the other tests. Table 12.1 compares balance and stability evaluations.

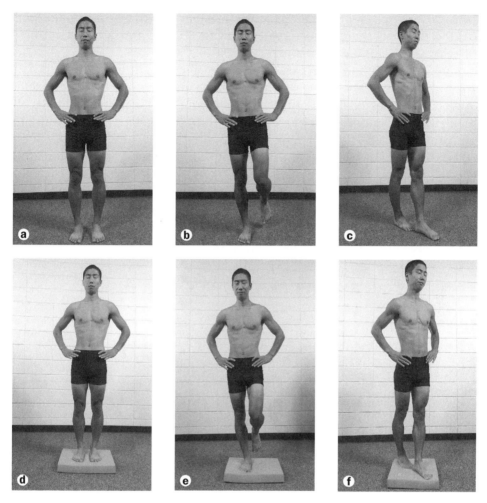

FIGURE 12.3   Balance error scoring system (BESS). Top row, firm surface condition. Bottom row, soft surface condition. Left column, parallel stance. Middle column, single-leg stance. Right column, tandem stance.

BALANCE ERROR SCORING SYSTEM (BESS)

EQUIPMENT

A foam balance pad. The foam pad is one piece of medium-density foam (45 cm² × 13 cm thick, density 60 kg/m³, load deflection 80-90).

PROCEDURE

The six positions of the balance error scoring system test are depicted in figure 12.3. Three stances (double-leg support, single-leg support, and tandem) are held for 20 seconds on two surfaces (firm floor and foam pad) for six permutations (Riemann, Guskiewicz, and Shields 1999). During the tandem stance, the dominant foot is in front of the nondominant foot.

During the single-leg stance, the subject stands on the nondominant foot. During the test, the eyes are closed and the hands are held on the hips (iliac crests).

Subjects are told to keep as steady as possible, and if they lose their balance, they are to try to regain the initial position as quickly as possible. Subjects are assessed one point for the following errors: lifting the hands off the iliac crests; opening the eyes; stepping, stumbling, or falling; remaining out of the test position for five seconds; moving the hip into more than 30° of hip flexion or abduction; or lifting the forefoot or heel (Riemann, Guskiewicz, and Shields 1999). A trial is considered incomplete if the subject cannot hold the position without error for at least five seconds. The maximal number of errors per condition is 10. An incomplete condition is given the maximal number of points (10). The numbers of errors for all six conditions are summed into a single score.

STAR EXCURSION BALANCE TEST (SEBT)

EQUIPMENT

Athletic or masking tape

PROCEDURE

The SEBT requires the floor to be marked with a star pattern in eight directions, 45° apart from each other: anterior, posterior, medial, lateral, posterolateral, posteromedial, anterolateral, and anteromedial (see figure 12.4). One foot is placed in the middle of the star pattern. The subject is instructed to reach as far as possible, sequentially (either clockwise or counter clockwise), in all eight directions.

The directions are not labeled consistently in the

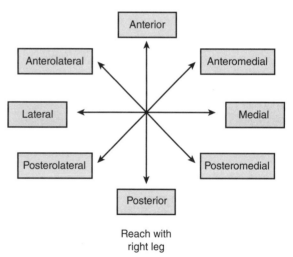

FIGURE 12.4 Directions of the star excursion balance test (SEBT) for the left support leg and right reaching leg. Note that the directions would be mirror images for the right support leg and left reaching leg.

Reprinted, by permission, from M.P. Reiman, 2009, *Functional testing in performance* (Champaign, IL: Human Kinetics), 109.

literature. For example, when balancing on the left leg and reaching to the right with the right leg, some authors call this direction medial (Gribble and Hertel 2003; Hertel et al. 2006), whereas others call it lateral (Bressel et al. 2007). This text adopts the convention that, when standing on the left leg, reaching to the right of the left leg is in the medial direction, whereas reaching to the left (and behind the stance leg) is in the lateral direction (see figure 12.4).

The subject makes a light tap on the floor, and then returns the leg to the center of the star. The distance from the center of the star to the tap is measured. The trial is nullified and has to be repeated if the subject commits any of the following errors: makes a heavy touch, rests the foot on the ground, loses balance, or cannot return to the starting position under control (Gribble 2003). The starting direction and support leg are chosen randomly. Three trials are performed and then averaged.

Because of the significant correlation between SEBT and leg length ($.02 \leq r^2 \leq .23$) in a majority of the directions, excursion values should be normalized to leg length, measured from the ASIS to the medial malleolus (Gribble and Hertel 2003). Additionally, Hertel and colleagues (2006) suggested that testing in eight directions is redundant, and that testing only the posteromedial direction is sufficient for most situations. To decrease the effect of learning, Kinzey and Armstrong (1998) suggested that subjects be given at least six practice trials before being tested, although other authors suggested reducing the number of practice trials to four (Robinson and Gribble 2008).

MODIFIED BASS TEST

EQUIPMENT

Athletic or masking tape

PROCEDURE

This multiple hop test requires that 1-inch (2.5 cm) tape squares be laid out in a course as shown in figure 12.5 (Riemann, Caggiano, and Lephart 1999). The subject is required to jump from square to square, in numbered sequence, using only one leg. The hands should remain on the hips. On landing, the subject remains looking facing straight ahead, without moving the support leg, for five seconds before jumping to the next square.

There are two types of errors: landing errors and balance errors. A landing error occurs if the subject's foot does not cover the tape, if the foot is not facing forward, if the subject stumbles on landing, or if the subject takes the hands off the hips. A balance error occurs if the subject takes the hands off the hips or if the nontesting leg touches down, touches the

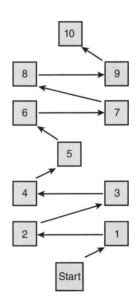

FIGURE 12.5 Course for a modified Bass test.

Reprinted, by permission, from M.P. Reiman, 2009, *Functional testing in performance* (Champaign, IL: Human Kinetics), 115.

opposite leg, or moves into excessive flexion, extension, or abduction. The subjects may look at the next square before jumping to it.

The examiner should count aloud the five seconds the subject is to maintain the position before moving to the next square. At the conclusion of the test, 10 points are given for each five-second period in which there was a landing error and 3 points for each period in which there was a balance error. The sum of the two is the total score. At least two practice sessions should be given before testing for score.

Interpreting the Results

When interpreting the results of balance or stability tests, values can be compared to normative data, the other leg (if performed on a single leg), or the same person over time. Normative data are presented for the BESS, SEBT, and modified Bass in tables 12.2 through 12.4, respectively. Currently, no data exist to suggest either a cutoff score for these tests or, in the case of the SEBT or modified Bass test, a bilateral difference that would be a cause for concern. These are areas for future investigations. Balance scores tend to be better in the morning than in the afternoon or evening (Gribble, Tucker, and White 2007), suggesting that if multiple tests are to be compared over time, the time of day needs to be standardized.

TABLE 12.2   Normative Data for the Balance Error Scoring System Test

Age	n	M	Median	SD	PERCENTILE RANK RANGES FROM THE NATURAL DISTRIBUTION OF SCORES					
					>90th	76–90th	25–75th	10–24th	2–9th	<2nd
20–39	104	10.97	10	5.05	0–3	4–6	7–14	15–17	18–22	23+
40–49	172	11.88	11	5.40	0–5	6–7	8–15	16–19	20–25	26+
50–54	96	12.73	11	6.07	0–6	7–8	9–15	16–20	21–31	32+
55–59	89	14.85	13	7.32	0–7	8–9	10–17	18–24	25–33	34+
60–64	80	17.20	16	7.83	0–7	8–11	12–21	22–28	29–35	36+
65–69	48	20.38	18	7.78	0–11	12–14	15–23	24–31	32–39	40+

Note: The BESS scores are not normally distributed. Therefore, the percentile ranks corresponding to the natural distribution of scores are presented. For example, for 20- to 39-year-olds, a score of 2 falls in the top 10% and a score of 19 falls in the bottom 10% of the 104 subjects.

Reprinted, by permission, from G.L. Iverson, M.L. Kaarto, and M.S. Koehle, 2008, "Normative data for the balance error scoring system: Implications for brain injury evaluation," *Brain Injury* 22:147-152.

TABLE 12.3 Normative Data for the Star Excursion Balance Test

STUDY	LANNING		GRIBBLE	
Population	Collegiate athletes		Recreationally trained	
Gender	Male	Female	Male	Female
Anterior			79.2 ± 7.0	76.9 ± 6.2
Posterior			93.9 ± 10.5	85.3 ± 12.9
Medial			97.7 ± 9.5	90.7 ± 10.7
Lateral			80.0 ± 17.5	79.8 ± 13.7
Anterolateral			73.8 ± 7.7	74.7 ± 7.0
Anteromedial	103 ± 3	102 ± 6	85.2 ± 7.5	83.1 ± 7.3
Posterolateral			90.4 ± 13.5	85.5 ± 13.2
Posteromedial	112 ± 4	111 ± 5	95.6 ± 8.3	89.1 ± 11.5

Data from Lanning et al. 2006 and Gribble and Hertel 2003, expressed as a percentage of leg length.

TABLE 12.4 Normative Data for the Modified Bass Test

Error	Mean (± standard deviation)
Balance error	7.3 (5.9)
Landing error	43.7 (23.3)

Data from Riemann et al. 1999.

Like many other abilities, balance is necessary for purposeful movement. An inability to remain balanced can disrupt force production and limit performance. Undoubtedly, different sports require different balance and stability profiles. Sports that require movements on one leg (such as gymnastics and soccer) would require better performance and robustness than sports that are predominately performed on both legs (such as basketball) (Hrysomallis 2011), because of the smaller base of support. In contrast to balance, stability is the ability to return to a desired position or trajectory following a disturbance. Sports performed on unstable surfaces (such as skiing or surfing) or that involve contact with an opponent (American football, wrestling) would have greater performance and robustness requirements than sports performed on a firm surface with no such contact.

There is a stronger (and arguably more important) link between various measures of balance or stability and injury than the link between balance or stability and performance. Sporting activities require that energy be generated, absorbed, and transferred between the segments in the kinetic chain. This requires proper alignment of the joints (Zajac, Neptune, and Kautz 2002). It stands to reason that if the athlete cannot maintain, or return to, the proper position, energy will

Professional Applications

(continued)

(continued)

be absorbed by tissues that may not be equipped to handle it. It is then easy to see how injuries, such as lateral ankle sprains, develop. The old adage "an ounce of prevention is worth a pound of cure" is very apropos when it comes to balance and stability.

All athletes should be screened for balance and stability. Because each test category evaluates a unique ability, a test from each category should be used when possible. Rather than attempting to maximize balance and stability traits in those of average abilities, fitness professionals should direct their efforts toward those who are considered poor performers and assign remedial work based on their deficiencies.

The BESS is a test of postural steadiness. People with poor postural steadiness, particularly those whose sports require time supported on a single leg, should engage in exercises that require them to support themselves on a single limb or unstable surface, such as a balance board or Dyna Disc. These exercises can be incorporated as part of the warm-up. Low levels of instability are probably sufficient for training; athletes need not be trained like circus performers.

The SEBT is a test of postural sway, or robustness. A more robust system can withstand a larger perturbation. Athletes deficient in this area can tolerate only minor perturbations. Attention should be paid not only to low performers, but also to those with large bilateral differences in performance. Drills that perturb athletes while they are maintaining a position on one leg can result in improvements. Tap drills, in which athletes are pushed in various directions, are one category. Another is to have the athlete catch a medicine ball while standing on one leg. Increasing the weight of the ball or the distance from the center of the body will increase the size of the perturbation and theoretically improve robustness.

The modified Bass test is a test of postural stability. This requires the athlete to land on one foot from various directions. Athletes who perform poorly on these types of tests should be regressed in their plyometric training and work on "sticking" the landing after the eccentric phase before progressing back to rapidly transitioning from the eccentric to concentric phase. Before progressing to the rapid reversal from the eccentric phase to the concentric phase of the exercise, athletes should be able to stick the landing (stop in a stable position after the eccentric phase). Poor performers on the modified Bass test will not be able to do so, at least on one foot when landing from multiple directions. Enforcing this requirement, and requiring athletes to perform plyometrics on one leg and in multiple directions, should help correct this deficiency.

The essence of balance and stability training is exposing athletes to a variety of tasks with different objectives and perturbations. Many athletes will already possess the necessary abilities to minimize injury risk and succeed in their sports. As with many other abilities, more is not better; if a recipe calls for two cups of sugar, adding four cups will not make a better cake. But adding only one cup will surely affect the cake. Athletes need a minimal amount of balance and stability, and adequate testing and training will ensure that they do. Anything less in an overall program is a recipe for disaster.

SUMMARY

- Balance is the ability to maintain the body's center of gravity over its base of support.
- Stability is the ability to return to a desired position or trajectory following a disturbance.
- Balance and stability are different motor qualities, and require different types of tests.
- The balance error scoring system (BESS), star excursion balance test (SEBT), and modified Bass test measure postural steadiness, limits of sway, and postural stability, respectively. All three should be included as part of a comprehensive testing program.
- Although more is not always better in terms of balance and stability training, poor performers on these tests should be given programs to improve their abilities.

References

Chapter 1

Cohen, J. 1988. *Statistical Power Analysis for the Behavioral Sciences,* 2nd ed. Hillsdale, NJ: L. Erlbaum Associates.

Jaric, S., D. Mirkov, and G. Markovic. 2005. Normalizing physical performance tests for body size: A proposal for standardization. *Journal of Strength and Conditioning Research* 19 (2): 467-474.

Morrow, J.R., A.W. Jackson, J.G. Disch, and D.P. Mood. 2000. *Measurement and Evaluation in Human Performance.* Champaign, IL: Human Kinetics.

National Strength and Conditioning Association. 2000. *Essentials of Strength Training and Conditioning,* 2nd ed. Edited by T.R. Baechle and R.W. Earle. Champaign, IL: Human Kinetics.

Nevill, A., R. Ramsbottom, and C. Williams. 1992. Scaling physiological measurements for individuals of different body size. *European Journal of Applied Physiology* 65: 110-117.

Peterson, M.D., B.A. Alvar, and M.R. Rhea. 2006. The contribution of maximal force production to explosive movement among young collegiate athletes. *Journal of Strength and Conditioning Research* 20: 867-873.

Rhea, M.R. 2004. Determining the magnitude of treatment effects in strength training research through the use of the effect size. *Journal of Strength and Conditioning Research* 18: 918-920.

Chapter 2

American College of Sports Medicine. 2007. *ACSM's Health-Related Physical Fitness Assessment Manual,* 2nd ed. Philadelphia: Lippincott Williams & Wilkins.

American College of Sports Medicine. 2008. *ACSM's Guidelines for Exercise Testing and Prescription,* 8th ed. Philadelphia: Lippincott Williams & Wilkins.

Ballard, T.P., L. Fafara, and M.D. Vukovich. Comparison of Bod Pod and DXA in female collegiate athletes. *Medicine & Science in Sports & Exercise* 36: 731-735.

Broeder, C.E., K.A. Burrhus, L.S. Svanevik, J. Volpe, and J.H. Wilmore. 1997. Assessing body composition before and after resistance or endurance training. *Medicine & Science in Sports & Exercise* 29: 705-712.

Brozek J., F. Grande, J. Anderson, et al. 1963. Densitometric analysis of body composition: Revision of some quantitative assumptions. *Annals of the New York Academy of Sciences* 110: 113-140.

Clasey, J.L., J.A. Kanaley, J. Wideman, et al. 1999. Validity of methods of body composition assessment in young and older men and women. *Journal of Applied Physiology* 86: 1728-1738.

Collins, M.A., M.L. Millard-Stafford, P.B. Sparling, et al. 1999. Evaluation of the BOD POD for assessing body fat in collegiate football players. *Medicine & Science in Sports & Exercise* 31: 1350-1356.

Despres, J.P., and I. Lemieux. 2006. Abdominal obesity and metabolic syndrome. *Nature* 444: 881-887.

Dixon, C.B., R.W. Deitrick, J.R. Pierce, P.T. Cutrufello, and L.L. Drapeau. 2005. Evaluation of the BOD POD and leg-to-leg bioelectrical impedance analysis for estimating percent body fat in National Collegiate Athletic Association Division III collegiate wrestlers. *Journal of Strength and Conditioning Research* 19: 85-91.

Durnin, J.V.G.A., and J. Womersley. 1974. Body fat assessed from total body density and its estimation from skinfold thickness: Measurements on 481 men and women aged from 16 to 72 years. *British Journal of Nutrition* 32: 77-97.

Fornetti, W.C., J.M. Pivarnik, J.M. Foley, and J.J. Fiechtner. 1999. Reliability and validity of body composition measures in female athletes. *Journal of Applied Physiology* 87: 1114-1122.

Graves, J.E., J.A. Kanaley, L. Garzarella, and M.L. Pollock. 2006. Anthropometry and body composition assessment. In *Physiological Assessment of Human Fitness*, 2nd ed. Edited by P.J. Maud and C. Foster, 185-225. Champaign, IL: Human Kinetics.

Harman E., and J. Garhammer. 2008. Administration, scoring, and interpretation of selected tests. In *Essentials of Strength Training and Conditioning*, 3rd ed. Edited by T.R. Baechle and R.W. Earle, 249-292. Champaign, IL: Human Kinetics.

Heyward, V.H., and L.M. Stolarczyk. 1996. *Applied Body Composition Assessment*. Champaign, IL: Human Kinetics.

Higgins, P.B., D.A. Fields, G.R. Hunter, and B.A. Gower. 2001. Effect of scalp and facial hair on air displacement plethysmography estimates of percentage of body fat. *Obesity Research* 9: 326-330.

Housh, T.J., G.O. Johnson, D.J. Housh, et al. 2004. Accuracy of near-infrared interactance instruments and population-specific equations for estimating body composition in young wrestlers. *Journal of Strength and Conditioning Research* 18: 556-560.

Housh, T.J., J.R. Stout, G.O. Johnson, D.J. Housh, and J.M. Eckerson. 1996. Validity of near-infrared interactance instruments for estimating percent body fat in youth wrestlers. *Pediatric Exercise Science* 8: 69-76.

Jackson, A.S., and M.L. Pollock. 1978. Generalized equations for predicting body density of men. *British Journal of Nutrition* 40: 497-504.

Jackson, A.S., and M.L. Pollock. 1985. Practical assessment of body composition. *Physician and Sportsmedicine* 13: 76-90.

Jackson, A.S., M.L. Pollock, and A. Ward. 1980. Generalized equations for predicting body density of women. *Medicine & Science in Sports & Exercise* 12: 175-181.

Kaiser, G.E., J.W. Womack, J.S. Green, B. Pollard, G.S. Miller, and S.F. Crouse. 2008. Morphological profiles for first-year National Collegiate Athletic Association Division I football players. *Journal of Strength and Conditioning Research* 22: 243-249.

Kohrt, W.M. 1998. Preliminary evidence that DEXA provides an accurate assessment of body composition. *Journal of Applied Physiology* 84: 372-377.

Kraemer, W.J., J.C. Torine, R. Silvestre, et al. 2005. Body size and composition of National Football League players. *Journal of Strength and Conditioning Research* 19: 485-489.

Liuke, M., S. Solovieva, A. Lamminen, K. Luoma, P. Leino-Arjas, R. Luukkonen, and H. Riihimaki. 2005. Disc degeneration of the lumbar spine in relation to overweight. *International Journal of Obesity* 29: 903-908.

Mathews, E.M., and D.R. Wagner. 2008. Prevalence of overweight and obesity in collegiate American football players, by position. *Journal of American College Health* 57: 33-38.

McArdle, W.D., F.I. Katch, and V.L. Katch. 2007. *Exercise Physiology: Energy, Nutrition, and Human Performance,* 6th ed. Philadelphia: Lippincott Williams & Wilkins, pp. 773-809, Appendix I.

Norcross, J., and Van Loan, M.D. 2004. Validation of fan beam dual energy x ray absorptiometry for body composition assessment in adults aged 18-45 years. *British Journal of Sports Medicine* 38: 472-476.

Pollock, M.L., D.H. Schmidt, and A.S. Jackson. 1980. Measurement of cardiorespiratory fitness and body composition in the clinical setting. *Comprehensive Therapy* 6: 12-27.

Siri, W.E. 1956. The gross composition of the body. *Advances in Biological and Medical Physiology* 4: 239-280.

Sloan, A.W., and J.B. Weir. 1970. Nomograms for prediction of body density and total body fat from skinfold measurements. *Journal of Applied Physiology* 28: 221-222.

Tataranni, P.A., D.J. Pettitt, and E. Ravussin. 1996. Dual energy X-ray absorptiometry: Inter-machine variability. *International Journal of Obesity and Related Metabolic Disorders* 20: 1048-1050.

Vescovi, J.D., L. Hildebrandt, W. Miller, R. Hammer, and A. Spiller. 2002. Evaluation of the BOD POD for estimating percent fat in female college athletes. *Journal of Strength and Conditioning Research* 16: 599-605.

Wearing, S.C., E.M. Hennig, N.M. Byrne, J.R. Steele, and A.P. Hills. 2006. Musculoskeletal disorders associated with obesity: A biomechanical perspective. *Obesity Review* 7: 239-250.

Chapter 3

Adams, G., and W. Beam. 2008. *Exercise physiology laboratory manual,* 5th ed. Boston: McGraw Hill.

Boudet, G., and A. Chaumoux. 2001. Ability of new heart rate monitors to measure normal and abnormal heart rate. *The Journal of Sports Medicine and Physical Fitness* 41 (4) (12): 546-553.

Canzanello, V.J., P.L. Jensen, and G.L. Schwartz. 2001. Are aneroid sphygmomanometers accurate in hospital and clinic settings? *Archives of Internal Medicine* 161 (5) (03/12): 729-731.

Chobanian, A.V., G.L. Bakris, H.R. Black, W.C. Cushman, L.A. Green, J.L Izzo Jr., D.W. Jones, B.J. Materson, S. Oparil, J.T. Wright Jr., E.J. Roccella, and the National High Blood Pressure Education Program Coordinating Committee. 2003. Seventh report of the Joint National Committee on Prevention, Detection, Evaluation, and Treatment of High Blood Pressure. *Journal of the American Heart Association* 42: 1206-1252.

Clement, D.L., M.L. De Buyzere, D.A. De Bacquer, P.W. de Leeuw, D.A. Duprez, R.H. Fagard, P.J. Gheeraert, et al. 2003. Prognostic value of ambulatory blood-pressure recordings in patients with treated hypertension. *The New England Journal of Medicine* 348 (24) (06/12): 2407-2415.

Ehrman, J., P. Gordon, P. Visich, and S. Keteyian. 2009. *Clinical Exercise Physiology,* 2nd ed. Champaign, IL: Human Kinetics.

Franklin, B.A., ed. 2000. *ACSM's Guidelines for Exercise Testing and Prescription.* Philadelphia: Lippincott Williams & Wilkins.

Goldberg, A., and E. Goldberg. 1994. *Clinical Electrocardiography: A Simplified Approach,* 5th ed. Baltimore: Mosby.

Guyton, A. 1991. *Textbook of Medical Physiology,* 8th ed. Philadelphia: W.B. Saunders.

Kapit, W., R. Macey, and E. Meisami. 1987. *The Physiology Coloring Book.* New York: Harper-Collins.

Karvonen, J., and T. Vuorimaa. 1988. Heart rate and exercise intensity during sports activities. Practical application. *Sports Medicine* (Auckland, NZ) 5 (5) (05): 303-311.

MacDougall, J.D., R.S. McKelvie, D.E. Moroz, D.G. Sale, N. McCartney, and F. Buick. 1992. Factors affecting blood pressure during heavy weight lifting and static contractions. *Journal of Applied Physiology* (Bethesda, MD: 1985) 73 (4) (10): 1590-1597.

MacDougall, J.D., D. Tuxen, D.G. Sale, J.R. Moroz, and J.R. Sutton. 1985. Arterial blood pressure response to heavy resistance exercise. *Journal of Applied Physiology* (Bethesda, MD: 1985) 58 (3) (03): 785-790.

Mancia, G., G. De Backer, A. Dominiczak, R. Cifkova, et al. 2007. 2007 guidelines for the management of arterial hypertension: The Task Force for the Management of Arterial Hypertension of the European Society of Hypertension (ESH) and of the European Society of Cardiology (ESC). *European Heart Journal* 28 (12): 1462-1536.

Marieb, E., and K. Hoehn. 2010. *Human Anatomy and Physiology,* 8th ed. New York: Benjamin Cummings.

O'Brien, E., G. Beevers, and G.Y. Lip. 2001. ABC of hypertension: Blood pressure measurement. Part IV-automated sphygmomanometry: Self blood pressure measurement. *British Medical Journal* (Clinical Research Ed.) 322 (7295) (05/12): 1167-1170.

Perloff, D., C. Grim, J. Flack, E.D. Frohlich, M. Hill, M. McDonald, and B.Z. Morgenstern. 1993. Human blood pressure determination by sphygmomanometry. *Circulation* 88 (5) (11): 2460-2470.

Pickering, T.G. 2002. Principles and techniques of blood pressure measurement. *Cardiology Clinics* 20 (2) (05): 207-223.

Pickering, T.G., J.E. Hall, L.J. Appel, B.E. Falkner, J. Graves, M.N. Hill, D.W. Jones, T. Kurtz, S.G. Sheps, and E.J. Roccella. 2005a. Recommendations for blood pressure measurement in humans and experimental animals: Part 1: Blood pressure measurement in humans: A statement for professionals from the subcommittee of professional and public education of the American Heart Association Council on High Blood Pressure Research. *Circulation* 111 (5) (02/08): 697-716.

Pickering, T.G., J.E. Hall, L.J. Appel, B.E. Falkner, J. Graves, M.N. Hill, D.W. Jones, T. Kurtz, S.G. Sheps, and E.J. Roccella. 2005b. Recommendations for blood pressure measurement in humans and experimental animals: Part 1: Blood pressure measurement in humans: A statement for professionals from the subcommittee of professional and public education of the American Heart Association Council on High Blood Pressure Research. *Hypertension* 45 (1) (01/20): 142-161.

Pickering, T.G., J.E. Hall, L.J. Appel, B.E. Falkner, J. Graves, M.N. Hill, D.W. Jones, T. Kurtz, S.G. Sheps, and E.J. Roccella. 2005c. Recommendations for blood pressure measurement in humans: An AHA scientific statement from the Council on High Blood Pressure Research Professional and Public Education Subcommittee. *Journal of Clinical Hypertension* (Greenwich, CT) 7 (2) (02): 102-109.

Powers, S., and E. Howley. 2007. *Exercise Physiology: Theory Application to Fitness and Performance,* 6th ed. Boston: McGraw-Hill.

Roberds, R., and S. Roberts. 1987. *Exercise Physiology: Exercise Performance and Clinical Applications.* New York: Mosby.

Sale, D.G., D.E. Moroz, R.S. McKelvie, J.D. MacDougall, and N. McCartney. 1994. Effect of training on the blood pressure response to weight lifting. *Canadian Journal of Applied Physiology (Revue Canadienne De Physiologie Appliquée)* 19 (1) (03): 60-74.

Sjøgaard, G., and B. Saltin. 1982. Extra- and intracellular water spaces in muscles of man at rest and with dynamic exercise. *American Journal of Physiology* 243 (3) (09): R271-R280.

Smith, J., and J. Kampine. 1984. *Circulatory Physiology: The Essentials,* 2nd ed. Philadelphia: Williams & Wilkins.

Tanaka, H., C.A. DeSouza, and D.R. Seals. 1998. Absence of age-related increase in central arterial stiffness in physically active women. *Arteriosclerosis, Thrombosis, and Vascular Biology* 18 (1) (01): 127-132.

Thompson, P.D., B.A. Franklin, G.J. Balady, S.N. Blair, D. Corrado, N. Estes, N.A. Mark III, J.E. Fulton, et al. 2007. Exercise and acute cardiovascular events placing the risks into perspective: A scientific statement from the American Heart Association Council on Nutrition, Physical Activity, and Metabolism and the Council on Clinical Cardiology. *Circulation* 115 (17) (05/01): 2358-2368.

Venes, D., ed. 2009. *Taber's Cyclopedic Medical Dictionary,* 21st ed. Philadelphia: F.A. Davis.

Whitworth, J.A., N. Kaplan, S. Mendis, and N. Poulter. 2003. World Health Organization (WHO)/International Society of Hypertension (ISH) statement on management of hypertension. *Journal of Hypertension* 21 (11): 1983-1992.

Wilmore, J., D. Costill, and L. Kenney. 2008. *Physiology of Sport and Exercise,* 4th ed. Champaign, IL: Human Kinetics.

Chapter 4

American College of Sports Medicine. 1997. Collection of questionnaires for health-related research. *Medicine & Science in Sports & Exercise* 29: S1-S208.

American College of Sports Medicine. 2010. *ACSM's Guidelines for Exercise Testing and Prescription,* 8th ed. Baltimore: Lippincott Williams & Wilkins.

Bray, G.A. 1983. The energetics of obesity. *Medicine & Science in Sports & Exercise* 15: 32-40.

Brown, S.P., W.C. Miller, and J. Eason. 2006. *Exercise Physiology: Basis of Human Movement in Health and Disease.* Baltimore: Lippincott Williams & Wilkins.

Byrne, H.K., and J.H. Wilmore. 2001. The relationship of mode and intensity of training on resting metabolic rate in women. *International Journal of Sport Nutrition and Exercise Metabolism* 11: 1-14.

Children's Physical Activity Research Group. 2011. Previous Day Physical Activity Recall (PDPAR). Accessed February 1. www.sph.sc.edu/USC_CPARG/tool_detail.asp?id=1.

Craig, C.L., A.L. Marshall, M. Sjostrom, A.E. Bauman, M.L. Booth, B. Ainsworth, M. Pratt, U. Ekelund, A. Yngve, J. Sallis, and P. Oja. 2002. International Physical Activity Questionnaire: 12-country reliability and validity. *Medicine & Science in Sports & Exercise* 35: 1381-1395.

Cunningham, J.J. 1982. Body composition and resting metabolic rate: The myth of feminine metabolism. *American Journal of Clinical Nutrition* 36: 721-726.

Forman, J.N., W.C. Miller, L.M. Szymanski, and B. Fernhall. 1998. Differences in resting metabolic rates of inactive obese African-American and Caucasian women. *International Journal of Obesity* 22: 215-221.

Fricker, J., R. Rozen, J.C. Melchior, and M. Apfelbaum. 1991. Energy-metabolism adaptation in obese adults on a very-low-calorie diet. *American Journal of Clinical Nutrition* 53: 826-830.

Gaesser, G., and G.A. Brooks. 1984. Metabolic basis of excess postexercise oxygen consumption: A review. *Medicine & Science in Sports & Exercise* 16: 29-43.

Geliebter, A., M.M. Maher, L. Gerace, G. Bernard, S.B. Heymsfield, and S.A. Hashim. 1997. Effects of strength or aerobic training on body composition, resting metabolic rate, and peak oxygen consumption in obese dieting subjects. *American Journal of Clinical Nutrition* 66: 557-563.

Glass, J.N., W.C. Miller, L.M. Szymanski, B. Fernhall, and J.L. Durstine. 2002. Physiological responses to weight-loss intervention in inactive obese African-American and Caucasian women. *Journal of Sports Medicine and Physical Fitness* 42: 56-64.

Harris, J.A., and F.G. Benedict. 1919. *A Biometric Study of Basal Metabolism in Man.* Publication No. 279. Washington, DC: Carnegie Institute of Washington.

Harris, T.J., C.G. Owen, C.R. Victor, R. Adams, U. Ekelund, and D.G. Cook. 2009. A comparison of questionnaire, accelerometer, and pedometer: Measures in older people. *Medicine & Science in Sports & Exercise* 41: 1392-1402.

Heil, D.P. 2006. Predicting activity energy expenditure using the Actical activity monitor. *Research Quarterly for Exercise & Sport* 77: 64-80.

Hunter, G.R., N.M. Byrne, B. Sirikul, J.R. Fernandez, P.A. Zuckerman, B.E. Darnell, and B.A. Gower. 2008. Resistance training conserves fat-free mass and resting energy expenditure following weight loss. *Obesity* 16: 1045-1051.

IPAQ. International Physical Activity Questionnaire. 2011. Accessed February 1. www .ipaq.ki.se.

Kleiber, M. 1932. Body size and metabolism. *Hilgardia* 6: 315-353.

Livingston, E.H., and I. Kohlstadt. 2005. Simplified resting metabolic rate-predicting formulas for normal-sized and obese individuals. *Obesity Research* 13: 1255-1262.

McArdle, E.D., F.I. Katch, and V.L. Katch. 2001. *Exercise Physiology: Energy, Nutrition, and Human Performance,* 5th ed. Baltimore: Lippincott Williams & Wilkins.

Mifflin, M.D., S.T. Joer, L.A. Hill, B.J. Scott, S.A. Daugherty, and Y.O. Koh. 1990. A new predictive equation for resting energy expenditure in healthy individuals. *American Journal of Clinical Nutrition* 51: 241-247.

Miller, W.C. 2006. Energy balance. In *Scientific Evidence for Musculoskeletal, Bariatric, and Sports Nutrition,* edited by I. Kohlstadt, 193-209. Boca Raton, FL: CRC Press.

Respironics. 2008. *Actical Physical Activity Monitoring System.* Bend, OR: Respironics.

Sharp, T.A., M.L. Bell, G.K. Grunwald, K.H. Schmitz, S. Sidney, C.E. Lewis, K. Tolan, and J.O. Hill. 2002. Differences in resting metabolic rate between White and African-American young adults. *Obesity Research* 10: 726-732.

Stiegler, P., and A. Cunliff. 2006. The role of diet and exercise for the maintenance of fat-free mass and resting metabolic rate during weight loss. *Sports Medicine* 36: 239-262.

Van Pelt, R.E., P.P. Jones, K.P. Davy, C.A. Desouza, H. Tanaka, B.M. Davy, and D.R. Seals. 1997. Regular exercise and the age-related decline in resting metabolic rate in women. *Journal of Clinical Endocrinology & Metabolism* 10: 3208-3212.

Weston, A.T., R. Petosa, and R.R. Pate. 1997. Validation of an instrument for measurement of physical activity in youth. *Medicine & Science in Sports & Exercise* 29: 138-143.

Wilmore, J.H., P.R. Stanforth, L.A. Hudspeth, J. Gagnon, E.W. Daw, A.S. Leon, D.C. Rao, J.S. Skinner, and C. Bouchard. 1998. Alterations in resting metabolic rate as a consequence of 20 wk of endurance training: The HERITAGE Family Study. *American Journal of Clinical Nutrition* 68: 66-71.

Chapter 5

American College of Sports Medicine. 2000. *ACSM's Guidelines for Exercise Testing and Prescription,* 6th ed. Philadelphia: Lippincott Williams & Wilkins.

American College of Sports Medicine. 2006. *ACSM's Guidelines for Exercise Testing and Prescription,* 7th ed. Philadelphia: Lippincott Williams & Wilkins.

American College of Sports Medicine. 2010. *ACSM's Guidelines for Exercise Testing and Prescription,* 8th ed. Philadelphia: Lippincott Williams & Wilkins.

Andersen, L.B. 1995. A maximal cycle exercise protocol to predict maximal oxygen uptake. *Scandinavian Journal of Medicine and Science in Sports* 5: 143-146.

Åstrand, I. 1960. Aerobic work capacity in men and women with special reference to age. *ACTA Physiologica Scandinavica* 49: 51.

Åstrand, P.O., and K. Rodahl. 1986. *Textbook of Work Physiology.* New York: McGraw-Hill.

Åstrand, P.O., and I. Ryhming. 1954. A nomogram for calculation of aerobic capacity (physical fitness) from pulse rate during submaximal work. *Journal of Applied Physiology* 7: 218-221.

Baechle, T.R., and R.W. Earle. 2008. *Essentials of Strength Training and Conditioning,* 3rd ed. Champaign, IL: Human Kinetics.

Balke, B., and R.W. Ware. 1959. An experimental study of physical fitness of Air Force personnel. *United Stated Armed Forces Medical Journal* 10: 675-688.

Baumgartner, T.A., and A.S. Jackson. 1991. *Measurement for Evaluation in Physical Education and Exercise Science,* 4th ed. Dubuque, IA: Wm. C. Brown.

Berthon, P., M. Dabonneville, N. Fellmann, M. Bedu, and A. Chamoux. 1997a. Maximal aerobic velocity measured by the 5-min running field test on two different fitness level groups. *Archives of Physiology and Biochemistry* 105: 633-639.

Berthon, P., N. Fellmann, M. Bedu, B. Beaune, M. Dabonneville, J. Coudert, and A. Chamoux. 1997b. A 5-min running field test as a measurement of maximal aerobic velocity. *European Journal of Applied Physiology* 75: 233-238.

Bosquet, L., L. Léger, and P. Legros. 2002. Methods to determine aerobic endurance. *Sports Medicine* 32: 675-700.

Bruce, R.A., F. Kusumi, and D. Hosmer. 1973. Maximal oxygen intake and nomographic assessment of functional aerobic impairment in cardiovascular disease. *American Heart Journal* 85: 546-562.

Buchfuhrer, M.J., J.E. Hansen, T.E. Robinson, et al. 1983. Optimizing the exercise protocol for cardiopulmonary assessment. *Journal of Applied Physiology* 55: 1558-1564.

Buono, M.J., T.L. Borin, N.T. Sjoholm, and J.A. Hodgdon. 1996. Validity and reliability of a timed 5 km cycle ergometer ride to predict maximum oxygen uptake. *Physiological Measurement* 17: 313-317.

Buono, M.J., J.J. Roby, F.G. Micale, J.F. Sallis, and W.E. Shepard. 1991. Validity and reliability of predicting maximum oxygen uptake via field tests in children and adolescents. *Pediatric Exercise Science* 3: 250-255.

Castro-Pinero, J., J. Mora, J.L. Gonzalez-Montesinos, M. Sjostrom, and J.R. Ruiz. 2009. Criterion-related validity of the one-mile run/walk test in children aged 8-17 years. *Journal of Sports Sciences* 27: 405-413.

Cink, C.E., and T.R. Thomas. 1981. Validity of the Astrand-Ryhming nomogram for predicting maximal oxygen intake. *British Journal of Sports Medicine* 15: 182-185.

Conley, D.S., K.J. Cureton, D.R. Denger, and P.G. Weyand. 1991. Validation of the 12-min swim as a field test of peak aerobic power in young men. *Medicine & Science in Sports & Exercise* 23: 766-773.

Conley, D.S., K.J. Cureton, B.T. Hinson, E.J. Higbie, and P.G. Weyand. 1992. Validation of the 12-minute swim as a field test of peak aerobic power in young women. *Research Quarterly for Exercise and Sport* 63: 153-161.

Cooper, K.H. 1968. A means of assessing maximal oxygen intake. *Journal of the American Medical Association* 203: 201-204.

Cooper, K.H. 1982. *The Aerobics Program for Total Well-Being.* Toronto: Bantam Books.

Cureton, K.J., M.A. Sloniger, J.P. O'Bannon, D.M. Black, and W.P. McCormack. 1995. A generalized equation for prediction of $\dot{V}O_2$peak from 1-mile run/walk performance. *Medicine & Science in Sports & Exercise* 27: 445-451.

Dabney, U., and M. Butler. 2006. The predictive ability of the YMCA test and Bruce test for triathletes with different training backgrounds. *Emporia State Research Studies* 43: 38-44.

Dabonneville, M., P. Berthon, P. Vaslin, and N. Fellmann. 2003. The 5 min running field test: Test and retest reliability on trained men and women. *European Journal of Applied Physiology* 88: 353-360.

Disch, J.R., R. Frankiewicz, and A. Jackson. 1975. Construct validation of distance run tests. *Research Quarterly* 2: 169-176.

Dolgener, F.A., L.D. Hensley, J.J. Marsh, and J.K. Fjelstul. 1994. Validation of the Rockport fitness walking test in college males and females. *Research Quarterly for Exercise and Sport* 65: 152-158.

Donnelly, J.E., D.J. Jacobsen, J.M. Jakicic, J. Whatley, S. Gunderson, W.J. Gillespie, G.L. Blackburn, and Z.V. Tran. 1992. Estimation of peak oxygen consumption from a submaximal half mile walk in obese females. *International Journal of Obesity* 16: 585-589.

Ebbeling, C.B., A. Ward, E.M. Puleo, J. Widrick, and J.M. Rippe. 1991. Development of a single-stage submaximal treadmill walking test. *Medicine & Science in Sports & Exercise* 23: 966-973.

Fernhall, B., K. Pittetti, N. Stubbs, and L. Stadler Jr. 1996. Validity and reliability of the ½ mile run-walk as an indicator of aerobic fitness with mental retardation. *Pediatric Exercise Science* 8: 130-142.

Foster, C., A.S. Jackson, M.L. Pollock, M.M. Taylor, J. Hare, S.M. Sennett, J.L. Rod, M. Sarwar, and D.H. Schmidt. 1984. Generalized equations for predicting functional capacity from treadmill performance. *American Heart Journal* 107: 1229-1234.

Gellish, R.L., B.R. Goslin, R.E. Olson, A. McDonald, G.D. Russi, and V.K. Moudgil. 2007. Longitudinal modeling of the relationship between age and maximal heart rate. *Medicine & Science in Sports & Exercise* 39: 822-829.

George, J.D. 1996. Alternative approach to maximal exercise testing and $\dot{V}O_2$max prediction in college students. *Research Quarterly for Exercise and Sport* 67: 452-457.

George, J.D., G.W. Fellingham, and A.G. Fisher. 1998. A modified version of the Rockport fitness walking test for college men and women. *Research Quarterly for Exercise and Sport* 69: 205-209.

George, J.D., S.L. Paul, A. Hyde, D.I. Bradshaw, P.R. Vehrs, R.L. Hager, and F.G. Yanowitz. 2009. Prediction of maximum oxygen uptake using both exercise and non-exercise data. *Measurement in Physical Education and Exercise Science* 13: 1-12.

George, J.D., W.J. Stone, and L.N. Burkett. 1997. Non-exercise $\dot{V}O_2$max estimation for physically active college students. *Medicine & Science in Sports & Exercise* 29: 415-423.

George, J.D., P.R. Vehrs, P.E. Allsen, G.W. Fellingham, and A.G. Fisher. 1993a. $\dot{V}O_2$max estimation from a submaximal 1-mile track jog for fit college-age individuals. *Medicine & Science in Sports & Exercise* 25: 401-406.

George, J.D., P.R. Vehrs, P.E. Allsen, G.W. Fellingham, and A.G. Fisher. 1993b. Development of a submaximal treadmill jogging test for fit college-aged individuals. *Medicine & Science in Sports & Exercise* 25: 643-647.

Golding, L.A., C.R. Myers, and W.E. Sinning. 1989. *Y 's Way to Physical Fitness,* 3rd ed. Champaign, IL: Human Kinetics.

Greenhalgh, H.A., J.D. George, and R.L. Hager. 2001. Cross-validation of a quarter-mile walk test using two $\dot{V}O_2$max regression models. *Measurement in Physical Education and Exercise Science* 5: 139-151.

Hambrecht, R., G.C. Schuler, T. Muth, et al. 1992. Greater diagnostic sensitivity of treadmill versus cycle ergometry exercise testing of asymptomatic men with coronary artery disease. *American Journal of Cardiology* 70: 141-146.

Huse, D., P. Patterson, and J. Nichols. 2000. The validity and reliability of the 12-minute swim test in male swimmers ages 13-17. *Measurement in Physical Education and Exercise Science* 4: 45-55.

Jung, A.P., D.C. Nieman, and M.W. Kernodle. 2001. Prediction of maximal aerobic power in adolescents from cycle ergometry. *Pediatric Exercise Science* 13: 167-172.

Kline, G.M., J.P. Porcari, R. Hintermeister, P.S. Freedson, A. Ward, R.F. McCarron, J. Ross, and J.M. Rippe. 1987. Estimation of $\dot{V}O_2$max from a one-mile track walk, gender, age, and body weight. *Medicine & Science in Sports & Exercise* 19: 253-259.

Kovaleski, J.E., W.E. Davis, R.J. Heitman, P.M. Norrell, and S.F. Pugh. 2005. Concurrent validity of two submaximal bicycle exercise tests in predicting maximal oxygen consumption (Abstract). *Research Quarterly for Exercise and Sport* 76: A29.

Larsen, G.E., J.D. George, J.L. Alexander, G.W. Fellingham, S.G. Aldana, and A.C. Parcell. 2002. Prediction of maximum oxygen consumption from walking, jogging, or running. *Research Quarterly for Exercise and Sport* 73: 66-72.

Londeree, B.R. 1997. Effect of training on lactate/ventilatory thresholds: A meta-analysis. *Medicine & Science in Sports & Exercise* 29: 837-843.

MacNaughton, L., R. Croft, J. Pennicott, and T. Long. 1990. The 5 and 15 minute runs as predictors of aerobic capacity in high school students. *Journal of Sports Medicine and Physical Fitness* 30: 24-28.

Maeder, M., T. Wolber, R. Atefy, M. Gadza, P. Ammann, J. Myers, and H. Rickli. 2005. Impact of the exercise mode on exercise capacity. *Chest* 128: 2804-2811.

Massicotte, D.R., R. Gauthier, and P. Markon. 1985. Prediction of $\dot{V}O_2$max from the running performance in children aged 10-17 years. *Journal of Sports Medicine* 25: 10-17.

Mayhew, J.L., and P.B. Gifford. 1975. Prediction of maximal oxygen uptake in preadolescent boys from anthropometric parameters. *Research Quarterly* 46: 302-311.

McSwegin, P.J., S.A. Plowman, G.M. Wolff, and G.L. Guttenberg. 1998. The validity of a one-mile walk test for high school age individuals. *Measurement in Physical Education and Exercise Science* 2: 47-63.

Mello, R.P., M.M. Murphy, and J.A. Vogel. 1988. Relationship between a two mile run for time and maximal oxygen uptake. *Journal of Applied Sport Science Research* 2: 9-12.

Murray, T.D., J.L. Walker, A.S. Jackson, J.R. Morrow, J.A. Eldridge, and D.L. Rainey. 1993. Validation of a 20-minute steady-state jog as an estimate of peak oxygen uptake in adolescents. *Research Quarterly for Exercise and Sport* 64: 75-82.

Myers, J., N. Buchanan, D. Walsh, et al. 1991. Comparison of the ramp versus standard exercise protocols. *Journal of the American College of Cardiology* 17: 1334-1342.

Oja, P., R. Laukkanen, M. Pasanen, T. Tyry, and I. Vuori. 1991. A 2-km walking test for assessing the cardiorespiratory fitness of healthy adults. *International Journal of Sports Medicine* 12: 356-362.

Pettersen, S.A., P.M. Fredrikson, and F. Ingjer. 2001. The correlation between peak O_2 uptake ($\dot{V}O_2$peak) and running performance in children and adolescents; aspects of different units. *Scandinavian Journal of Medicine and Science in Sports* 11: 223-228.

Plowman, S.A., and N.Y.S. Liu. 1999. Norm-referenced and criterion-referenced validity of the one-mile run and PACER in college age individuals. *Measurement in Physical Education and Exercise Science* 3: 63-84.

Pollock, M.L., R.L. Bohannon, K.H. Cooper, J.J. Ayres, A. Ward, S.R. White, and A.C. Linnerud. 1976. A comparative analysis of four protocols for maximal treadmill stress testing. *American Heart Journal* 92: 39-46.

Pollock, M.L., C. Foster, D. Schmidt, C. Hellman, A.C. Linnerud, and A. Ward. 1982. Comparative analysis of physiologic responses to three different maximal graded exercise test protocols in healthy women. *American Heart Journal* 103: 363-373.

Sharkey, B.J. 1988. Specificity of testing. In *Advances in Sports Medicine and Fitness*, edited by W.A. Grana. Chicago: Year Book Medical Publishers.

Siconolfi, S.F., E.M. Cullinane, R.A. Carleton, and P.D. Thompson. 1982. Assessing $\dot{V}O_2$max in epidemiologic studies: Modification of the Astrand-Rhyming test. *Medicine & Science in Sports & Exercise* 4: 335-338.

Spackman, M.B., J.D. George, T.R. Pennington, and G.W. Fellingham. 2001. Maximal graded exercise test protocol preferences of relatively fit college students. *Measurement in Physical Education & Exercise Science* 5: 1-12.

Storer, T.W., J.A. Davis, and V.J. Caiozzo. 1990. Accurate prediction of $\dot{V}O_2$max in cycle ergometry. *Medicine & Science in Sports & Exercise* 22: 704-712.

Tokmakidis, S.P., L. Léger, D. Mercier, F. Peronnet, and G. Thibault. 1987. New approaches to predict $\dot{V}O_2$max and endurance from running performance. *Journal of Sports Medicine* 27: 401-409.

Vehrs, P.R., J.D. George, G.W. Fellingham, S.A. Plowman, and K. Dustman-Allen. 2007. Submaximal treadmill exercise test to predict $\dot{V}O_2$max in fit adults. *Measurement in Physical Education and Exercise Science* 11: 61-72.

Weltman, A., R. Seip, A.J. Bogardus, D. Snead, E. Dowling, S. Levine, J. Weltman, and A. Rogol. 1990. Prediction of lactate threshold (LT) and fixed blood lactate concentrations (FBLC) from 3200-m running performance in women. *International Journal of Sports Medicine* 11: 373-378.

Weltman, A., D. Snead, R. Seip, R. Schurrer, S. Levine, R. Rutt, T. Reilly, J. Weltman, and A. Rogol. 1987. Prediction of lactate threshold and fixed blood lactate concentrations from 3200-m running performance in male runners. *International Journal of Sports Medicine* 8: 401-406.

Wicks, J.R., J.R. Sutton, N.B. Oldridge, et al. 1978. Comparison of the electrocardiographic changes induced by maximum exercise testing with treadmill and cycle ergometer. *Circulation* 57: 1066-1069.

Wyndham, C.H., N.B. Strydom, C.H. VanGraan, A.J. VanRensburg, G.G. Rogers, J.S. Greyson, and W.H. VanDerWalt. 1971. Estimating the maximum aerobic capacity for exercise. *South African Medical Journal* 45: 53-57.

Chapter 6

Beneke, R. 2003. Methodological aspects of maximal lactate steady state-implications for performance testing. *European Journal of Applied Physiology* 89: 95-99.

Bentley, D., L. McNaughton, D. Thompson, V. Vleck, and A. Batterham. 2001. Peak power output, the lactate threshold, and time trial performance in cyclists. *Medicine & Science in Sports & Exercise* 33: 2077-2081.

Bishop, D., D. Jenkins, and L. Mackinnon. 1998. The relationship between plasma lactate parameters, Wpeak and 1-h cycling performance in women. *Medicine & Science in Sports & Exercise* 30: 1270-1275.

Bouchard, C., R. Lesage, G. Lortie, J.A. Simoneau, P. Hamel, M.R. Boulay, L. Pérusse, G. Thériault, and C. Leblanc. 1986. Aerobic performance in brothers, dizygotic and monozygotic twins. *Medicine & Science in Sports & Exercise* 18: 639-646.

Cheng, B., H. Kuipers, A.C. Snyder, H.A. Keizer, A. Jeukendrup, and M. Hesselink. 1992. A new approach for the determination of ventilatory and lactate thresholds. *International Journal of Sports Medicine* 13: 518-522.

Davis, J.A., R. Rozenek, D.M. DeCicco, M.T. Carizzi, and P.H. Pham. 2007. Comparison of three methods for detection of the lactate threshold. *Clinical Physiological and Functional Imaging* 27: 381-384.

El-Sayed, M.S., K.P. George, and K. Dyson. 1993. The influence of blood sampling site on lactate concentration during submaximal exercise at 4 mmol·l⁻¹ lactate level. *European Journal of Applied Physiology* 67: 518-522.

Foxdal, P., B. Sjödin, A. Sjödin, and B. Östman. 1994. The validity and accuracy of blood lactate measurements for prediction of maximal endurance running capacity. *International Journal of Sports Medicine* 15: 89-95.

Henriksson, J., and J.S. Reitman. 1976. Quantitative measures of enzyme activities in type I and type II muscle fibres of man after training. *Acta Physiologica Scandinavica* 97: 394-397.

Henritze, J., A. Weltman, R.L. Schurrer, and K. Barlow. 1985. Effects of training at and above the lactate threshold on the lactate threshold and maximal oxygen uptake. *European Journal of Applied Physiology* 54: 84-88.

Holloszy, J.O., and E.F. Coyle. 1984. Adaptations of skeletal muscle to endurance exercise and their metabolic consequences. *Journal of Applied Physiology* 56: 831-838.

Joyner, M.J., and E.F. Coyle. 2008. Endurance exercise performance: The physiology of champions. *Journal of Physiology* 586 (1): 35-44.

Kenefick, R.W., C.O. Mattern, N.V. Mahood, and T.J. Quinn. 2002. Physiological variables at lactate threshold under-represent cycling time-trial intensity. *Journal of Sports Medicine and Physical Fitness* 42: 396-402.

Morris, D.M., J.T. Kearney, and E.R. Burke. 2000. The effects of breathing supplemental oxygen during altitude training on cycling performance. *Journal of Science and Medicine in Sport* 3: 165-175.

Morris, D.M., and R.S. Shafer. 2010. Comparison of power output during time trialing and power outputs eliciting metabolic variables in cycling ergometry. *International Journal of Sport Nutrition and Exercise Metabolism* 20: 115-121.

Nicholson, R.M., and G.G. Sleivert. 2001. Indices of lactate threshold and their relationship with 10-km running velocity. *Medicine & Science in Sports & Exercise* 33: 339-342.

Robergs, R.A., F. Ghiasvand, and D. Parker. 2004. Biochemistry of exercise induced acidosis. *American Journal of Physiology* 287: R502-R516.

Schmidt, W., N. Maassen, F. Trost, and D. Böning. 1988. Training induced effects on blood volume, erythrocyte turnover and haemoglobin oxygen binding properties. *European Journal of Applied Physiology and Occupational Physiology* 57: 490-498.

Tanaka, K. 1990. Lactate-related factors as a critical determinant of endurance. *Annals of Physiological Anthropology* 9: 191-202.

Thoden, J.S. 1991. Testing aerobic power. In *Physiological Testing of the High-Performance Athlete*, edited by H.A. Wenger, J.D. MacDougall, and H.J. Green. Champaign, IL: Human Kinetics.

Urhausen, A., B. Coen, B. Weiler, and W. Kinderman. 1993. Individual anaerobic threshold and maximum lactate steady state. *International Journal of Sports Medicine* 14: 134-139.

Weltman, A., R.L. Seip, D. Snead, J.Y. Weltman, E.M. Hasvitz, W.S. Evans, J.D. Veldhuis, and A.D. Rogul. 1992. Exercise training at and above the lactate threshold in previously untrained women. *International Journal of Sports Medicine* 13: 257-263.

Zhou, S., and S.B. Weston. 1997. Reliability of using the *D*-max method to define physiological responses to incremental exercise testing. *Physiological Measures* 18: 145-154.

Zoladz, J., A.C. Rademaker, and A.J. Sargeant. 1995. Non-linear relationship between O_2 uptake and power output at high intensities of exercise in humans. *Journal of Physiology* 488: 211-217.

Chapter 7

Aagaard, P., and J.L. Andersen. 1998. Correlation between contractile strength and myosin heavy chain isoform composition in human skeletal muscle. *Medicine & Science in Sports & Exercise* 30: 1217-1222.

Abernethy, P.J., and J. Jürimäe. 1996. Cross-sectional and longitudinal uses of isoinertial, isometric, and isokinetic dynamometry. *Medicine & Science in Sports & Exercise* 28: 1180-1187.

Abernethy, P., G. Wilson, and P. Logan. 1995. Strength and power assessment: Issues, controversies and challenges. *Sports Medicine* 19: 401-417.

Adams, K.J., A.M. Swank, K.L. Barnard, J.M. Bering, and P.G. Stevene-Adams. 2000. Safety of maximal power, strength, and endurance testing in older African American women. *Journal of Strength and Conditioning Research* 14: 254-260.

Ahtiainen, J.P., A. Parkarinen, M. Alen, W.J. Kraemer, and K. Häkkinen. 2005. Short vs. long rest period between the sets in hypertrophic resistance training: Influence on muscle strength, size, and hormonal adaptations in trained men. *Journal of Strength and Conditioning Research* 19: 572-582.

Allen, D.G., G.D. Lamb, and H. Westerblad. 2008. Skeletal muscle fatigue: Cellular mechanisms. *Physiology Reviews* 88: 287-332.

Amiridis, I.G., A. Martin, B. Morlon, L. Martin, G. Cometti, M. Pousson, and J. van Hoecke. 1996. Co-activation and tension-regulating phenomena during isokinetic knee extension in sedentary and highly skilled humans. *European Journal of Applied Physiology* 73: 149-156.

Augustsson, J., A. Esko, R. Thomeé, and U. Svantesson. 1998. Weight training of the thigh muscles using closed vs. open kinetic chain exercises: A comparison of performance enhancement. *Journal of Sports Physical Therapy* 27: 3-8.

Baechle, T.R., R.W. Earle, and D. Wathen. 2008. Resistance training. In *Essentials of Strength Training and Conditioning*, edited by T.R. Baechle and R.W. Earle, 381-412. Champaign, IL: Human Kinetics.

Baker, D. 2001. Comparison of upper-body strength and power between professional and college-aged rugby league players. *Journal of Strength and Conditioning Research* 15: 30-35.

Baker, D.G., and R.U. Newton. 2006. Discriminative analysis of various upper body tests in professional rugby league players. *International Journal of Sports Physiology and Performance* 1: 347-360.

Baker, D., G. Wilson, and R. Carlyon. 1994. Generality versus specificity: A comparison of dynamic and isometric measures of strength and speed-strength. *European Journal of Applied Physiology* 68: 350-355.

Baldwin, K.M., and F. Haddad. 2001. Effects of different activity and inactivity paradigms on myosin heavy chain gene expression in striated muscle. *Journal of Applied Physiology* 90: 345-357.

Baltzopoulos, V. 2008. Isokinetic dynamometry. In *Biomechanical Evaluation of Movement in Sport and Exercise,* edited by C.J. Payton and R.M. Bartlett, 103-128. London: Routledge.

Bartlett, L.R., M.D. Storey, and B.D. Simons. 1989. Measurement of upper extremity torque production and its relationship to throwing speed in the competitive athlete. *American Journal of Sports Medicine* 17: 89-91.

Bartlett, R. 2007. *Introduction to Sports Biomechanics. Analysing Human Movement Patterns.* London: Routledge.

Bazett-Jones, D.M., J.B. Winchester, and J.M. McBride. 2005. Effect of potentiation and stretching on maximal force, rate of force development, and range of motion. *Journal of Strength and Conditioning Research* 19: 421-426.

Behm, D.G., D.C. Button, and J.C. Butt. 2001. Factors affecting force loss with prolonged stretching. *Canadian Journal of Applied Physiology* 26: 262-272.

Bergh, U., and B. Ekblom. 1979. Influence of muscle temperature on maximal muscle strength and power output in human skeletal muscle. *Acta Physiologica Scandinavica* 107: 33-37.

Bishop, D. 2003a. Warm up I. Potential mechanisms and the effects of passive warm-up on exercise performance. *Sports Medicine* 33: 439-454.

Bishop, D. 2003b. Warm up II. Performance changes following active warm-up and how to structure the warm-up. *Sports Medicine* 33: 483-498.

Blazevich, A.J., N. Gill, and R.U. Newton. 2002. Reliability and validity of two isometric squat tests. *Journal of Strength and Conditioning Research* 16: 298-304.

Blazevich, A.J., and D.G. Jenkins. 2002. Effect of the movement speed of resistance training exercises on sprint and strength performance in concurrently training elite junior sprinters. *Journal of Sports Sciences* 20: 981-990.

Bompa, T.O., and G.G. Haff. 2009. *Periodization: Theory and Methodology of Training.* Champaign, IL: Human Kinetics.

Bottinelli, R., and C. Reggiani. 2000. Human skeletal muscle fibers: Molecular and functional diversity. *Progress in Biophysics and Molecular Biology* 73: 195-262.

Braith, R.W., J.E. Graves, S.H. Leggett, and M.L. Pollock. 1993. Effect of training on the relationship between maximal and submaximal strength. *Medicine & Science in Sports & Exercise* 25: 132-138.

Brock Symons, T., A.A. Vandervoort, C.L. Rice, T.J. Overend, and G.D. Marsh. 2004. Reliability of isokinetic and isometric knee-extensor force in older women. *Journal of Aging and Physical Activity* 12: 525-537.

Brown, D.A., S.A. Kautz, and C.A. Dairaghi. 1996. Muscle activity patterns altered during pedaling at different body orientations. *Journal of Biomechanics* 29: 1349-1356.

Carbuhn, A.F., J.M. Womack, J.S. Green, K. Morgan, G.S. Miller, and S.F. Crouse. 2008. Performance and blood pressure characteristics of first-year National Collegiate Athletic Association Division I football players. *Journal of Strength and Conditioning Research* 22: 1347-1354.

Carroll, T.J., P.J. Abernethy, P.A. Logan, M. Barber, and M.T. McEniery. 1998. Resistance training frequency: strength and myosin heavy chain responses to two and three bouts per week. *European Journal of Applied Physiology* 78: 270-275.

Carter, A.B., T.W. Kaminski, A.T. Douex, C.A. Knight, and J.G. Richards. 2007. Effects of high volume upper extremity plyometric training on throwing velocity and functional strength ratios of the shoulder rotators in collegiate baseball players. *Journal of Strength and Conditioning Research* 21: 208-215.

Chaouachi, A., M. Brughelli, K. Chamari, G.T. Levin, N.B. Abdelkrim, L. Laurencelle, and C. Castagna. 2009. Lower limb maximal dynamic strength and agility determinants in elite basketball players. *Journal of Strength and Conditioning Research* 23: 1570-1577.

Chapman, A. 2008. *Biomechanical Analysis of Fundamental Human Movements.* Champaign, IL: Human Kinetics.

Cheng, A.J., and C.L. Rice. 2005. Fatigue and recovery of power and isometric torque following isotonic knee extensions. *Journal of Applied Physiology* 99: 1446-1452.

Christ, C.B., R.A. Boileau, M.H. Slaughter, R.J. Stillman, and J.A. Cameron. 1993. The effect of test protocol instructions on the measurement of muscle function in adult women. *Journal of Orthopaedic and Sports Physical Therapy* 18: 502-510.

Chu, Y., G.S. Fleisig, K.J. Simpson, and J.R. Andrews. 2009. Biomechanical comparison between elite female and male baseball pitchers. *Journal of Applied Biomechanics* 25: 22-31.

Cometti, G., N.A. Maffiuletti, M. Pousson, J.C. Chatard, and N. Maffulli. 2001. Isokinetic strength and anaerobic power of elite, subelite and amateur French soccer players. *International Journal of Sports Medicine* 22: 45-51.

Cotterman, M.L., L.A. Darby, and W.A. Skelly. 2005. Comparison of muscle force production using the Smith machine and free weights for bench press and squat exercises. *Journal of Strength and Conditioning Research* 19: 169-176.

Dapena, J., and C.S. Chung. 1988. Vertical and radial motions of the body during the take-off phase of high jumping. *Medicine & Science in Sports & Exercise* 20: 290-302.

de Ruiter, C.J., D.A. Jones, A.J. Sargeant, and A. de Haan. 1999. Temperature effect on the rates of isometric force development and relaxation in the fresh and fatigued adductor pollicis muscle. *Experimental Physiology* 84: 1137-1150.

Deighan, M.A., M.B.A. De Ste Croix, and N. Armstrong. 2003. Reliability of isokinetic concentric and eccentric knee and elbow extension and flexion in 9/10 year old boys. *Isokinetics and Exercise Science* 11: 109-115.

Dorchester, F.E. 1944. *Muscle Action and Health.* Vancouver, BC: Mitchell.

Dowson, M.N., M.E. Neville, H.K.A. Lakomy, A.M. Neville, and R.J. Hazeldine. 1998. Modeling the relationship between isokinetic muscle strength and sprint running performance. *Journal of Sports Sciences* 16: 257-265.

Drury, D.G., K.J. Stuempfle, C.W. Mason, and J.C. Girman. 2006. The effects of isokinetic contraction velocity on concentric and eccentric strength of the biceps brachii. *Journal of Strength and Conditioning Research* 20: 390-395.

Duchateau, J., J.G. Semmler, and R.M. Enoka. 2006. Training adaptations in the behavior of human motor units. *Journal of Applied Physiology* 101: 1766-1775.

Dudley, G.A., R.T. Harris, M.R. Duvoisin, B.M. Hather, and P. Buchanan. 1990. Effect of voluntary vs. artificial activation on the relationship of muscle torque to speed. *Journal of Applied Physiology* 69: 2215-2221.

Earle, R.W., and T.R. Baechle. 2008. Resistance training and spotting techniques. In *Essentials of Strength Training and Conditioning,* edited by T.R. Baechle and R.W. Earle, 325-376. Champaign, IL: Human Kinetics.

Faigenbaum, A.D., L.A. Milliken, and W.L. Wescott. 2003. Maximal strength testing in healthy children. *Journal of Strength and Conditioning Research* 17: 162-166.

Falvo, M.J., B.K. Schilling, R.J. Bloomer, W.A. Smith, and A.C. Creasey. 2007. Efficacy of prior eccentric exercise in attenuating impaired exercise performance after muscle injury in resistance trained men. *Journal of Strength and Conditioning Research* 21: 1053-1060.

Faulkner, J.A. 2003. Terminology for contractions of muscles during shortening, while isometric, and during lengthening. *Journal of Applied Physiology* 95: 455-459.

Finni, T., S. Ikegawa, and P.V. Komi. 2001. Concentric force enhancement during human movement. *Acta Physiologica Scandinavica* 173: 369-377.

Flanagan, E.P., L. Galvin, and A.J. Harrison. 2008. Force production and reactive strength capabilities after anterior cruciate ligament reconstruction. *Journal of Athletic Training* 43: 249-257.

Foldvari, M., M. Clark, L.C. Laviolette, M.A. Bernstein, D. Kaliton, C. Castaneda, C.T. Pu, J.M. Hausdorff, R.A. Fielding, and M.A. Fiatarone Singh. 2000. Association of muscle power with functional status in community-dwelling elderly women. *Journal of Gerontology. Series A, Biological and Medical Sciences* 22: M192-M199.

Forte, R., and A. Macaluso. 2008. Relationship between performance-based and laboratory tests for lower-limb strength and power assessment in healthy older women. *Journal of Sports Sciences* 26: 1431-1436.

Forthomme, B., J.M. Crielaard, L. Forthomme, and J.L. Croisier. 2007. Field performance of javelin throwers: Relationship with isokinetic findings. *Isokinetics and Exercise Science* 15: 195-202.

Frohm, A., K. Halvorsen, and A. Thorstensson. 2005. A new device for controlled eccentric overloading in training and rehabilitation. *European Journal of Applied Physiology* 94: 168-174.

Fry, A.C., and W.J. Kraemer. 1991. Physical performance characteristics of American collegiate football players. *Journal of Applied Sport Science Research* 5: 126-138.

Green, H.J. 1992. Myofibrillar composition and mechanical function in mammalian skeletal muscle. *Sport Science Review* 1: 43-64.

Guette, M., J. Gondin, and A. Martin. 2005. Time-of-day effect on the torque and neuromuscular properties of the dominant and non-dominant quadriceps femoris. *Chronobiology International* 22: 541-558.

Haff, G.G., M. Stone, H.S. O'Bryant, E. Harman, C. Dinan, R. Johnson, and K-H. Han. 1997. Force-time characteristics of dynamic and isometric muscle actions. *Journal of Strength and Conditioning Research* 11: 269-272.

Häkkinen, K., M. Kallinen, V. Linnamo, U-M. Pastinen, R.U. Newton, and W.J. Kraemer. 1996. Neuromuscular adaptations during bilateral versus unilateral strength training in middle-aged and elderly men and women. *Acta Physiologica Scandinavica* 158: 77-88.

Häkkinen, K., and P.V. Komi. 1983. Electromyographic changes during strength training and detraining. *Medicine & Science in Sports & Exercise* 15: 455-460.

Harman, E. 2008. Principles of test selection and administration. In *Essentials of Strength Training and Conditioning,* edited by T.R. Baechle and R.W. Earle, 237-247. Champaign, IL: Human Kinetics.

Harry, J.D., A.W. Ward, N.C. Heglund, D.L. Morgan, and T.A. McMahon. 1990. Cross-bridge cycling theories cannot explain high-speed lengthening behavior in frog muscle. *Biophysics Journal* 57: 201-208.

Heinonen, A., H. Sievanen, J. Viitasalo, M. Pasanen, P. Oja, and I. Vuori. 1994. Reproducibility of computer measurement of maximal isometric strength and electromyography in sedentary middle-aged women. *European Journal of Applied Physiology* 68: 310-314.

Henwood, T.R., S. Riek, and D.R. Taafe. 2008. Strength versus power-specific resistance training in community-dwelling older adults. *Journal of Gerontology. Series A, Biological and Medical Sciences* 63: 83-91.

Hodgson, M., D. Docherty, and D. Robbins. 2005. Post-activation potentiation: Underlying physiology and implications for motor performance. *Sports Medicine* 35: 585-595.

Hoeger, W.W.K., D.R. Hopkins, S.L. Barette, and D.F. Hale. 1990. Relationship between repetitions and selected percentages of one-repetition maximum: A comparison between untrained and trained males and females. *Journal of Applied Sport Science Research* 4: 47-54.

Hoffman, J. 2006. *Norms for Fitness, Performance, and Health.* Champaign, IL: Human Kinetics.

Hoffman, J.R., G. Tenenbaum, C.M. Maresh, and W.J. Kraemer. 1996. Relationship between athletic performance tests and playing time in elite college basketball players. *Journal of Strength and Conditioning Research* 10: 67-71.

Hollander, D.B., R.R. Kraemer, M.W. Kilpatrick, Z.G. Ramadan, G.V. Reeves, M. Francois, E.P. Herbert, and J.L. Tryniecki. 2007. Maximal eccentric and concentric strength discrepancies between young men and women for dynamic resistance exercise. *Journal of Strength and Conditioning Research* 21: 34-40.

Hopkins, W.G. 2000. Measures of reliability in sports medicine and science. *Sports Medicine* 30: 1-15.

Humphries, B., T. Triplett-McBride, R.U. Newton, S. Marshall, R. Bronks, J. McBride, K. Häkkinen, and W.J. Kraemer. 1999. The relationship between dynamic, isokinetic and isometric strength and bone mineral density in a population of 45 to 65 year old women. *Journal of Science and Medicine in Sport* 2: 364-374.

Ichinose, Y., H. Kanehisa, M. Ito, Y. Kawakami, and T. Fukunaga. 1998. Relationship between muscle fiber pennation and force generation capabilities in Olympic athletes. *International Journal of Sports Medicine* 19: 541-546.

Ichinose, Y., Y. Kawakami, M. Ito, H. Kanehisa, and T. Fukunaga. 2000. In vivo estimation of contraction velocity of human vastus lateralis muscle during "isokinetic" action. *Journal of Applied Physiology* 88: 851-856.

Iki, M., Y. Saito, E. Kajita, H. Nishino, and Y. Kusaka. 2006. Trunk muscle strength is a strong predictor of bone loss in post-menopausal women. *Clinical Orthopedic Related Research* 443: 66-72.

Izquierdo, M., J. Ibañez, E. Gorostiaga, M. Garrues, A. Zúñiga, A. Antón, J.L. Larrión, and K. Häkkinen. 1999. Maximal strength and power characteristics in isometric and dynamic actions of the upper and lower extremities in middle-aged and older men. *Acta Physiologica Scandinavica* 167: 57-68.

Jaric, S., D. Mirkov, and G. Markovic. 2005. Normalizing physical performance tests for body size: A proposal for standardization. *Journal of Strength and Conditioning Research* 19: 467-474.

Jeffreys, I. 2008. Warm-up and stretching. In *Essentials of Strength Training and Conditioning,* edited by T.R. Baechle and R.W. Earle, 295-324. Champaign, IL: Human Kinetics.

Johnson, M.D., and J.G. Buckley. 2001. Muscle power patterns in the mid-acceleration phase of sprinting. *Journal of Sports Sciences* 19: 263-272.

Kawakami, Y., T. Abe, and T. Fukunaga. 1993. Muscle-fiber pennation angles are greater in hypertrophied than in normal muscle. *Journal of Applied Physiology* 74: 2740-2744.

Kawakami, Y., Y. Ichinose, K. Kubo, M. Ito, M. Imai, and T. Fukunaga. 2000. Architecture of contracting human muscles and its functional significance. *Journal of Applied Biomechanics* 16: 88-98.

Kawamori, N., S.J. Rossi, B.D. Justice, E.E. Haff, E.E. Pistilli, H.S. O'Bryant, M.H. Stone, and G.G. Haff. 2006. Peak force and rate of force development during isometric and dynamic mid-thigh clean pulls performed at various intensities. *Journal of Strength and Conditioning Research* 20: 483-491.

Kemmler, W.K., D. Lauber, A. Wassermann, and J.L. Mayhew. 2006. Predicting maximal strength in trained postmenopausal women. *Journal of Strength and Conditioning Research* 20: 838-842.

Kivi, D.M.R., B.K.V. Maraj, and P. Gervais. 2002. A kinematic analysis of high-speed treadmill sprinting over a range of velocities. *Medicine & Science in Sports & Exercise* 34: 662-666.

Knutzen, K.M., L.R. Brilla, and D. Caine. 1999. Validity of 1RM prediction equations for older adults. *Journal of Strength and Conditioning Research* 13: 242-246.

Kokkonen, J., A.G. Nelson, and A. Cornwell. 1998. Acute muscle stretching inhibits maximal strength performance. *Research Quarterly for Exercise and Sport* 69: 411-415.

Komi, P.V. 1984. Physiological and biomechanical correlates of muscle function: Effects of muscle structure and stretch-shortening cycle on force and speed. *Exercise and Sport Sciences Reviews* 12: 81-121.

Komi, P.V. 2003. Stretch-shortening cycle. In *Strength and Power in Sport*, edited by P.V. Komi. Oxford, UK: Blackwell Science Ltd.

Kraemer, W.J., P.A. Piorkowski, J.A. Bush, A.L. Gomez, C.C. Loebel, J.S. Volek, R.U. Newton, S.A. Mazzetti, S.W. Etzweiler, M. Putukian, and W.J. Sebastianelli. 2000. The effects of NCAA division I intercollegiate competitive tennis match play on the recovery of physical performance in women. *Journal of Strength and Conditioning Research* 14: 265-272.

Kravitz, L., C. Akalan, K. Nowicki, and S.J. Kinzey. 2003. Prediction of 1 repetition maximum in high-school power lifters. *Journal of Strength and Conditioning Research* 17: 167-172.

Kuitunen, S., P.V. Komi, and H. Kyrolainen. 2002. Knee and ankle joint stiffness in sprint running. *Medicine & Science in Sports & Exercise* 34: 166-173.

LaStayo, P.C., J.M. Woolf, M.D. Lewek, L. Snyder-Mackler, T. Reich, and S.L. Lindstedt. 2003. Eccentric muscle contractions: Their contribution to injury, prevention, rehabilitation, and sport. *Journal of Orthopaedic and Sports Physical Therapy* 33: 557-571.

Latin, R.W., K. Berg, and T. Baechle. 1994. Physical and performance characteristics of NCAA Division I male basketball players. *Journal of Strength and Conditioning Research* 8: 214-218.

Leiber, L. 2002. *Skeletal Muscle Structure, Function, and Plasticity. The Physiological Basis of Rehabilitation.* Baltimore: Lippincott Williams & Wilkins.

LeSuer, D.A., J.H. McCormick, J.L. Mayhew, R.L. Wasserstein, and M.D. Arnold. 1997. The accuracy of prediction equations for estimating 1RM performance in the bench press, squat, and deadlift. *Journal of Strength and Conditioning Research* 11: 211-213.

Luhtanen, P., and P.V. Komi. 1979. Mechanical power and segmental contribution to force impulses in long jump take-off. *European Journal of Applied Physiology* 41: 267-274.

MacIntosh, B.R., P.F. Gardiner, and A.J. McComas. 2006. *Skeletal Muscle: Form and Function.* Champaign, IL: Human Kinetics.

Maffiuletti, N.A., M. Bizzini, K. Desbrosses, N. Babault, and M. Munzinger. 2007. Reliability of knee extension and flexion measurements using the Con-Trex isokinetic dynamometer. *Clinical Physiology and Functional Imaging* 27: 346-353.

Marques, M.C., R. van den Tillaar, J.D. Vescovi, and J.J. González-Badillo. 2007. Relationship between throwing velocity, muscle power, and bar velocity during bench press in elite handball players. *International Journal of Sports Physiology and Performance* 2: 414-422.

Marsh, A.P., M.E. Miller, W.J. Rejeski, S.L. Hutton, and S.B. Kritchevsky. 2009. Lower extremity muscle function after strength or power training in older adults. *Journal of Aging and Physical Activity* 17: 416-443.

Mayhew, J.L., J.A. Jacques, J.S. Ware, P.P. Chapman, M.G. Bemben, T.E. Ward, and J.P. Slovak. 2004. Anthropometric dimensions do not enhance one repetition maximum prediction from the NFL-225 test in college football players. *Journal of Strength and Conditioning Research* 18: 572-578.

McBride, J.M., T. Triplett-McBride, A. Davie, and R.U. Newton. 2002. The effect of heavy- vs. light-load jump squats on the development of strength, power, and speed. *Journal of Strength and Conditioning Research* 16: 75-82.

McComas, A.J. 1996. *Skeletal Muscle: Form and Function.* Champaign, IL: Human Kinetics.

McCurdy, K., G.A. Langford, A.L. Cline, M. Doscher, and R. Hoff. 2004. The reliability of 1- and 3RM tests of unilateral strength in trained and untrained men and women. *Journal of Sports Science and Medicine* 3: 190-196.

Meckel, Y., H. Atterbom, A. Grodjinovsky, D. Ben-Sira, and A. Rostein. 1995. Physiological characteristics of female 100 metre sprinters of different performance levels. *Journal of Sports Medicine and Physical Fitness* 35: 169-175.

Meller, R., C. Krettek, T. Gösling, K. Wähling, M. Jagodzinski, and J. Zeichen. 2007. Recurrent shoulder instability among athletes: Changes in quality of life, sports activity, and muscle function following open repair. *Knee Surgery, Sports Traumatology, Arthroscopy* 15: 295-304.

Miller, L.E., L.M. Pierson, M.E. Pierson, G.M. Kiebzak, W.K. Ramp, W.G. Herbert, and J.W. Cook. 2009. Age influences anthropometric and fitness-related predictors of bone mineral in men. *The Aging Male* 12: 47-53.

Moir, G., R. Sanders, C. Button, and M. Glaister. 2005. The influence of familiarization on the reliability of force variables measured during unloaded and loaded vertical jumps. *Journal of Strength and Conditioning Research* 19: 140-145.

Moir, G., R. Sanders, C. Button, and M. Glaister. 2007. The effect of periodised resistance training on accelerative sprint performance. *Sports Biomechanics* 6: 285-300.

Morgan, D. 1990. New insights into the behavior of muscle during active lengthening. *Biophysics Journal* 57: 209-221.

Moritz, C.T., B.K. Barry, M.A. Pascoe, and R.M. Enoka. 2005. Discharge rate variability influences the variation in force fluctuations across the working range of a hand muscle. *Journal of Neurophysiology* 94: 2449-2459.

Moss, B.M., P.E. Refsnes, A. Abildgaard, K. Nicolaysen, and J. Jensen. 1997. Effects of maximal effort training with different loads on dynamic strength, cross-sectional area, load-power and load-velocity relationships. *European Journal of Applied Physiology* 75: 193-199.

Müller, S., H. Baur, T. König, A. Hirschmüller, and F. Mayer. 2007. Reproducibility of single- and multi-joint strength measures in healthy and injured athletes. *Isokinetics and Exercise Science* 15: 295-302.

Murphy, A.J., and G.J. Wilson. 1996. Poor correlations between isometric tests and dynamic performance: Relationship to muscle activation. *European Journal of Applied Physiology* 73: 353-357.

Murphy, A.J., and G.J. Wilson. 1997. The ability of tests of muscular function to reflect training induced changes in performance. *Journal of Sports Sciences* 15: 191-200.

Murphy, A.J., G.J. Wilson, and J.F. Pryor. 1994. Use of iso-inertial force mass relationship in the prediction of dynamic human performance. *European Journal of Applied Physiology* 69: 250-257.

Murphy, A.J., G.J. Wilson, J.F. Pryor, and R.U. Newton. 1995. Isometric assessment of muscular function: The effect of joint angle. *Journal of Applied Biomechanics* 11: 205-215.

Murray, J., and P.V. Karpovich. 1956. *Weight Training in Athletics.* Englewood Cliffs, NJ: Prentice Hall.

Nesser, T.W., R.W. Latin, K. Berg, and E. Prentice. 1996. Physiological determinants of 40-meter sprint performance in young male athletes. *Journal of Strength and Conditioning Research* 10: 263-267.

Newton, R.U., K. Häkkinen, A. Häkkinen, M. McCormick, J. Volek, and W.J. Kraemer. 2002. Mixed-methods resistance training increases power and strength of young and older men. *Medicine & Science in Sports & Exercise* 34: 1367-1375.

Nicol, C., J. Avela, and P.V. Komi. 2006. The stretch-shortening cycle. A model to study naturally occurring neuromuscular fatigue. *Sports Medicine* 36: 977-999.

Nicolas, A., A. Gauthier, N. Bessot, S. Moussay, D. Davenne. 2005. Time-of-day effects on myoelectric and mechanical properties of muscle during maximal and prolonged isokinetic exercises. *Chronobiology International* 22: 997-1011.

Ojanen, T., T. Rauhala, and K. Häkkinen. 2007. Strength and power profiles of the lower and upper extremities in master throwers at different ages. *Journal of Strength and Conditioning Research* 21: 216-222.

Oya, T., S. Riek, and A.G. Cresswell. 2009. Recruitment and rate coding organization for soleus motor units across entire range of voluntary isometric plantar flexions. *Journal of Physiology* 587: 4737-4748.

Paschall, H.B. 1954. *Development of Strength.* London: Vigour Press.

Paillard, T., F. Noé, P. Passelergue, and P. Dupui. 2005. Electrical stimulation superimposed onto voluntary muscular contraction. *Sports Medicine* 35: 951-966.

Perry, M.C., S.F. Carville, I.C. Smith, O.M. Rutherford, and D.J. Newham. 2007. Strength, power output and symmetry of leg muscles: Effect of age and history of falling. *European Journal of Applied Physiology* 100: 553-561.

Person, R.S. 1974. Rhythmic activity of a group of human motoneurones during voluntary contractions of a muscle. *Electroencephalography and Clinical Neurophysiology* 36: 585-595.

Peterson, M.D., B.A. Alvar, and M.R. Rhea. 2006. The contributions of maximal force production to explosive movement among young collegiate athletes. *Journal of Strength and Conditioning Research* 20: 867-873.

Phillips, W.T., A.M. Batterham, J.E. Valenzuela, and L.N. Burkett. 2004. Reliability of maximal strength testing in older adults. *Archives of Physical Medicine and Rehabilitation* 85: 329-334.

Pienaar, A.E., M.J. Spamer, and H.S. Steyn. 1998. Identifying and developing rugby talent among 10-year-old boys: A practical model. *Journal of Sports Sciences* 16: 691-699.

Ploutz-Snyder, L.L., and E.L. Giamis. 2001. Orientation and familiarization to 1RM strength testing in old and young women. *Journal of Strength and Conditioning Research* 15: 519-523.

Rassier, D.E. 2000. The effects of length on fatigue and twitch potentiation in human skeletal muscle. *Clinical Physiology* 20: 474-482.

Rassier, D.E., B.R. MacIntosh, and W. Herzog. 1999. Length dependence of active force production in skeletal muscle. *Journal of Applied Physiology* 86: 1445-1457.

Reeves, N.D., and M.V. Narici. 2003. Behavior of human muscle fascicles during shortening and lengthening contractions in vivo. *Journal of Applied Physiology* 95: 1090-1096.

Reilly, T., J. Bangsbo, and A. Franks. 2000. Anthropometric and physiological predisposition for elite soccer. *Journal of Sports Sciences* 18: 669-683.

Requena, B., J.J. González-Badillo, E.S.S. de Villareal, J. Ereline, I. García, H. Gapeyeva, and M. Pääsuke. 2009. Functional performance, maximal strength, and power characteristics in isometric and dynamic actions of lower extremities in soccer players. *Journal of Strength and Conditioning Research* 23: 1391-1401.

Reynolds, J.M., T.J. Gordon, and R.A. Robergs. 2006. Prediction of one repetition maximum strength from multiple repetition maximum testing and anthropometry. *Journal of Strength and Conditioning Research* 20: 584-592.

Robbins, D. 2005. Postactivation potentiation and its practical applicability: A brief review. *Journal of Strength and Conditioning Research* 19: 453-458.

Rubini, E.C., A.L.L. Costa, and S.C. Gomes. 2007. The effects of stretching on strength performance. *Sports Medicine* 37: 213-224.

Rutherford, O.M., and D.A. Jones. 1986. The role of learning and coordination in strength training. *European Journal of Applied Physiology* 55: 100-105.

Rydwik, E., C. Karlsson, K. Frändin, and G. Akner. 2007. Muscle strength testing with one repetition maximum in the arm/shoulder for people aged 75+—test-retest reliability. *Clinical Rehabilitation* 21: 258-265.

Sampon, C.A. 1895. *Strength: A Treatise on the Development and Use of Muscle.* London: Edward Arnold.

Sanborn, K., R. Boros, J. Hruby, B. Schilling, H.S. O'Bryant, R.L. Johnson, T. Hoke, M.E. Stone, and M.H. Stone. 2000. Short-term performance effects of weight training with multiple sets not to failure vs a single set to failure in women. *Journal of Strength and Conditioning Research* 14: 328-331.

Schmidtbleicher, D. 1992. Training for power events. In *Strength and Power in Sport,* edited by P.V. Komi. Oxford, UK: Blackwell Science Ltd.

Shellock, F.G., and W.E. Prentice. 1985. Warming-up and stretching for improved physical performance and prevention of sports-related injuries. *Sports Medicine* 2: 267-278.

Shimano, T., W.J. Kraemer, B.A. Spiering, J.S. Volek, D.L. Hatfield, R. Silvestre, J.L. Vingren, M.S. Fragala, C.M. Maresh, S.J. Fleck, R.U. Newton, L.P.B. Spreuwenberg, and K. Häkkinen. 2006. Relationship between the number of repetitions and selected percentages of one repetition maximum in free weight exercises in trained and untrained men. *Journal of Strength and Conditioning Research* 20: 819-823.

Siff, M.C. 2000. *Supertraining.* Denver: Supertraining Institute.

Smith, K., K. Winegard, A.L. Hicks, and N. McCartney. 2003. Two years of resistance training in older men and women: The effects of three years of detraining on the retention of dynamic strength. *Canadian Journal of Applied Physiology* 28: 462-474.

Stewart, R.D., T.A. Duhamel, S. Rich, A.R. Tupling, and H.J. Green. 2008. Effects of consecutive days of exercise and recovery on muscle mechanical function. *Medicine & Science in Sports & Exercise* 40: 316-325.

Stienen, G.J.M., J.L. Kiers, R. Bottinelli, and C. Reggiani. 1996. Myofibrillar ATPase activity in skinned human skeletal muscle fibres: Fibre type and temperature dependence. *Journal of Physiology* 493: 299-307.

Stone, M.H., K. Sanborn, H.S. O'Bryant, M. Hartman, M.E. Stone, C. Proulx, B. Ward, and J. Hruby. 2003. Maximum strength-power-performance relationships in collegiate throwers. *Journal of Strength and Conditioning Research* 17: 739-745.

Stone, M.H., W.A. Sands, J. Carlock, S. Callan, D. Dickie, K. Daigle, J. Cotton, S.L. Smith, and M. Hartman. 2004. The importance of isometric maximum strength and peak rate-of-force development in sprint cycling. *Journal of Strength and Conditioning Research* 18: 878-884.

Stone, M.H., M. Stone, and W.A. Sands. 2007. *Principles and Practice of Resistance Training.* Champaign, IL: Human Kinetics.

Tan, B. 1999. Manipulating resistance training program variables to optimize maximum strength in men: A review. *Journal of Strength and Conditioning Research* 13: 289-304.

Ter Haar Romney, B.M., J.J. van der Gon, and C.C.A.M. Gielen. 1982. Changes in recruitment order of motor units in the human biceps muscle. *Experimental Neurology* 78: 360-368.

Ter Haar Romney, B.M., J.J. van der Gon, and C.C.A.M. Gielen. 1984. Relation between location of a motor unit in the human biceps brachii and its critical firing levels for different tasks. *Experimental Neurology* 85: 631-650.

Tidow, G. 1990. Aspects of strength training in athletics. *New Studies in Athletics* 1: 93-110.

Vandervoort, A.A., and T.B. Symons. 1997. Functional and metabolic consequences of sarcopenia. *Canadian Journal of Applied Physiology* 26: 90-101.

Wilson, G. 2000. Limitations of the use of isometric testing in athletic assessment. In *Physiological Tests for Elite Athletes,* edited by C.J. Gore, 151-154. Champaign, IL: Human Kinetics.

Wilson, G.J., A.J. Murphy, and A. Giorgi. 1996. Weight and plyometric training: Effects on eccentric and concentric force production. *Canadian Journal of Applied Physiology* 21: 301-315.

Wrigley, T., and G. Strauss. 2000. Strength assessment by isokinetic dynamometry. In *Physiological Tests for Elite Athletes,* edited by C.J. Gore, 155-199. Champaign, IL: Human Kinetics.

Wyszomierski, S.A., A.J. Chambers, and R. Cham. 2009. Knee strength capabilities and slip severity. *Journal of Applied Biomechanics* 25: 140-148.

Young, W.B., and D.G. Behm. 2002. Should static stretching be used during a warm-up for strength and power activities? *Strength and Conditioning Journal* 24: 33-37.

Young, W.B., and G.E. Bilby. 1993. The effect of voluntary effort to influence speed of contraction on strength, muscular power, and hypertrophy development. *Journal of Strength and Conditioning Research* 7: 172-178.

Zajac, F.E., and M.E. Gordon. 1989. Determining muscle's force and action in multi-articular movement. *Exercise and Sport Science Reviews* 17: 187-230.

Zatsiorsky, V.M. 1995. *Science and Practice of Strength Training.* Champaign, IL: Human Kinetics.

Chapter 8

Abernethy, P., G. Wilson, and P. Logan. 1995. Strength and power assessment: Issues, controversies and challenges. *Sports Medicine* 19: 401-417.

Adams, K.J., A.M. Swank, K.L. Barnard, J.M. Bering, and P.G. Stevene-Adams. 2000. Safety of maximal power, strength, and endurance testing in older African American women. *Journal of Strength and Conditioning Research* 14: 254-260.

Allen, D.G., G.D. Lamb, and H. Westerblad. 2008. Skeletal muscle fatigue: Cellular mechanisms. *Physiology Reviews* 88: 287-332.

Baker, D. 2009. Ability and validity of three different methods of assessing upper-body strength endurance to distinguish playing rank in professional rugby league players. *Journal of Strength and Conditioning Research* 23: 1578-1582.

Baker, D.G., and R.U. Newton. 2006. Discriminative analysis of various upper body tests in professional rugby league players. *International Journal of Sports Physiology and Performance* 1: 347-360.

Baumgartner, T.A., A.S. Jackson, M.T. Mahar, and D.A. Rowe. 2007. *Measurement and Evaluation in Physical Education and Exercise Science.* New York: McGraw-Hill.

Baumgartner, T.A., S. Oh, H. Chung, and D. Hales. 2002. Objectivity, reliability, and validity for a revised push-up test protocol. *Measurement in Physical Education and Exercise Science* 6: 225-242.

Boland, E., D. Boland, T. Carroll, and W.R. Barfield. 2009. Comparison of the Power Plate and free weight exercises on upper body muscular endurance in college age subjects. *International Journal of Exercise Science* 2: 215-222.

Chapman, P.P., J.R. Whitehead, and R.H. Binkert. 1998. The 225-lb reps-to-fatigue test as a submaximal estimate of 1-RM bench press performance in college football players. *Journal of Strength and Conditioning Research* 12: 258-261.

Clemons, J.M., C.A. Duncan, O.E. Blanchard, W.H. Gatch, D.B. Hollander, and J.L. Doucet. 2004. Relationships between the flexed-arm hang and selected measures of muscular fitness. *Journal of Strength and Conditioning Research* 18: 630-636.

Earle, R.W., and T.R. Baechle. 2008. Resistance training and spotting techniques. In *Essentials of Strength Training and Conditioning*, edited by T.R. Baechle and R.W. Earle, 325-376. Champaign, IL: Human Kinetics.

Eisenmann, J.C., and R.M. Malina. 2003. Age- and sex-associated variation in neuromuscular capacities of adolescent distance runners. *Journal of Sports Sciences* 21: 551-557.

Engelman, M.E., and J.R. Morrow. 1991. Reliability and skinfold correlates for traditional and modified pull-ups in children greade 3–5. *Research Quarterly for Exercise and Sports* 62: 88-91.

Foldvari, M., M. Clark, L.C. Laviolette, M.A. Bernstein, D. Kaliton, C. Castaneda, C.T. Pu, J.M. Hausdorff, R.A. Fielding, and M.A. Fiatarone Singh. 2000. Association of muscle power with functional status in community-dwelling elderly women. *Journal of Gerontology. Series A, Biological and Medical Sciences* 22: M192-M199.

Grant, S., T. Hasler, C. Davies, T.C. Aitchison, J. Wilson, and A. Whittaker. 2001. A comparison of the anthropometric, strength, endurance and flexibility characteristics of female elite and recreational climbers and non-climbers. *Journal of Sports Sciences* 19: 499-505.

Grant, S., V. Hynes, A. Whittaker, and T. Aitchison. 1996. Anthropometric, strength, endurance and flexibility characteristics of elite and recreational climbers. *Journal of Sports Sciences* 14: 301-309.

Halet, K.A., J.L. Mayhew, C. Murphy, and J. Fanthorpe. 2009. Relationship of 1 repetition maximum lat-pull to pull-up and lat-pull repetitions in elite collegiate women swimmers. *Journal of Strength and Conditioning Research* 23: 1496-1502.

Harman, E. 2008. Principles of test selection and administration. In *Essentials of Strength Training and Conditioning*, edited by T.R. Baechle and R.W. Earle, 237-247. Champaign, IL: Human Kinetics.

Henwood, T.R., S. Riek, and D.R. Taafe. 2008. Strength versus power-specific resistance training in community-dwelling older adults. *Journal of Gerontology. Series A, Biological and Medical Sciences* 63: 83-91.

Hoffman, J. 2006. *Norms for Fitness, Performance, and Health*. Champaign, IL: Human Kinetics.

Hoffman, J.R., W.J. Kraemer, A.C. Fry, M. Deschenes, and M. Kemp. 1990. The effects of self-selection for frequency of training in a winter conditioning program for football. *Journal of Applied Sport Science Research* 4: 76-82.

Kraemer, W.J., K. Adams, E. Cafarelli, G.A. Dudley, C. Dooly, et al. 2002. American College of Sports Medicine position stand: Progression models in resistance training for healthy adults. *Medicine & Science in Sports & Exercise* 34: 364-380.

LaChance, P.F., and T. Hortobagyi. 1994. Influence of cadence on muscular performance during push-up and pull-up exercise. *Journal of Strength and Conditioning Research* 8: 76-79.

Maffiuletti, N.A., M. Bizzini, K. Desbrosses, N. Babault, and M. Munzinger. 2007. Reliability of knee extension and flexion measurements using the Con-Trex isokinetic dynamometer. *Clinical Physiology and Functional Imaging* 27: 346-353.

Mayhew, J.L., J.A. Jacques, J.S. Ware, P.P. Chapman, M.G. Bemben, T.E. Ward, and J.P. Slovak. 2004. Anthropometric dimensions do not enhance one repetition maximum prediction from the NFL-225 test in college football players. *Journal of Strength and Conditioning Research* 18: 572-578.

Mazzetti, S.A., W.J. Kraemer, J.S. Volek, N.D. Duncan, N.A. Ratamess, R.U. Newton, K. Häkkinen, and S.J. Fleck. 2000. The influence of direct supervision of resistance training on strength performance. *Medicine & Science in Sports & Exercise* 32: 1175-1184.

Meir, R., R. Newton, E. Curtis, M. Fardell, and B. Butler. 2001. Physical fitness qualities of professional rugby league football players: Determination of positional differences. *Journal of Strength and Conditioning Research* 15: 450-458.

Murphy, A.J., and G.J. Wilson. 1997. The ability of tests of muscular function to reflect training induced changes in performance. *Journal of Sports Sciences* 15: 191-200.

Rana, S.R., G.S. Chleboun, R.M. Gilders, F.C. Hagerman, J.R. Herman, R.S. Hikida, M.R. Kushnick, R.S. Staron, and K. Toma. 2008. Comparison of early phase adaptations for traditional strength and endurance, and low velocity resistance training programs in college-aged women. *Journal of Strength and Conditioning Research* 22: 119-127.

Rassier, D.E., B.R. MacIntosh, and W. Herzog. 1999. Length dependence of active force production in skeletal muscle. *Journal of Applied Physiology* 86: 1445-1457.

Reynolds, J.M., T.J. Gordon, and R.A. Robergs. 2006. Prediction of one repetition maximum strength from multiple repetition maximum testing and anthropometry. *Journal of Strength and Conditioning Research* 20: 584-592.

Rivera, M.A., A.M. Rivera-Brown, and W.R. Frontera. 1998. Health related physical fitness characteristics of elite Puerto Rican athletes. *Journal of Strength and Conditioning Research* 12: 199-203.

Saint Romain, B., and M.T. Mahar. 2001. Norm-referenced and criterion-referenced reliability of the push-up and modified pull-up. *Measurement in Physical Education and Exercise Science* 5: 67-80.

Sherman, T., and J.P. Barfield. 2006. Equivalence reliability among the FITNESSGRAM® upper-body tests of muscular strength and endurance. *Measurement in Physical Education and Exercise Science* 10: 241-254.

Siegel, J.A., D.N. Camaione, and T.G. Manfredi. 1989. The effects of upper body resistance training on prepubescent children. *Pediatric Exercise Science* 1: 145-154.

Siff, M.C. 2000. *Supertraining*. Denver: Supertraining Institute.

Stone, M.H., M. Stone, and W.A. Sands. 2007. *Principles and Practice of Resistance Training*. Champaign, IL: Human Kinetics.

Stone, M.H., M. Stone, W.A. Sands, K.C. Pierce, R.U. Newton, G.G. Haff, and J. Carlock. 2006. Maximum strength and strength training—A relationship to endurance? *Strength and Conditioning Journal* 28: 44-53.

Vescovi, J.D., T.M. Murray, and J.L. Van Heest. 2007. Positional performance profiling of elite ice hockey players. *International Journal of Sports Physiology and Performance* 1: 84-94.

Williford, H.N., W.J. Duey, M.S. Olson, R. Howard, and N. Wang. 1999. Relationship between fire fighting suppression tasks and physical fitness. *Ergonomics* 42: 1179-1186.

Woods, J.A., R.R. Pate, and M.L. Burgess. 1992. Correlates to performance on field tests of muscular strength. *Pediatric Exercise Science* 4: 302-311.

Zatsiorsky, V.M. 1995. *Science and Practice of Strength Training*. Champaign, IL: Human Kinetics.

Chapter 9

Aagaard, P., E.B. Simonsen, J.L. Andersen, P. Magnusson, and P. Dyhre-Poulsen. 2002. Increased rate of force development and neural drive of human skeletal muscle following resistance training. *Journal of Applied Physiology* 93: 1318-1326.

Alexander, R.M. 2000. Storage and release of elastic energy in the locomotor system and the stretch-shortening cycle. In *Biomechanics and Biology of Movement,* edited by B.M. Nigg, B.R. MacIntosh, and J. Mester. Champaign, IL: Human Kinetics.

Atha, J. 1981. Strengthening muscle. *Exercise and Sport Science Reviews* 9: 1-73.

Ayalon, A., O. Inbar, and O. Bar-Or. 1974. Relationship among measurements of explosive strength and aerobic power. In *International Series on Sport Sciences, Vol I,* edited by R.C. Nelson, and C.A. Morehouse. New York: MacMillan.

Baker, D., S. Nance, and M. Moore. 2001. The load that maximizes the average mechanical power output during jump squats in power trained athletes. *Journal of Strength and Conditioning Research* 15: 92-97.

Bannister, E.W. 1991. Modeling elite athletic performance. In *Physiological Testing of the High Performance Athlete,* edited by J.D. MacDougall, H.A. Wenger, and H.J. Green. Champaign, IL: Human Kinetics.

Bar-Or, O. 1987. The Wingate Anaerobic Test: An update on methodology. Validity and reliability. *Sports Medicine* 4: 381-394.

Bar-Or, O. 1992. An abbreviated Wingate Anaerobic Test for women and men of advanced age. *Medicine & Science in Sports & Exercise* 24: S22.

Bartlett, R. 2007. *Introduction to Sports Biomechanics: Analysing Human Movement Patterns,* 2nd ed. London: Routledge.

Baudry, S., and J. Duchateau. 2007. Postactivation potentiation in a human muscle: Effect on the rate of torque development of tetanic and voluntary isometric contractions. *Journal of Applied Physiology* 102: 1394-1401.

Bean, J.F., D.K. Kiely, S. Herman, S.G. Leveille, K. Mizer, W.R. Frontera, and R.A. Fielding. 2002. The relationship between leg power and physical performance in mobility-limited older people. *Journal of the American Geriatric Society* 50: 461-467.

Bobbert, M.F., K.G. Gerritsen, M.C. Litjens, and A.J. Van Soest. 1996. Why is countermovement jump height greater than squat jump height? *Medicine & Science in Sports & Exercise* 28: 1402-1412.

Carlock, J.M., S.L. Smith, M.J. Hartman, R.T. Morris, D.A. Ciroslan, K.C. Pierce, R.U. Newton, E.A. Harman, W.A. Sands, and M.H. Stone. 2004. The relationship between vertical jump power estimates and weightlifting ability: A field-test approach. *Journal of Strength and Conditioning Research* 18: 534-539.

Chatzopoulos, D.E., C.J. Michailidis, A.K. Giannakos, K.C. Alexiou, D.A. Patikas, C.B. Antonopoulos, and C.M. Kotzamanidis. 2007. Postactivation potentiation effects after heavy resistance exercise. *Journal of Strength and Conditioning Research* 21 (4): 1278-1281.

Chelly, S.M., and C. Denis. 2001. Leg power and hopping stiffness: Relationship with sprint running performance. *Medicine & Science in Sports & Exercise* 33 (2): 326-333.

Chiu, L.Z.F., and J.L. Barnes. 2003. The fitness fatigue model revisited: Implications for planning short- and long-term training. *Strength and Conditioning Journal* 25 (6): 42-51.

Chmielewski, T.L., G.D. Myer, D. Kauffman, and S.M. Tillman. 2006. Plyometric exercise in the rehabilitation of athletes: Physiological responses and clinical application. *Journal of Orthopaedic & Sports Physical Therapy* 36 (5): 308-319.

Chu, D.A. 1996. *Explosive Power and Strength.* Champaign, IL: Human Kinetics.

Clemons, J., and M. Harrison. 2008. Validity and reliability of a new stair sprinting test of explosive power. *Journal of Strength and Conditioning Research* 22 (5): 1578-1583.

Clemons, J.M., B. Campbell, and C. Jeansonne. 2010. Validity and reliability of a new test of upper body power. *Journal of Strength and Conditioning Research* 24 (6): 1559-1565.

Cormie, P., and S.P. Flanagan. 2008. Does an optimal load exist for power training? Point-counterpoint. *Strength and Conditioning Journal* 30 (2): 67-69.

Cormie, P., G.O. McCaulley, and J.M. McBride. 2007. Power versus strength-power jump squat training: Influence on the load-power relationship. *Medicine & Science in Sports & Exercise* 39 (6): 996-1003.

Cormie, P., G.O. McCaulley, T.N. Triplett, and J.M. McBride. 2007. Optimal loading for maximal power output during lower-body resistance exercises. *Medicine & Science in Sports & Exercise* 39 (2): 340-349.

Cormie, P., McGuigan, M.R., and R.U. Newton. 2011a. Developing maximal neuromuscular power. Part 1 – Biological basis of maximal power production. *Sports Medicine* 41 (1): 17-38.

Cormie, P., McGuigan, M.R., and R.U. Newton. 2011b. Developing maximal neuromuscular power. Part 2 – Training considerations for improving maximal power production. *Sports Medicine* 41 (2): 125-146.

Cronin, J., and G. Sleivert. 2005. Challenges in understanding the influence of maximal power training on improving athletic performance. *Sports Medicine* 35 (3): 213-234.

Earles, D.R., J.O. Judge, and O.T. Gunnarsson. 1997. Power as a predictor of functional ability in community dwelling older persons. *Medicine & Science in Sports & Exercise* 29: S11.

Evans, W.J. 2000. Exercise strategies should be designed to increase muscle power. *Journal of Gerontology: Medical Science* 55A: M309-M310.

Faulkner, J.A., D.R. Claflin, and K.K. McCully. 1986. Power output of fast and slow fibers from human skeletal muscles. In *Human Power Output*, edited by N.L. Jones, N. McCartney, and A.J. McComas. Champaign, IL: Human Kinetics.

Flanagan, E.P., W.P. Ebben, and R.L. Jensen. 2008. Reliability of the reactive strength index and time to stabilization during depth jumps. *Journal of Strength and Conditioning Research* 22 (5): 1677-1682.

Flanagan, E.P., and A.J. Harrison. 2007. Muscle dynamics differences between legs, in healthy adults. *Journal of Strength and Conditioning Research* 21: 67-72.

Fox, E., R. Bowers, and M. Foss. 1993. *The Physiological Basis for Exercise and Sport.* Madison, WI: Brown & Benchmark.

Friedman, J.E., P.D. Neufer, and L.G. Dohm. 1991. Regulation of glycogen synthesis following exercise. *Sports Medicine* 11 (4): 232-243.

Garhammer, J. 1993. A review of power output studies of Olympic and power lifting: Methodology, performance prediction, and evaluation tests. *Journal of Strength and Conditioning Research* 7 (2): 76-89.

Gibala, M., J. Little, M. van Essen, G. Wilkin, K. Burgomaster, A. Safdar, S. Raha, and M. Tarnopolsky. 2006. Short-term sprint interval versus traditional endurance training: Similar initial adaptations in human skeletal muscle and exercise performance. *Journal of Physiology* 575 (Pt. 3): 901-911.

Gollnick, P.D., and A.W. Bayly. 1986. Biochemical training adaptations and maximal power. In *Human Muscle Power*, edited by N.L. Jones, N. McCartney, and A.J. McComas. Champaign, IL: Human Kinetics.

Ham, D.J., W.L. Knez, and W.B. Young. 2007. A deterministic model of the vertical jump: Implications for training. *Journal of Strength and Conditioning Research* 21 (3): 967-972.

Harman, E., and J. Garhammer. 2008. Administration, scoring, and interpretation of selected tests. In *NSCA's Essentials of Strength Training and Conditioning*, 3rd ed., edited by T.R. Baechle and R.W. Earle. Champaign, IL: Human Kinetics.

Harman, E.A., M.T. Rosenstein, P.N. Frykman, R.M. Rosenstein, and W.J. Kraemer. 1991. Estimation of human power output from vertical jump. *Journal of Applied Sport Science Research* 5 (3): 116-120.

Harris, R.C., R.H.T. Edwards, E. Hultman, L.O. Nordesjo, B. Nylind, and K. Sahlin. 1976. The time course of phosphorylcreatine resynthesis during recovery of the quadriceps muscle in man. *Pflugers Archives* 367: 137-142.

Hill, A.V. 1938. The heat of shortening and the dynamic constants of muscle. *Proceedings of the Royal Society of London* 126: 136.

Hill, A.V. 1964. The effect of load on the heat of shortening of muscle. *Proceedings of the Royal Society of London* 159: 297.

Hoffman, J. 2006. *Norms for Fitness, Performance and Health*. Champaign, IL: Human Kinetics.

Inbar, O., O. Bar-Or, and J.S. Skinner. 1996. *The Wingate Anaerobic Test*. Champaign, IL: Human Kinetics.

Josephson, R.K. 1993. Contraction dynamics and power output of skeletal muscle. *Annual Review of Physiology* 55: 527-546.

Kalamen, J.L. 1968. Measurement of maximum muscular power in man. PhD diss., The Ohio State University, Columbus, OH.

Kaneko, M., T. Fuchimoto, H. Toji, and K. Suei. 1983. Training effect of different loads on the force-velocity relationship and mechanical power output in human muscle. *Scandinavian Journal of Medicine & Science in Sports* 5: 50-55.

Krogh, A., and J. Lindhard. 1913. The regulation of respiration and circulation during the initial stages of muscular work. *Journal of Physiology* 47: 112-136.

Lunn, W.R., J.A. Finn, and R.S. Axtell. 2009. Effects of sprint interval training and body weight reduction on power to weight ratio in experienced cyclists. *Journal of Strength and Conditioning Research* 23 (4): 1217-1224.

Margaria, R., P. Aghemo, and E. Rovelli. 1966. Measurement of muscular power (anaerobic) in man. *Journal of Applied Physiology* 21: 1662-1664.

Maud, P.J., and B.B. Shultz. 1989. Norms for the Wingate Anaerobic Test with comparison to another similar test. *Research Quarterly for Exercise & Sport* 60 (2): 144-151.

McArdle, W.D., F.I. Katch, and V.L. Katch. 2007. *Exercise Physiology: Energy, Nutrition, and Human Performance*, 6th ed. Philadelphia: Lippincott Williams & Wilkins.

McGuigan, M.R., T.L.A. Doyle, M. Newton, D.J. Edwards, S. Nimphius, and R.U. Newton. 2006. Eccentric utilization ratio: Effect of sport and phase of training. *Journal of Strength and Conditioning Research* 20 (4): 992-995.

Nindl, B.C., M.T. Mahar, E.A. Harman, and J.F. Patton. 1995. Lower and upper body anaerobic performance in male and female adolescent athletes. *Medicine & Science in Sports & Exercise* 27: 235-241.

Nordlund, M.M., A. Thorstensson, and A.G. Cresswell. 2004. Central and peripheral contributions to fatigue in relation to level of activation during repeated maximal voluntary isometric plantar flexions. *Journal of Applied Physiology* 96: 218-225.

Patterson, D.D., and D.H. Peterson. 2004. Vertical jump and leg power norms for young adults. *Measurement in Physical Education and Exercise Science* 8: 33-41.

Poussen, M., J. Van Hoeke, and F. Goubel. 1990. Changes in elastic characteristics of human muscle induced by eccentric exercise. *Journal of Biomechanics* 23: 343-348.

Puthoff, M.L., and D.H. Nielsen. 2007. Relationships among impairments in lower-extremity strength and power, functional limitations, and disability in older adults. *Physical Therapy* 87 (10): 1334-1347.

Racinais, S., D. Bishop, R. Denis, G. Lattier, A. Mendez-Villaneuva, and S. Perrey. 2007. Muscle deoxygenation and neural drive to the muscle during repeated sprint cycling. *Medicine & Science in Sports & Exercise* 39: 268-274.

Sayers, S.P., D.V. Harackiewicz, E.A. Harman, P.N. Frykman, and M.T. Rosenstein. 1999. Cross-validation of three jump power equations. *Medicine & Science in Sports & Exercise* 31: 572-577.

Stone, M.H., D. Collins, S. Plisk, G. Haff, and M.E. Stone. 2000. Training principles: Evaluation of modes and methods of resistance training. *Strength and Conditioning Journal* 22 (3): 65-76.

Suetta, C., P. Aagaard, S.P. Magnusson, L.L. Andersen, S. Sipila, A. Rosted, A.K. Jakobsen, B. Duus, and M. Kjaer. 2007. Muscle size, neuromuscular activation, and rapid force characteristics in elderly men and women: Effects of unilateral long-term disuse due to hip-osteoarthritis. *Journal of Applied Physiology* 102: 942-948.

Suetta, C., P. Aagaard, A. Rosted, A.K. Jakobsen, B. Duus, M. Kjaer, and S.P. Magnusson. 2004. Training-induced changes in muscle CSA, muscle strength, EMG, and rate of force development in elderly subjects after long-term unilateral disuse. *Journal of Applied Physiology* 97: 1954-1961.

Suzuki, T., J.F. Bean, and R.A. Fielding. 2001. Muscle power of the ankle flexors predicts functional performance in community-dwelling older women. *Journal of the American Geriatrics Society* 49: 1161-1167.

Thorstensson, A., J. Karlsson, H.T. Viitasalo, P. Luhtanen, and P.V. Komi. 1976. Effect of strength training on EMG of human skeletal muscle. *Acta Physiologica Scandinavica* 98: 232-236.

Walshe, A.D., G.J. Wilson, and A.J. Murphy. 1996. The validity and reliability of a test of lower body musculotendinous stiffness. *European Journal of Applied Physiology* 73: 332-339.

Wilson, G.J., A.J. Murphy, and J.F. Pryor. 1994. Musculotendinous stiffness: Its relationship to eccentric, isometric, and concentric performance. *Journal of Applied Physiology* 76 (6): 2714-2719.

Wu, J.Z., and W. Herzog. 1999. Modeling concentric contraction of muscle using an improved cross-bridge model. *Journal of Biomechanics* 32: 837-848.

Yucesoy, C.A., J.M. Koopman, P.A. Huijing, and H.J. Grootenboer. 2002. Three-dimensional finite element modeling of skeletal muscle using a two-domain approach: Linked fiber-matrix mesh model. *Journal of Biomechanics* 35 (9): 1253-1262.

Zupan, M.F., A.W. Arata, L.H. Dawson, A.L. Wile, T.L. Payn, and M.E. Hannon. 2009. Wingate Anaerobic Test peak power and anaerobic capacity classifications for men and women intercollegiate athletes. *Journal of Strength and Conditioning Research* 23 (9): 2598-2604.

Chapter 10

Altug, Z., T. Altug, and A. Altug. 1987. A test selection guide for assessing and evaluating athletes. *National Strength and Conditioning Association Journal* 9 (3): 62-66.

Bandy, W.D., J.M. Irion, and M. Briggler. 1998. The effect of static stretch and dynamic range of motion training on the flexibility of the hamstring muscles. *Journal of Orthopedic and Sports Physical Therapy* 4: 295-300.

Behm, D.G., D.C. Button, and J.C. Butt. 2001. Factors affecting force loss with prolonged stretching. *Canadian Journal of Applied Physiology* 26 (3): 261-272.

Church, J.B., M.S. Wiggins, F.M. Moode, and R. Crist. 2001. Effect of warm-up and flexibility treatments on vertical jump performance. *Journal of Strength and Conditioning Research* 15 (3): 332-336.

Cressey, E.M., C.A. West, D.P. Tiberio, W.J. Kraemer, and C.M. Maresh. 2007. The effects of ten weeks of lower-body unstable surface training on markers of athletic performance. *Journal of Strength and Conditioning Research* 21 (2): 561-567.

Farlinger, C.M., L.D. Kruisselbrink, and J.R. Fowles. 2007. Relationships to skating performance in competitive hockey players. *Journal of Strength and Conditioning Research* 21 (3): 915-922.

Fletcher, I.M., and B. Jones. 2004. The effect of different warm-up stretch protocols on 20 meter sprint performance in trained rugby union players. *Journal of Strength and Conditioning Research* 18 (4): 885-888.

Gabbett, T.J. 2007. Physiological and anthropometric characteristics of elite women rugby league players. *Journal of Strength and Conditioning Research* 21 (3): 875-881.

Gabbett, T., and B. Georgieff. 2007. Physiological and anthropometric characteristics of Australian junior national, state, and novice volleyball players. *Journal of Strength and Conditioning Research* 21 (3): 902-908.

Harman, E., and J. Garhammer. 2008. Administration, scoring, and interpretation of selected tests. In *Essentials of Strength Training and Conditioning,* 3rd ed., edited by T.R. Baechle, and R.W. Earle, 250-292. Champaign, IL: Human Kinetics.

Hedrick, A. 2000. Dynamic flexibility training. *Strength and Conditioning Journal* 22 (5): 33-38.

Hoffman, J. 2006. *Norms for Fitness, Performance, and Health.* Champaign, IL: Human Kinetics.

Hoffman, J.R., N.A. Ratamess, K.L. Neese, R.E. Ross, J. Kang, J.F. Nagrelli, and A.D. Faigenbaum. 2009. Physical performance characteristics in NCAA Division III champion female lacrosse athletes. *Journal of Strength and Conditioning Research* 23 (5): 1524-1539.

Kovacs, M.S., R. Pritchett, P.J. Wickwire, J.M. Green, P. Bishop. 2007. Physical performance changes after unsupervised training during the autumn/spring semester break in competitive tennis players. *British Journal of Sports Medicine* 41 (11): 705-710.

Mann, D.P., and M.T. Jones. 1999. Guidelines to the implementation of a dynamic stretching program. *Strength and Conditioning Journal* 21 (6): 53-55.

Nelson, A.G., and J. Kokkonen. 2001. Acute muscle stretching inhibits maximal strength performance. *Research Quarterly for Exercise and Sport* 72 (4): 415-419.

Plisk, S. 2008. Speed, agility, and speed-endurance development. In *Essentials of Strength Training and Conditioning,* 3rd ed., edited by T.R. Baechle, and R.W. Earle, 458-485. Champaign, IL: Human Kinetics.

Power, K., D. Behm, F. Cahill, M. Carroll, and W. Young. 2004. An acute bout of static stretching: Effects on force and jumping performance. *Medicine & Science in Sports & Exercise* 36 (8): 1389-1396.

Young, W.B., and D.G. Behm. 2003. Effects of running, static stretching, and practice jumps on explosive force production and jumping performance. *Journal of Sports Medicine and Physical Fitness* 43 (1): 21-27.

Chapter 11

Berryman Reese, N., and W.D. Bandy. 2002. *Joint Range of Motion and Muscle Length Testing.* Philadelphia: W.B. Saunders.

Bobbert, M.F., and G.J. van Ingen Schenau. 1988. Coordination in vertical jumping. *Journal of Biomechanics* 21: 249-262.

Brosseau, L., S. Balmer, M. Tousignant, J.P. O'Sullivan, C. Goudreault, M. Goudreault, and S. Gringras. 2001. Intra- and intertester reliability and criterion validity of the parallelogram and universal goniometers for measuring maximum active knee flexion and extension of patients with knee restrictions. *Archives of Physical Medicine and Rehabilitation* 82: 396-402.

Burkhart, S.S., C.D. Morgan, and W.B. Kibler. 2003. The disabled throwing shoulder: Spectrum of pathology part 1: Pathoanatomy and biomechanics. *Arthroscopy: The Journal of Arthroscopic and Related Surgery* 19: 404-420.

Cook, G. 2001. Baseline sports-fitness testing. In *High Performance Sports Conditioning: Modern Training for Ultimate Athletic Development,* edited by B. Foran, 19-48. Champaign, IL: Human Kinetics.

Corkery, M., H. Briscoe, N. Ciccone, G. Foglia, P. Johnson, S. Kinsman, L. Legere, B. Lum, and P.K. Canavan. 2007. Establishing normal values for lower extremity muscle length in college-age students. *Physical Therapy in Sport* 8: 66-74.

Croxford, P., K. Jones, and K. Barker. 1998. Inter-tester comparison between visual estimation and goniometric measurement of ankle dorsiflexion. *Physiotherapy Theory and Practice* 14: 107-113.

Fayad, F., S. Hanneton, M.M. Lefevre-Colau, S. Poiraudeau, M. Revel, and A. Roby-Brami. 2008. The trunk as a part of the kinematic chain for arm elevation in healthy subjects and in patients with frozen shoulder. *Brain Research* 1191: 107-115.

Fleisig, G.S., S.W. Barrentine, R.F. Escamilla, and J.R. Andrews. 1996. Biomechanics of overhand throwing with implications for injuries. *Sports Medicine* 21: 421-437.

Haff, G.G., J.T. Cramer, T.W. Beck, A.D. Egan, S.D. Davis, J. McBride, and D. Wathen. 2006. Roundtable discussion: Flexibility training. *Strength and Conditioning Journal* 28: 64-85.

Houglum, P.A. 2005. *Therapeutic Exercise for Musculoskeletal Injuries.* Champaign, IL: Human Kinetics.

Kadaba, M.P., H.K. Ramakrishnan, M.E. Wooten, J. Gainey, G. Gorton, and G.V.B. Cochran. 1989. Repeatability of kinematic, kinetic, and electromyographic data in normal adult gait. *Journal of Orthopaedic Research* 7: 849-860.

Kendall, F.P., E.K. McCreary, and P.G. Provance. 1993. *Muscles: Testing and Function.* Philadelphia: Lippincott Williams & Wilkins.

Kiesel, K., P.J. Plisky, and M.L. Voight. 2007. Can serious injury in professional football be predicted by a preseason functional movement screen? *North American Journal of Sports Physical Therapy* 2: 147-158.

Knapik, J.J., C.L. Bauman, B.H. Jones, J.M. Harris, and L. Vaughan. 1991. Preseason strength and flexibility imbalances associated with athletic injuries in female collegiate athletes. *American Journal of Sports Medicine* 19: 76-81.

Knudson, D.V., and C.S. Morrison. 1997. *Qualitative Analysis of Human Movement.* Champaign, IL: Human Kinetics.

Lett, K.K., and S.M. McGill. 2006. Pushing and pulling: Personal mechanics influence spine loads. *Ergonomics* 49: 895-908.

Levangie, P.K., and C.C. Norkin. 2001. *Joint Structure and Function: A Comprehensive Analysis.* Philadelphia: F.A. Davis.

Loudon, J.K., W. Jenkins, and K.L. Loudon. 1996. The relationship between static posture and ACL injury in female athletes. *Journal of Orthopaedic & Sports Physical Therapy* 24: 91-97.

Markolf, K.L., D.I. Burchfield, M.M. Shapiro, M.E. Shepard, G.A.M. Finerman, and J.L. Slauterbeck. 1995. Combined knee loading states that generate high anterior cruciate ligament forces. *Journal of Orthopaedic Research* 13: 930-935.

McGill, S.M., R.L. Hughson, and K. Parks. 2000. Changes in lumbar lordosis modify the role of the extensor muscles. *Clinical Biomechanics* 15: 777-780.

Norkin, C.C., and D.J. White. 1995. *Measurement of Joint Motion: A Guide to Goniometry.* Philadelphia: F.A. Davis.

Novacheck, T.F. 1998. The biomechanics of running. *Gait & Posture* 7: 77-95.

Robertson, V.J., A.R. Ward, and P. Jung. 2005. The effect of heat on tissue extensibility: A comparison of deep and superficial heating. *Archives of Physical Medicine and Rehabilitation* 86: 819-825.

Scannell, J.P., and S.M. McGill. 2003. Lumbar posture: Should it, and can it, be modified? A study of passive tissue stiffness and lumbar position during activities of daily living. *Physical Therapy* 83: 907-917.

Shultz, S.J., P.A. Houglum, and D.H. Perrin. 2005. *Examination of Musculoskeletal Injuries.* Champaign, IL: Human Kinetics.

Sigward, S.M., S. Ota, and C.M. Powers. 2008. Predictors of frontal plane knee excursion during a drop land in young female soccer players. *Journal of Orthopaedic & Sports Physical Therapy* 38: 661-667.

Silder, A., S.B. Reeder, and D.G. Thelen. 2010. The influence of prior hamstring injury on lengthening muscle tissue mechanics. *Journal of Biomechanics* 43: 2254-2260.

Starkey, C., and J. Ryan. 2002. *Evaluation of Orthopedic and Athletic Injuries.* Philadelphia: F.A. Davis.

Stone, M., M.W. Ramsey, A.M. Kinser, H.S. O'Bryant, C. Ayers, and W. Sands. 2006. Stretching: Acute and chronic? The potential consequences. *Strength and Conditioning Journal* 28: 66-74.

Thacker, S.B., J. Gilchrist, D.F. Stroup, and C.D. Kimsey. 2004. The impact of stretching on sports injury risk: A systematic review of the literature. *Medicine & Science in Sports & Exercise* 36: 371-378.

Thelen, D.G., E.S. Chumanov, M.A. Sherry, and B.C. Heiderscheit. 2006. Neuromusculoskeletal models provide insights into the mechanisms and rehabilitation of hamstring strains. *Exercise and Sport Sciences Reviews* 34: 135-141.

Weir, J., and N. Chockalingam. 2007. Ankle joint dorsiflexion: Assessment of true values necessary for normal gait. *International Journal of Therapy and Rehabilitation* 14: 76-82.

Wenos, D.L., and J.G. Konin. 2004. Controlled warm-up intensity enhances hip range of motion. *Journal of Strength and Conditioning Research* 18: 529-533.

Werner, S.L., M. Suri, J.A. Guido, K. Meister, and D.G. Jones. 2008. Relationships between ball velocity and throwing mechanics in collegiate baseball pitchers. *Journal of Shoulder and Elbow Surgery* 17: 905-908.

Whiteley, R. 2007. Baseball throwing mechanics as they relate to pathology and performance: A review. *Journal of Sports Science and Medicine* 6: 1-20.

Willson, J.D., M.L. Ireland, and I. Davis. 2006. Core strength and lower extremity alignment during single leg squats. *Medicine & Science in Sports & Exercise* 38: 945-952.

Youdas, J.W., C.L. Bogard, and V.J. Suman. 1993. Reliability of goniometric measurements and visual estimates of ankle joint active range of motion obtained in a clinical setting. *Archives of Physical Medicine and Rehabilitation* 74: 1113-1118.

Zatsiorsky, V.M. 1998. *Kinematics of Human Motion.* Champaign, IL: Human Kinetics.

Chapter 12

Aaltonen, S., H. Karjalainen, A. Heinonen, J. Parkkari, and U.M. Kujala. 2007. Prevention of sports injuries: Systematic review of randomized controlled trials. *Archives of Internal Medicine* 167: 1585-1592.

Arnold, B.L., and R.J. Schmitz. 1998. Examination of balance measures produced by the biodex stability system. *Journal of Athletic Training* 33: 323-327.

Ashton-Miller, J.A., E.M. Wojtys, L.J. Huston, and D. Fry-Welch. 2001. Can proprioception really be improved by exercises? *Knee Surgery Sports Traumatology Arthroscopy* 9: 128-136.

Behm, D.G., M.J. Wahl, D.C. Button, K.E. Power, and K.G. Anderson. 2005. Relationship between hockey skating speed and selected performance measures. *Journal of Strength and Conditioning Research* 19: 326-331.

Blackburn, T., K.M. Guskiewicz, M.A. Petschauer, and W.E. Prentice. 2000. Balance and joint stability: The relative contributions of proprioception and muscular strength. *Journal of Sport Rehabilitation* 9: 315-328.

Bressel, E., J.C. Yonker, J. Kras, and E.M. Heath. 2007. Comparison of static and dynamic balance in female collegiate soccer, basketball, and gymnastics athletes. *Journal of Athletic Training* 42: 42-46.

Broglio, S.P., J.J. Sosnoff, K.S. Rosengren, and K. McShane. 2009. A comparison of balance performance: Computerized dynamic posturography and a random motion platform. *Archives of Physical Medicine and Rehabilitation* 90: 145-150.

Burkhart, S.S., C.D. Morgan, and W.B. Kibler. 2000. Shoulder injuries in overhead athletes: The "dead arm" revisited. *Clinics in Sports Medicine* 19: 125-158.

Cressey, E.M., C.A. West, D.P. Tiberio, W.J. Kraemer, and C.M. Maresh. 2007. The effects of ten weeks of lower-body unstable surface training on markers of athletic performance. *Journal of Strength and Conditioning Research* 21: 561-567.

Docherty, C.L., T.C.V. McLeod, and S.J. Shultz. 2006. Postural control deficits in participants with functional ankle instability as measured by the balance error scoring system. *Clinical Journal of Sport Medicine* 16: 203-208.

Drouin, J.M., P.A. Houglum, D.H. Perrin, and B.M. Gansneder. 2003. Weight-bearing and non-weight-bearing knee-joint reposition sense and functional performance. *Journal of Sport Rehabilitation* 12: 54-66.

Duncan, P.W., D.K. Weiner, J. Chandler, and S. Studenski. 1990. Functional reach: A new clinical measure of balance. *Journals of Gerontology* 45: M192-M197.

Eechaute, C., P. Vaes, and W. Duquet. 2009. The dynamic postural control is impaired in patients with chronic ankle instability: Reliability and validity of the multiple hop test. *Clinical Journal of Sport Medicine* 19: 107-114.

Evans, T., J. Hertel, and W. Sebastianelli. 2004. Bilateral deficits in postural control following lateral ankle sprain. *Foot & Ankle International* 25: 833-839.

Gribble, P. 2003. The star excursion balance test as a measurement tool. *Athletic Therapy Today* 8: 46-47.

Gribble, P.A., and J. Hertel. 2003. Considerations for normalizing measures of the star excursion balance test. *Measurement in Physical Education and Exercise Science* 7: 89-100.

Gribble, P.A., W.S. Tucker, and P.A. White. 2007. Time-of-day influences on static and dynamic postural control. *Journal of Athletic Training* 42: 35-41.

Hamilton, R.T., S.J. Shultz, R.J. Schmitz, and D.H. Perrin. 2008. Triple-hop distance as a valid predictor of lower limb strength and power. *Journal of Athletic Training* 43: 144-151.

Herrington, L., J. Hatcher, A. Hatcher, and M. McNicholas. 2009. A comparison of Star Excursion Balance Test reach distances between ACL deficient patients and asymptomatic controls. *Knee* 16: 149-152.

Hertel, J., R.A. Braham, S.A. Hale, and L.C. Olmsted-Kramer. 2006. Simplifying the star excursion balance test: Analyses of subjects with and without chronic ankle instability. *Journal of Orthopaedic & Sports Physical Therapy* 36: 131-137.

Hertel, J., S.J. Miller, and C.R. Denegar. 2000. Intratester and intertester reliability during the Star Excursion Balance Tests. *Journal of Sport Rehabilitation* 9: 104-116.

Hertel, J., and L.C. Olmsted-Kramer. 2007. Deficits in time-to-boundary measures of postural control with chronic ankle instability. *Gait & Posture* 25: 33-39.

Hof, A.L. 2007. The equations of motion for a standing human reveal three mechanisms for balance. *Journal of Biomechanics* 40: 451-457.

Horak, F.B., and L.M. Nashner. 1986. Central programming of postural movements: Adaptation to altered support-surface configurations. *Journal of Neurophysiology* 55: 1369-1381.

Hrysomallis, C. 2011. Balance ability and athletic performance. *Sports Medicine* 41: 221-232.

Hrysomallis, C., P. McLaughlin, and C. Goodman. 2007. Balance and injury in elite Australian footballers. *International Journal of Sports Medicine* 28: 844-847.

Iverson, G. L., M. L. Kaarto, and M. S. Koehle. 2008. Normative data for the balance error scoring system: Implications for brain injury evaluations. *Brain Injury* 22:147-152.

Johnson, B.L., and J.K. Nelson. 1986. *Practical Measurements for Evaluation in Physical Education.* New York: MacMillan.

Kinzey, S.J., and C.W. Armstrong. 1998. The reliability of the star-excursion test in assessing dynamic balance. *Journal of Orthopaedic & Sports Physical Therapy* 27: 356-360.

Lafond, D., H. Corriveau, R. Hebert, and F. Prince. 2004. Intrasession reliability of center of pressure measures of postural steadiness in healthy elderly people. *Archives of Physical Medicine and Rehabilitation* 85: 896-901.

Lanning, C.L., T.L. Uhl, C.L. Ingram, C.G. Mattacola, T. English, and S. Newsom. 2006. Baseline values of trunk endurance and hip strength in collegiate athletes. *Journal of Athletic Training* 41:427-434.

Lee, A.J.Y., and W.H. Lin. 2008. Twelve-week biomechanical ankle platform system training on postural stability and ankle proprioception in subjects with unilateral functional ankle instability. *Clinical Biomechanics* 23: 1065-1072.

Mackey, D.C., and S.N. Robinovitch. 2005. Postural steadiness during quiet stance does not associate with ability to recover balance in older women. *Clinical Biomechanics* 20: 776-783.

MacKinnon, C.D., and D.A. Winter. 1993. Control of whole-body balance in the frontal plane during human walking. *Journal of Biomechanics* 26: 633-644.

Marsh, D.W., L.A. Richard, L.A. Williams, and K.J. Lynch. 2004. The relationship between balance and pitching error in college baseball pitchers. *Journal of Strength and Conditioning Research* 18: 441-446.

McCurdy, K., and G. Langford. 2006. The relationship between maximum unilateral squat strength and balance in young adult men and women. *Journal of Sports Science and Medicine* 5: 282-288.

McKeon, P.O., C.D. Ingersoll, D.C. Kerrigan, E. Saliba, B.C. Bennett, and J. Hertel. 2008. Balance training improves function and postural control in those with chronic ankle instability. *Medicine & Science in Sports & Exercise* 40: 1810-1819.

Nashner, L.M. 1997a. Computerized dynamic posturography. In *Handbook of Balance Function Testing,* edited by G.P. Jacobson, C.W. Newman, and J.M. Kartush, 280-307. San Diego: Singular Publishing Group.

Nashner, L.M. 1997b. Practical biomechanics and physiology of balance. In *Handbook of Balance Function Testing*, edited by G.P. Jacobson, C.W. Newman, and J.M. Kartush, 261-279. San Diego: Singular Publishing Group.

Olmsted, L.C., C.R. Carcia, J. Hertel, and S.J. Shultz. 2002. Efficacy of the star excursion balance tests in detecting reach deficits in subjects with chronic ankle instability. *Journal of Athletic Training* 37: 501-506.

Pai, Y.C., B.E. Maki, K. Iqbal, W.E. McIlroy, and S.D. Perry. 2000. Thresholds for step initiation induced by support-surface translation: A dynamic center-of-mass model provides much better prediction than a static model. *Journal of Biomechanics* 33: 387-392.

Plisky, P.J., M.J. Rauh, T.W. Kaminski, and F.B. Underwood. 2006. Star excursion balance test as a predictor of lower extremity injury in high school basketball players. *Journal of Orthopaedic & Sports Physical Therapy* 36: 911-919.

Reeves, N.P., K.S. Narendra, and J. Cholewicki. 2007. Spine stability: The six blind men and the elephant. *Clinical Biomechanics* 22: 266-274.

Riemann, B.L., N.A. Caggiano, and S.M. Lephart. 1999. Examination of a clinical method of assessing postural control during a functional performance task. *Journal of Sport Rehabilitation* 8: 171-183.

Riemann, B.L., K.M. Guskiewicz, and E.W. Shields. 1999. Relationship between clinical and forceplate measures of postural stability. *Journal of Sport Rehabilitation* 8: 71-82.

Robinson, R.H., and P.A. Gribble. 2008. Support for a reduction in the number of trials needed for the Star Excursion Balance Test. *Archives of Physical Medicine and Rehabilitation* 89: 364-370.

Ross, S.E., and K.M. Guskiewicz. 2003. Time to stabilization: A method for analyzing dynamic postural stability. *Athletic Therapy Today* 8: 37-39.

Ross, S.E., and K.M. Guskiewicz. 2004. Examination of static and dynamic postural stability in individuals with functionally stable and unstable ankles. *Clinical Journal of Sport Medicine* 14: 332-338.

Ross, S.E., K.M. Guskiewicz, M.T. Gross, and B. Yu. 2009. Balance measures for discriminating between functionally unstable and stable ankles. *Medicine & Science in Sports & Exercise* 41: 399-407.

Schmitz, R., and B. Arnold. 1998. Intertester and intratester reliability of a dynamic balance protocol using the Biodex stability system. *Journal of Sport Rehabilitation* 7: 95-101.

Shimada, H., S. Obuchi, N. Kamide, Y. Shiba, M. Okamoto, and S. Kakurai. 2003. Relationship with dynamic balance function during standing and walking. *American Journal of Physical Medicine & Rehabilitation* 82: 511-516.

Starkey, C., and J. Ryan. 2002. *Evaluation of Orthopedic and Athletic Injuries*. Philadelphia: F.A. Davis.

Whiting, W.C., and S. Rugg. 2006. *Dynatomy: Dynamic Human Anatomy*. Champaign, IL: Human Kinetics.

Yaggie, J.A., and B.M. Campbell. 2006. Effects of balance training on selected skills. *Journal of Strength and Conditioning Research* 20: 422-428.

Zajac, F.E., and M.E. Gordon. 1989. Determining muscles force and action in multi-articular movement. *Exercise and Sport Sciences Reviews* 17: 187-230.

Zajac, F.E., R.R. Neptune, and S.A. Kautz. 2002. Biomechanics and muscle coordination of human walking—Part I: Introduction to concepts, power transfer, dynamics and simulations. *Gait & Posture* 16: 215-232.

Index

Note: The italicized *f* and *t* following page numbers refer to figures and tables, respectively.

About the Editor

Todd Miller, PhD, CSCS*D, is an associate professor of exercise science at the George Washington University School of Public Health and Health Services in Washington, DC, where he is responsible for the development and oversight of the master's degree concentration in strength and conditioning. He has degrees in exercise physiology from Penn State and Texas A&M, and currently studies interactive video gaming as a means of increasing physical activity in children.

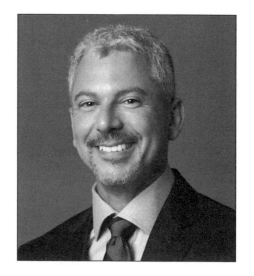

Contributors

Jonathan H. Anning, PhD, CSCS*D
Slippery Rock University, Pennsylvania

Daniel G. Drury, DPE, FACSM
Gettysburg College, Pennsylvania

Sean P. Flanagan, PhD, ATC, CSCS
California State University, Northridge

Todd Miller, PhD
George Washington University, District of Columbia

Wayne C. Miller, PhD, EMT
George Washington University, District of Columbia

Gavin L. Moir, PhD
East Stroudsburg, University of Pennsylvania

Dave Morris, PhD
Appalachian State University, Boone, North Carolina

Mark D. Peterson, PhD, CSCS*D
University of Michigan, Ann Arbor

Nicholas A. Ratamess, PhD, CSCS*D, FNSCA
The College of New Jersey, Ewing

Matthew R. Rhea, PhD, CSCS*D
Arizona State University, Mesa

N. Travis Triplett, PhD, CSCS*D, FNSCA
Appalachian State University, Boone, North Carolina

Science of Strength and Conditioning Series

The Science of Strength and Conditioning series was developed with the expertise of the National Strength and Conditioning Association (NSCA). This series of texts provides the guidelines for converting scientific research into practical application. The series covers topics such as tests and assessments, program design, and nutrition.

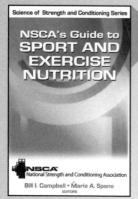

NSCA's Guide to Sport and Exercise Nutrition covers all aspects of food selection, digestion, metabolism, and hydration relevant to sport and exercise performance. This comprehensive resource will help you understand safe and effective ways to improve training and performance through natural nutrition-based ergogenic aids like supplementation and macronutrient intake manipulation. You will also learn guidelines about proper fluid intake to enhance performance and the most important criteria for effectively evaluating the quality of sport drinks and replacement beverages.

NSCA's Guide to Sport and Exercise Nutrition
National Strength and Conditioning Association
Bill I. Campbell, PhD, FISSN, CSCS, and Marie A. Spano, MS, RD/LD, FISSN, CSCS, CSSD, Editors
©2011 • Hardback • 320 pp

format also available

NSCA's Guide to Program Design moves beyond the simple template presentation of program design to help you grasp the why's and how's of organizing and sequencing training in a sport-specific, appropriate, and safe manner. The text offers 20 tables that are sample workouts or training plans for athletes in a variety of sports, technique photos and instructions for select drills, plus a sample annual training plan that shows how to assemble all the pieces previously presented. Plus, extensive references offer starting points for continued study and professional enrichment.

NSCA's Guide to Program Design
National Strength and Conditioning Association
Jay R. Hoffman, Editor
©2012 • Hardback • 336 pp

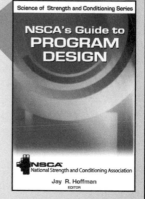

format also available

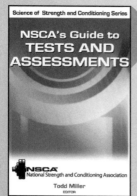

NSCA's Guide to Tests and Assessments presents the latest research from respected scientists and practitioners with expertise in exercise testing and assessment. The text begins with an introduction to testing, data analysis, and formulating conclusions. Then, you'll find a by-chapter presentation of tests and assessments for body composition, heart rate and blood pressure, metabolic rate, aerobic power, lactate threshold, muscular strength, muscular endurance, power, speed and agility, mobility, and balance and stability.

NSCA's Guide to Tests and Assessments
National Strength and Conditioning Association
Todd Miller, Editor
©2012 • Hardback • 376 pp

format also available

For more information, visit our website **www.HumanKinetics.com**.